Ultrasound Services in an Early Pregnancy and Acute Gynaecological Unit Book 2

Author:
Oluwakemi O. Ola - Ojo
MSc, GDU, BSc, DCR London (Diagnostics)
Ultrasonographer
Royal Free Hospital, London
United Kingdom

Editor:
Dr Dimitrios Spiliopoulos
MD, MSc
Obstetrician and Gynaecologist
Royal Free Hospital, London
United Kingdom

Dedication

This book is dedicated to:
You,
Our past and present students.
Thank you all for allowing my colleagues and me to share with you from our wealth of knowledge and experience
and
To all my colleagues from the multidisciplinary team,
it has been a blessing working with you all. Thanks.

Ultrasound Services in an Early Pregnancy and Acute Gynaecological Unit. Book 2

ii

'Ephraim'

"God has made me fruitful in the land of my suffering." NIV

Genesis 41: 52

**Ultrasound Services in an Early Pregnancy and
Acute Gynaecological Unit. Book 2**
© Oluwakemi O. Ola – Ojo MSc GDU BSc DCR(Diagnostic)
Radiographer/Ultrasonographer, London, UK
© Protokos Publishers. All rights reserved.
The right of Oluwakemi O. Ola-Ojo to be identified as author of this work has been
asserted by her in accordance with the Copyright, Designs and Patents Act 1988.

Edited by: Dr Dimitrios Spiliopoulos

First published 2019
ISBN: 978-1-908015-08-2
British Library Cataloguing in Publication Data
A catalogue record for this book is available from the British Library

Library of Congress Cataloguing in Publication Data

Design: Redsorel Designs

Ultrasound Services in an Early Pregnancy and Acute Gynaecological Unit. Book 2

iv

It is impossible to present in this book all the possible normal and abnormal findings seen in the EPAGU but these have been provided as examples. Sometimes it is not possible to obtain the standard views due to many factors. The ones presented in this book are the best obtainable views. Where the outcome is known in each of the case presented, it will be mentioned.

For the ease of writing and clarifications in this book, the Ultrasonographer will be referred to as he or him whilst the patient will be referred to as her or she.

Many protocols govern ultrasound examinations and practice from bodies such as NICE, BMUS, RCOG, COR, UKAS and the hospital including that of chaperoning etc. The Sonographer is encouraged to get familiar with his departmental protocols. Unlike in obstetrics, for gynecology examinations, the findings are communicated directly with the referring clinician so the ultrasonographer as such does not discuss the findings with the patient as the ultrasound findings many times are just a part of the jigsaw puzzle.

Ultrasound Services in an Early Pregnancy and Acute Gynaecological Unit. Book 2

v

Contents

Ultrasound Services in an Early Pregnancy and Acute Gynaecological Unit. Book 2

vi

Ultrasound Services in an Early Pregnancy and Acute Gynaecological Unit. Book 2

vii

BOOK 1

CONTENTS

Ultrasound Services in an Early Pregnancy and Acute Gynaecological Unit. Book 2

viii

Ultrasound Services in an Early Pregnancy and Acute Gynaecological Unit. Book 2

ix

Acknowledgements

- I would like to express my profound thanks to the following organisations: Royal Free Hospital NHS Trust London –my employer. Ectopic Trust for allowing me to use their illustration of ectopic pregnancy locations. I am grateful to Voluson for allowing me to use the images of their equipment and sterilisation process. I am grateful to HealthNetConnections and GE Healthcare for providing the access to the obstetrics charts reference data & respective authors; which are used within their Viewpoint ultrasound reporting software.

- A million thanks to Dr Peter Wylie, Consultant Radiologist for allowing me to use the MRI images and for reviewing book 2 of the series; Mr Khaled Zaedi, Consultant Obstetrician & Gynaecologist for reviewing book 1 of the series; Dr Phillis Serbang, then Radiology Registrar for reviewing both books. I am grateful for their professional wise counsel and encouragement. To my colleagues who shared their interesting cases with me, I am most grateful.

- To two of our 'then' newly qualified sonographers whose quest for excellence in EPAGU ultrasound led to the writing of these books, I am grateful for your trust, commitment to learning and good practice.

- Thank you to all the multidisciplinary team members involved in setting up and running the EPAGU services, for their dedication and commitment especially those of the Doctors, Nurses, Administrative, House Keeping, Laboratory and FMU staff.

- To all the students, colleagues and your good self who have made writing this book worthwhile. I am very grateful.

Ultrasound Services in an Early Pregnancy and Acute Gynaecological Unit. Book 2

x

- To the editor of book 2 of the series - Dr Dimitrios Spiliopoulos, I am most grateful for the encouragements and a job well done.

- To Adam Ben- Salem for the drawings done and at a very short notice. Thanks for your help and I am grateful.

- Finally and not in the least, to my family and friends – your understanding, prayers and support have been remarkable. Thank you all.

Ultrasound Services in an Early Pregnancy and Acute Gynaecological Unit. Book 2

xi

Abbreviations:

3-D – 3-dimensional

4-D – 4-dimensional

AC – Abdominal circumference

A&E – Accident & Emergency

AF – Amniotic fluid

AFI - Amniotic fluid index

AGEPU – Acute gynaecological and early pregnancy unit

AGU –Acute gynaecological unit

AM – Amniotic membrane

ANC – Antenatal clinic

a/40 a = gestational age; /40 = average length of a normal pregnancy

AP – Anteroposterior

b+c/40 – b=number of weeks; + c = days. 40 = length of a normal pregnancy

BMUS – British Medical Ultrasound Society

BPD – Biparietal diameter

bpm – beats per minute

CD – Compact disk

CH – Clinical history

CI – Cord insertion

CLC – Corpus luteal cyst

COR – College of Radiographers

Ultrasound Services in an Early Pregnancy and Acute Gynaecological Unit. Book 2

xii

CP – Choroid plexus

CRL – Crown-rump length

c/s – Caesarean section

CVS –Chorionic villus sampling

c/52 – c = number of weeks. 52 = weeks per year

DA – Diamniotic

DAU – Day assessment unit

DC – Dichorionic

DCDA – Dichorionic diamnotic

EDD – Expected date of delivery

EHR – Embryonic heart rate

EMP – Embryonic pole

EP – Ectopic pregnancy

EPAGU – Early pregnancy and acute gynaecology unit

EPU – Early pregnancy unit

FET – Frozen embryo transfer

FH – Fetal head

FHB – Fetal heart beats

FL – Femur length

FMU – Fetal medicine unit

FP – Fetal pole

GA – Gestational age

GH – Gut herniation

GIFT – Gamete intrafallopian transfer

Ultrasound Services in an Early Pregnancy and Acute Gynaecological Unit. Book 2

xiii

GIT – Gastrointestinal tract

GP – General practitioner

GS – Gestational sac

GSD – Gestational sac diameter

GSV – Gestational sac volume

HC – Head circumference

HCG – Human chorionic gonadotropin

ICSI – Intracytoplasmic sperm injection

IUCD – Intrauterine contraceptive device

IUD – Intrauterine death

IUGS – Intra uterine gestational sac

IUI – Intrauterine insemination

IUP – Intrauterine pregnancy

IVF – In vitro fertilisaton

KUB – Kidneys, ureters and bladder

LLB – Lower limb bud

LMP – Last menstrual period

LS – Longitudinal section

LT – Left

LO - Left Ovary

MA – Missed abortion or miscarriage

MC – Monochorionic

MCDA – Monochorionic diamniotic

MCMA – Monochorionic monoamniotic

Ultrasound Services in an Early Pregnancy and Acute Gynaecological Unit. Book 2

xiv

M mode – Motion mode

NHS – National Health Service

NICE – National Institute for Health and Care Excellence

NT – Nuchal translucency

OHSS –Ovarian hyperstimulation syndrome

PACS – Picture archiving computer system

PCOS – Polycystic ovary syndrome

PID – Pelvic inflammatory disease

PM – Postmenopausal

PMH – Past medical history

POD – Pouch of Douglas

PROM – Premature rupture of the membranes

PUL – Pregnancy of unknown location

PV – Per vagina

RCOG – Royal College of Obstetricians and Gynaecologists

RPOC – Retained products of conception

RSI – Repetitve strain injury

SROM – Spontaneous rupture of the membrane

RO - Right ovary

RT – Right

R/V – Retroverted

SUZI – Subzonal insemination

TA – Trans-abdominal

TS – Transverse section

Ultrasound Services in an Early Pregnancy and Acute Gynaecological Unit. Book 2

XV

TTTS – Twin-to-twin transfusion syndrome

TV – Trans-vaginal

UKAS – United Kingdom Association of Sonographers

ULB – Upper limb bud

VD – Vitelline duct

WC – Water closet

YS – Yolk sac

< – Less than

> – Greater than

= – Equal to

Ultrasound Services in an Early Pregnancy and Acute Gynaecological Unit. Book 2

xvi

Introduction

It is unrealistic to present in this book all the possible normal and abnormal findings seen in an early pregnancy and acute gynaecology unit (EPAGU), but these have been provided as examples. Sometimes it is not possible to obtain standard ultrasound views due to many factors, but those presented in this book are the best obtainable views. Where the outcome is known in each of the cases presented, it will be mentioned.

For ease of writing and clarifications in this book, the ultrasonographer or sonographer will be referred to as he or him, whilst the patient will be referred to as she or her. The term ultrasonographer is used to refer to the person performing and reporting the examination in respective of their medical background.

Many protocols govern ultrasound examination practices from organisations such as NICE, BMUS, RCOG, COR, UKAS, and hospitals including that of chaperoning etc. The sonographer is encouraged to get familiar with his departmental protocols. The charts used may not be the same for all departments. Please refer to your own departmental chart.

Ultrasound Services in an Early Pregnancy and Acute Gynaecological Unit. Book 2

17

Chapter 5

Acute Gynaecology

In this chapter we shall consider the following:

- **Normal menstrual cycle**
- **Normal ultrasound appearances of the female pelvis**
- **Ovarian appearance and the Menstrual cycle**
- **Oral Contraceptive Pills and the Menstrual Cycle**
- **Uterine Abnormalities**
- **HRT and the menstrual cycle**
- **Ovarian cysts**

Ultrasound equipment's resolution is getting better with many manufacturers offering the 3D/4D facilities which might make the purchase more expensive, it might require additional staff training but where it is available and used, it is worth the purchase. Whichever equipment is going to be used for emergency gynaecology ultrasound in EPAGU, it is essential that it has good image resolution and Dopplers facilities including Power and Coloured.

It is not unusual that there will be a need for follow ups where a pathology is suspected or confirmed. It is essential that good ultrasound views (as much as possible) of the pathology are obtained, documented and easily accessible so that a comparison can subsequently be made in the future.

Ultrasound Services in an Early Pregnancy and Acute Gynaecological Unit. Book 2

18

Immediately following the ultrasound examination an Ultrasound report should be generated containing the following information:

- Hospital details
- Patient's details
- LMP
- Date of Scan
- Reason for the scan or Clinical History
- Method of scanning TAS or and TVS
- Answer to examination request
- Quality of views obtained - good, poor or restricted and why?
- Ultrasound Equipment used e.g. Aloka, Toshiba, GE, Siemens etc.
- Any significant findings to the uterus, ovaries or adnexae
- Any other relevant comments
- Name and designation of the chaperone if present. If not this should be documented and why
- Any need for follow up or suggestion
- Name of the Ultrasonographer or Doctor

Women get referred to Acute Gynaecology Unit for many reasons. A sound knowledge of the menstrual cycle and corresponding normal ultrasound appearances at every menstrual phase is essential for the Sonographer.

At puberty there are significant changes to a woman including her now having a menstrual period. Most women have an average of 28-30 days menstrual cycle. This is what is generally used in calculating GA of any pregnancy or in saying where the woman is in her cycle e.g. Day 7 means the seventh day since her menstrual period began. Day 1 being the first full day of menstruation. In some women however the menstrual period could be shorter e.g. 21days or longer e.g. up to 35days or more.

Ultrasound Services in an Early Pregnancy and Acute Gynaecological Unit. Book 2

19

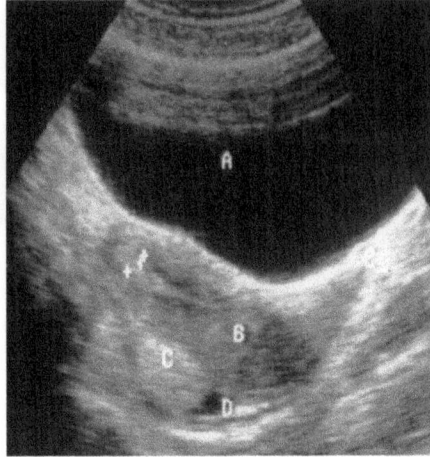

5.1a

LS view of the uterus. (TA scan)

A - Urinary bladder. B – cervical area. C- overlying bowel gas

D – Small quantity of fluid in the POD. ++ - endometrial thickness.

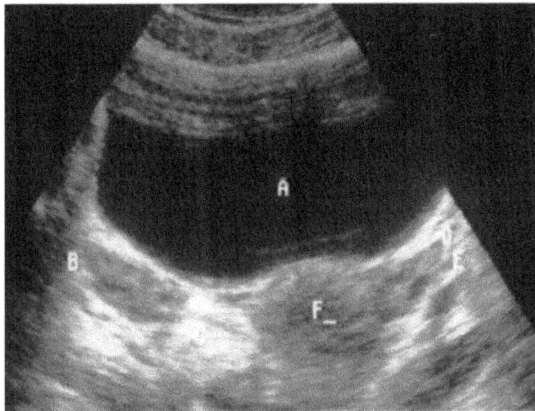

5.1b

TS view of the uterus and ovaries. (TA scan)

A – urinary bladder. B- right ovary. C- overlying bowel gas. D- left ovary

E – left iliac blood vessels. F- uterus .

Ultrasound Services in an Early Pregnancy and Acute Gynaecological Unit. Book 2

20

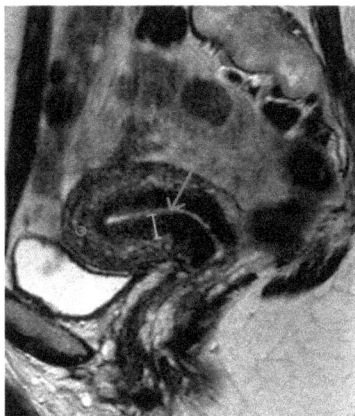

5.1c

TS normal sagittal anatomy

Normal MR Uterine anatomy – Sagittal image – Shows endometrium as high signal band (pink arrow), Junctional zone – inner myometrium – as very low signal stripe (blue callipers) and outer myometrium (green circle).

Normal Menstrual Cycle: It is a good idea to understand ultrasound appearances and changes that occur in a normal menstrual cycle. Most women who come into acute gynecology unit are women of child bearing age or post menopausal. Pre pubertal girls and post menopausal women don't have a menstrual cycle.

Some authors describe the 28 days menstrual cycle in four phases:
- menstrual phase - days 1-5.
- preovulatory or proliferative or follicular phase – days 6-13.
- ovulation – day 14 in a 28 days cycle.
- luteal or post ovulatory phase – days 15 -28.

Other authors describe it as in three phases:
- Follicular: days 1- 4. Day 1 being the first full day of bleeding. 25 – 65 mls of blood containing mucus, tissue fluid, the lining of the womb are shed. Movement within the endometrium is from the fundus to the cervix and the shed blood from the uterine cavity flows through the cervix and vagina.
- Days 6-13 – this is very variable in length as it is subject to considerable variation in the cycle length. During this time the follicles grow producing more oestrogen which in turn stimulate endometrial growth and thickening. In a natural menstrual cycle, one or two of the follicles outgrow

Ultrasound Services in an Early Pregnancy and Acute Gynaecological Unit. Book 2

21

the others thereby becoming the dominant follicles in that menstrual phase. See an example of such in figure 5.2b

- In a 28 days cycle, ovulation will normally take place on day 14 when the dominant follicle ruptures such that the oocyte and follicular fluid are released.
- Luteal or post ovulatory phase: This phase is usually constant in length irrespective of the cycle length.

Luteinizing hormone (LH) secretion stimulates the development of the corpus luteum which secrets increasing quantity of oestrogen and progesterone.

An example of TVS scan done on day 7

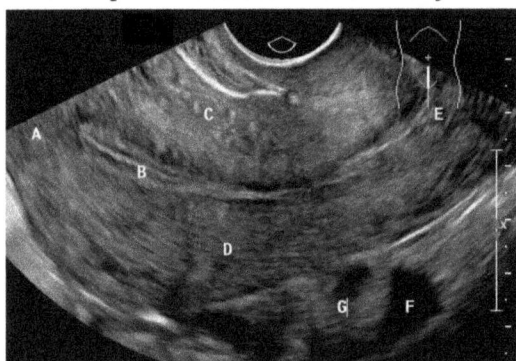

5.1d   **5.1e**

51d – *A-Fundus, B- Triple line endometrium, C- Anterior myometrium, D -Posterior myometrium, E -Cervix, F/G – Bowel*
51e- A&B – Bowel

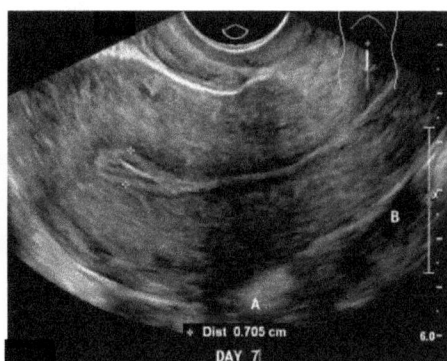

Normal Ultrasound Appearances

In this section we shall consider normal ultrasound appearances and other ultrasound findings that are specific to certain medical conditions.

Early in the normal cycle e.g. Day 3-5: The endometrium will be thin and the ovaries will be "quiet" with no dominant follicle.

Mid cycle: The endometrium will be thick and have a triple line appearance. One or both ovaries will be active and a dominant follicle will be seen. If it is after ovulation, there will be some fluid in the POD in (an antevetered uterus) or around the uterine fundus (in a retroverted uterus).

Ultrasound Services in an Early Pregnancy and Acute Gynaecological Unit. Book 2

22

The scan below was performed on day 6 of a normal 26 - 28 days cycle.

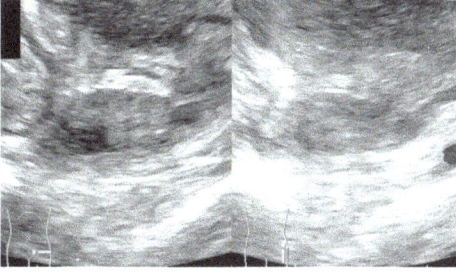 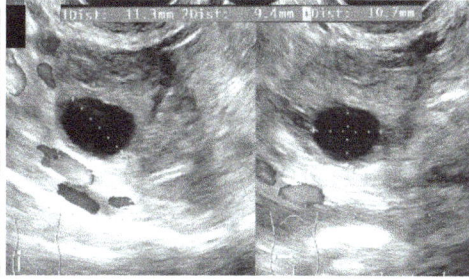

5.2a   **5.2b**

Note the growing follicle in the right ovary (5.2b)

The scan below was performed on day 12 of a normal 26 - 28 days cycle.

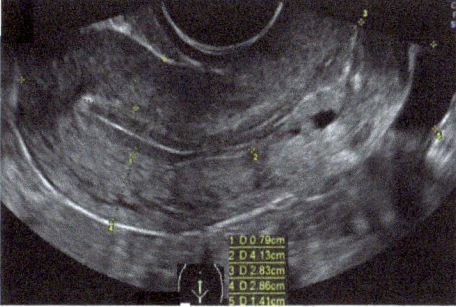 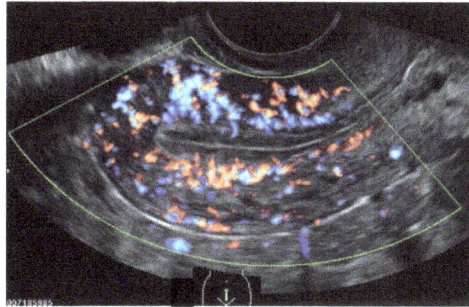

5.3a   **5.3b**

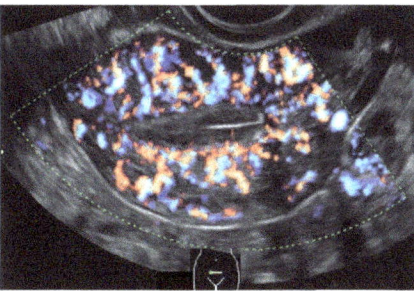

5.3c

(TV scan) Normal mid cycle appearance of the endometrium. Note the fluid in the POD and the triple line appearances of the endometrium.

Ultrasound Services in an Early Pregnancy and Acute Gynaecological Unit. Book 2

23

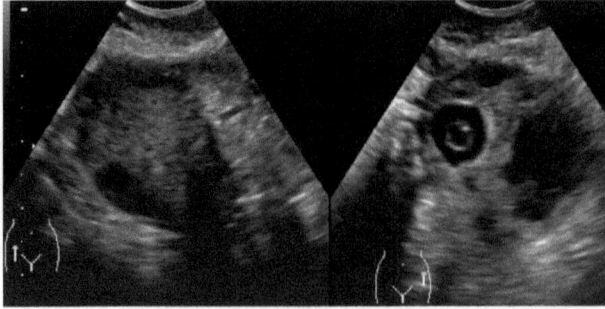

5.3d

Note the corpus luteum in the left ovary. Measurements not included (were much over 10mls each per ovary – an indication of PCO).

This is a scan of another patient in her mid cycle.

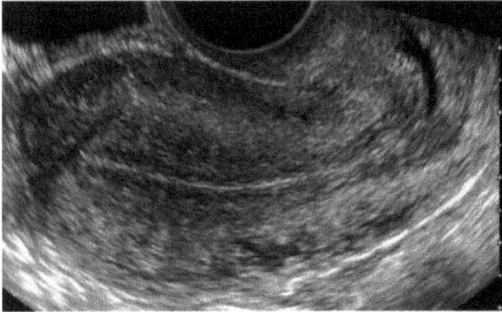 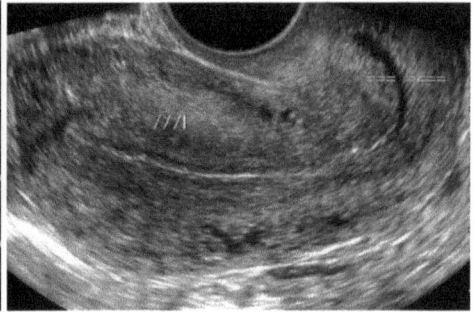

5.4a   **5.4b**

/// - triple line endometrium. === fluid in the cervical canal.

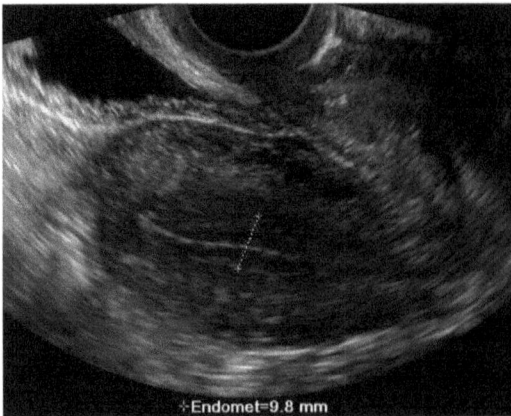 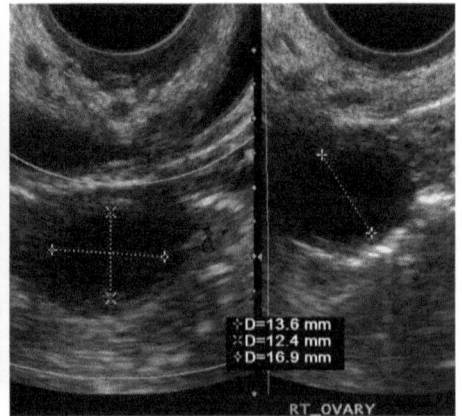

5.4c   **5.4d**

Ultrasound Services in an Early Pregnancy and Acute Gynaecological Unit. Book 2

24

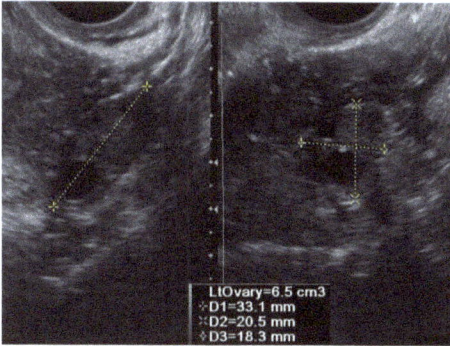

5.4e

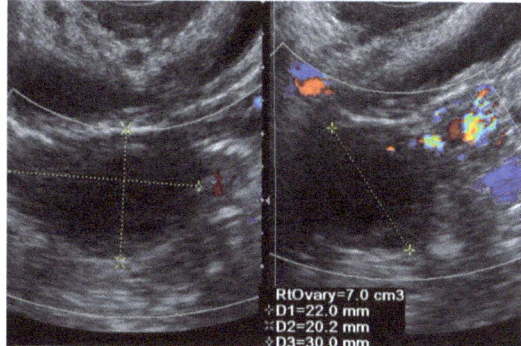

5.4f

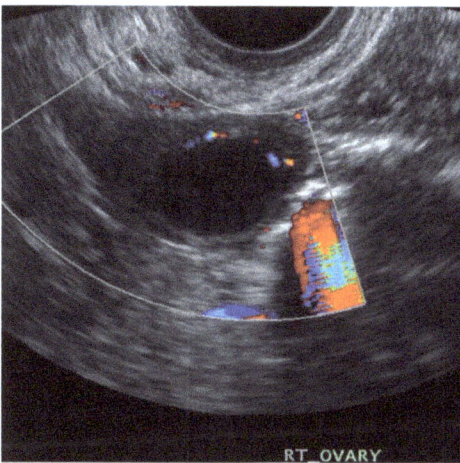

5.4g

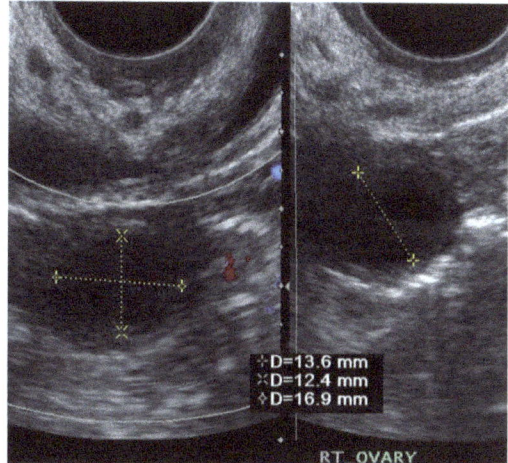

5.4h

Ultrasound findings: An anteverted uterus with a 9.8mm triple line endometrium (5.4a – c). There is some fluid in the cervical canal (5.4a-c). The right ovary is 7mls (5.4f) and the left ovary is 6.5mls(5.4e). There is an approx. 14 x 12 x 17mm corpus luteum in the right ovary (5.4 d & g- h).

Impression: Normal post ovulation ultrasound findings.

Luteal Phase: This is the period before menstruation. The endometrium should be thick and hyperechoic in echo texture. A corpus luteal cyst will be seen. There may be some fluid in the POD.

Ultrasound Services in an Early Pregnancy and Acute Gynaecological Unit. Book 2

25

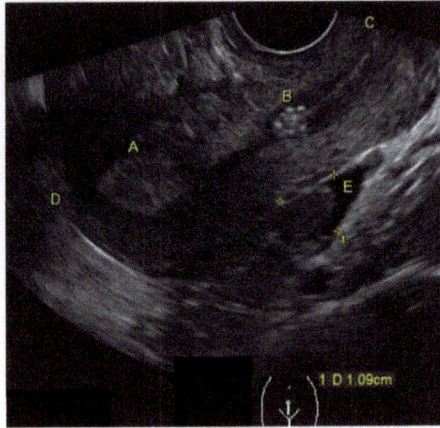

5.5a

A – thickened endometrium, B – internal os, C – cervix   D– uterine fundus, E – POD.

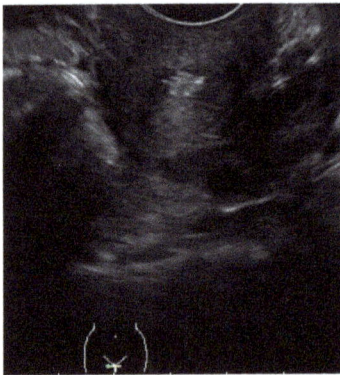

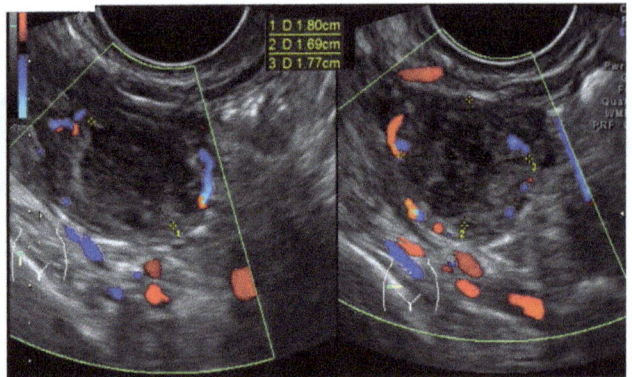

5.5b   **5.5c**

Note the 'ring of fire' around the corpus luteum (5.5c).

If the patient does not get pregnant then the endometrial lining gets shed off and appear as next menstrual bleeding.

Another example of a luteal phase endometrium. Same appearance could be seen before an IUGS is seen in early pregnancy.

Ultrasound Services in an Early Pregnancy and Acute Gynaecological Unit. Book 2

26

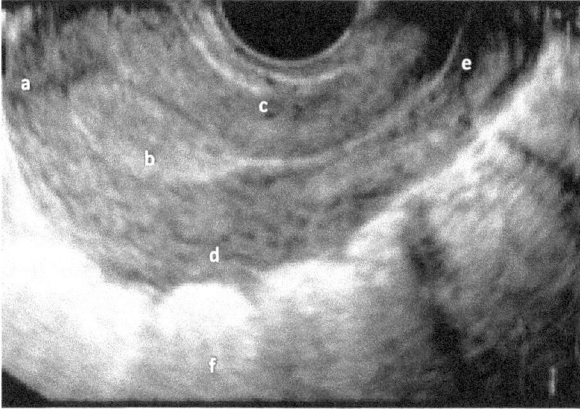

5.5d
LS section of an anteverted uterus

a – fundal myometrium, b – endometrium, c – anterior myometrium
d- posterior myometrium, e – cervix, f – overlying bowel gas

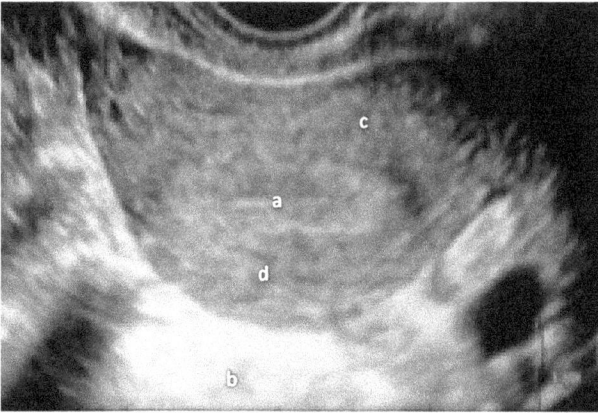

5.5e
TS view of the same uterus before

a – endometrium b – overlying bowel gas, c – anterior myometrium d – posterior myometrium

Ultrasound Services in an Early Pregnancy and Acute Gynaecological Unit. Book 2

27

TVS IN GYNAECOLOGY ULTRASOUND

In gynaecology especially in emergency settings, TVS provides a closer and more detailed information in cases including:

- Ovarian screening
- Assessment of PID
- Assessment of ?PCO
- Endometrial assessment in PMB
- Confirming or otherwise of ovarian torsion
- Endometrial assessment for polyps or fibroids
- Assessment of pelvic masses, cysts and fibroids
- Clarifying of TAS images that are due to poor resolution
- Assessment of pelvic pain and other gynaecological symptoms

However TVS is contraindicated in :

- Paediatric age group as in the next case
- Virgo intacta
- Patient who refuses for personal or religious reasons

In addition to TAS or and TVS, there might be need for further diagnostic tests such as

- Blood tests for assessing the Ca 125 (tumour markers)
- CT for staging known gynaecological malignancy
- MRI for staging of gynaecological malignancy

This 15 year old patient was referred with a clinical history of ?PCO. Below are the ultrasound findings.

Ultrasound Services in an Early Pregnancy and Acute Gynaecological Unit. Book 2

28

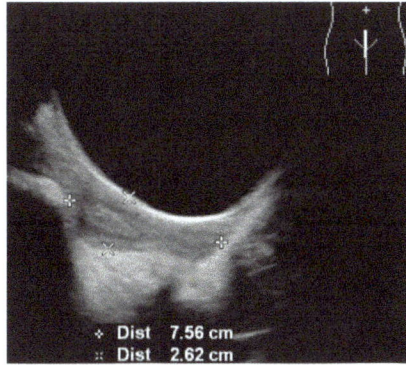

5.5f

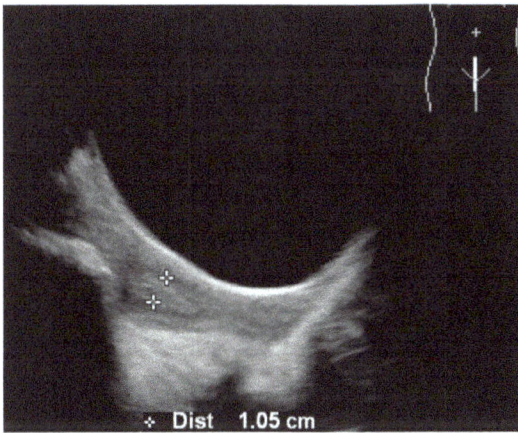

5.5g

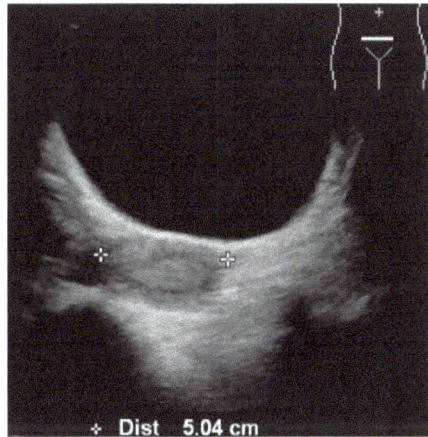

5.5h

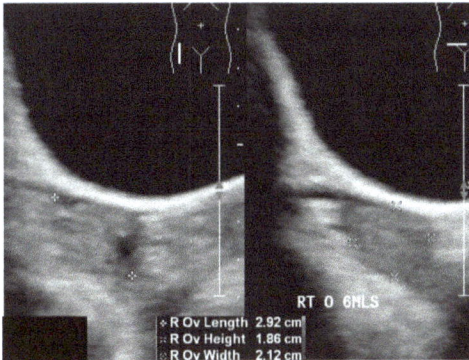

5.5i

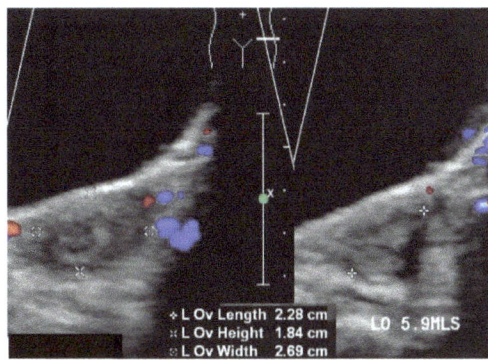

5.5h

Ultrasound findings: An anteverted uterus measuring 7.6 x 2.6 x 5cm with a 10.5mm luteal phase like smooth and regular endometrium. Both ovaries appear sonographically normal with the right ovarian volume of 6mls and the left ovarian volume of 5.9mls.

Ultrasound Services in an Early Pregnancy and Acute Gynaecological Unit. Book 2

29

note only TAS scan was performed in this patient
** This case has been included to show a normal paediatric pelvis but patient was not scanned in the EPAGU*

Post Hysterectomy

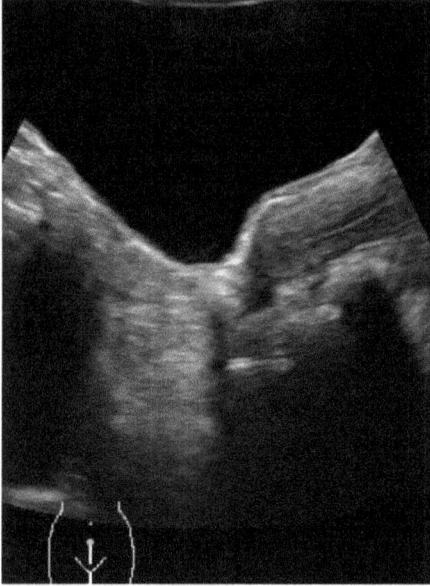 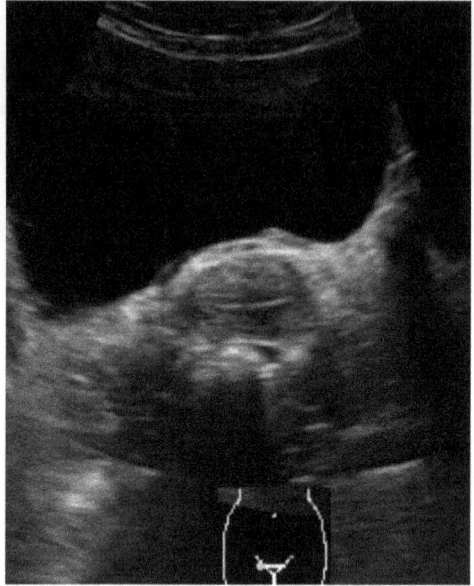

| 5.6a | 5.6b |

The above shows a normal Vaginal stump post hysterectomy.
It is essential to confirm from a woman with a history of post hysterectomy if the ovaries were also removed or left in place..

Vaginal Pessary

This is a device inserted in the vagina to treat a uterine prolapse. This helps to hold the prolapsed organ in place.

Ultrasound Services in an Early Pregnancy and Acute Gynaecological Unit. Book 2

30

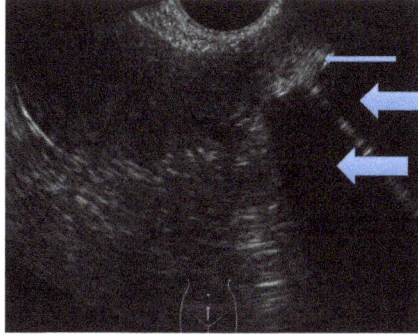

5.7a

Thin arrow – vaginal pessary. Thick arrows – shadows from the pessary

Ovarian appearance and the Menstrual cycle

The ovaries are usually found lying anterior to the iliac blood vessels in the LS section. In the TS section they are found at the level of the uterine fundus where the uterus becomes triangular. Ovarian measurement in a menstruating woman is approximately 40 x 29 x 10mm – ovarian volume 4.0 x 2.9 x 1.0cm x 0.5233 = 6.07mls.

Ovarian volume is influenced by factors such as the hormonal status of the patient, the patient's age – ovarian volume is known to be largest in the 30 -39year olds and normally decreases post menopausal. Use of fertility drugs, polycystic ovaries (PCO) or (PCOD) and presence of 'cysts' can make the overy bigger. The removal of one ovary may make the remaining ovary get bigger and the presence of 'cysts' might also increase the size of the ovary.

The location of the ovary can be affected by the position of the uterus e.g. in pregnancy the uterus ascends into the abdominal cavity and the ovaries get pulled along and become elongated. Post delivery the ovaries return to the pelvis but are now more horizontal in position. The bowels, fibroids, the degree of urinary bladder filling, Wertheim's hysterectomy and use of fertility treatment can also affect the location of the ovaries.

* It is possible for a woman to have one normal ovary in size and appearance and the other ovary can have the size and appearance of PCO.

Ultrasound Services in an Early Pregnancy and Acute Gynaecological Unit. Book 2

31

Just as the endometrial appearance changes during a normal cycle so does the ovary. In the menstrual phase - days 1-5, the ovary should be 'quiet' with no follicular growth. In the preovulatory or proliferative or follicular phase – days 6- 13, one or two follicles will begin to grow and at a point one of the follicles will become the dominant follicle growing between 14 -25mm in diameter. At ovulation, the matured follicle ruptures and the oocyte and some fluid are released. In the luteal phase the empty sac can become irregular in outline, fluid or blood filled and is now called a corpus luteum. Following menstruation, the corpus luteum disappears.

The scan below was performed on day 6 of a normal 26 - 28 days cycle.

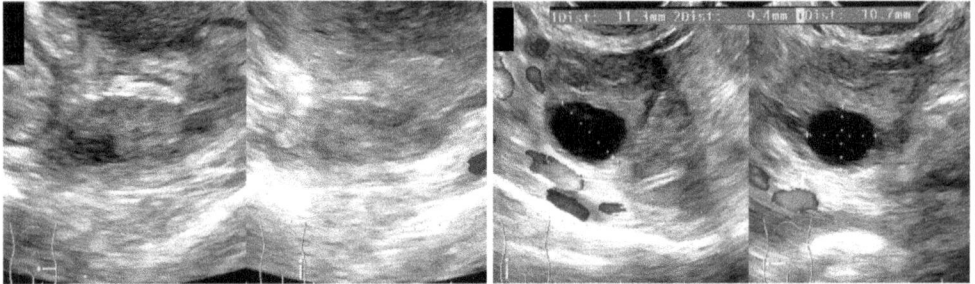

5.8a   **5.8b**

Note the growing follicle in the right ovary

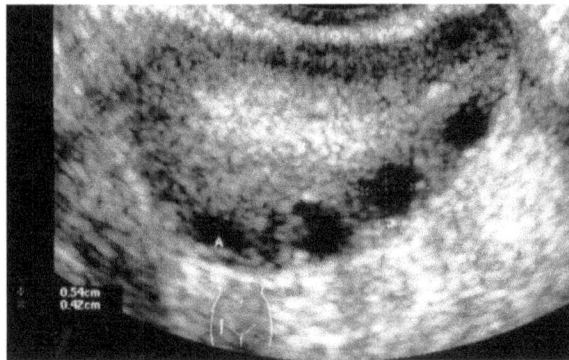

5.8c Right ovary – longitudinal section
A – follicle, B – stroma ++ - follicular measurement

Other ultrasound appearances

Previous C/S Scar: If it is in the A/V uterus, a cut in the anterior wall of the myometrium often appears as a thin line that does not cut across the mid line of the endometrial cavity.

Ultrasound Services in an Early Pregnancy and Acute Gynaecological Unit. Book 2

32

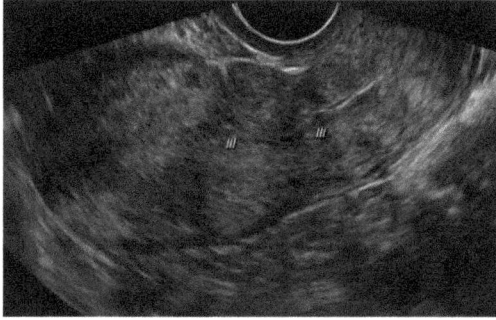

5.9a

/// Represent previous caesarean scar in an A/V uterus

This patient has had 3 previous C/S

Previous scar in a R/V uterus

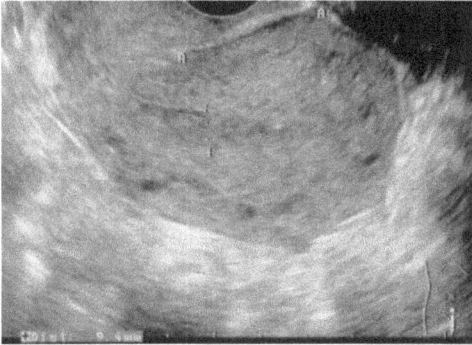

5.9b

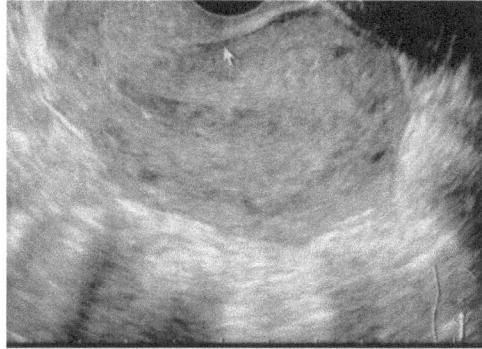

5.9c

a and the arrow head above shows a previous scar in a R/V uterus

Ultrasound Services in an Early Pregnancy and Acute Gynaecological Unit. Book 2

33

Day 8 scan

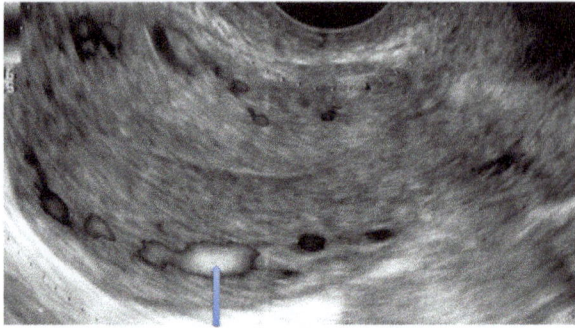

5.10 a

Arrow showing the arcuate vessel

(TV SCAN) LS view of the uterus

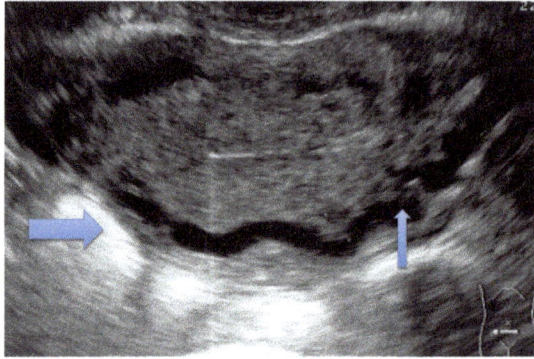

5.10b

Horizontal arrow – overlying bowel gas | *Upright arrow* – arcuate vessel

(TV scan) TS view of the uterus. Notice normal blood flow/ appearance in the arcuate vessels of the uterus.

Ultrasound Services in an Early Pregnancy and Acute Gynaecological Unit. Book 2

34

Another Patient

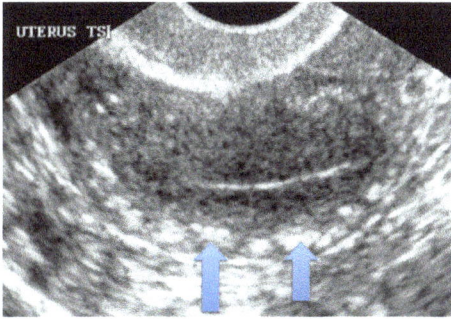

5.10c *Arrows show calcified arcuate vessels*

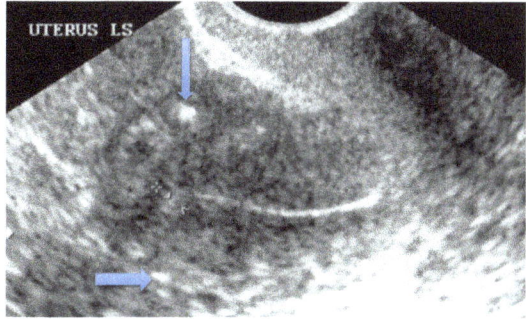

5.10d *Arrows show calcified arcuate vessel*

This ultrasound appearance is suggestive of calcified arcuate artery.

- Calcified arcuate artery usually involves multiple vessels at about the same level in the myometrium forming a circular configuration in the TS view and linear configuration in a longitudinal image of an AP pelvis. With fibroids, the calcification is seen randomly distributed in the fibroid or at the periphery and outlining the fibroid.
- It has been suggested that there is an association between calcified arcuate artery and diabetes, hypertension and atherosclerotic disease. Further clinical investigation for any of such conditions is advisable or recommended.

Oral Contraceptive Pill (OCP) and the Menstrual Cycle

Women who are on OCP tend to have very thin and smooth endometrium irrespective of the menstrual cycle day at the time of the ultrasound examination. Their ovaries are usually quiet with not much activity going on. The longer a patient has been on the OCP, the smaller in size the ovary is likely going to be on ultrasound.

Ultrasound Services in an Early Pregnancy and Acute Gynaecological Unit. Book 2

35

Day 17 on the Pill

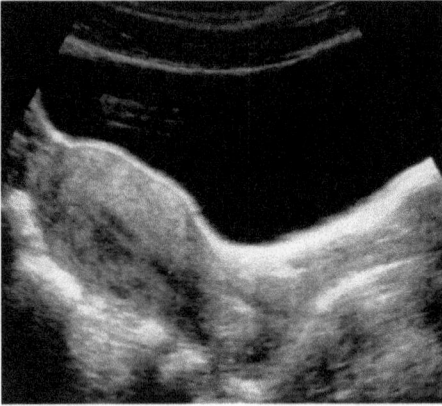

5.11a

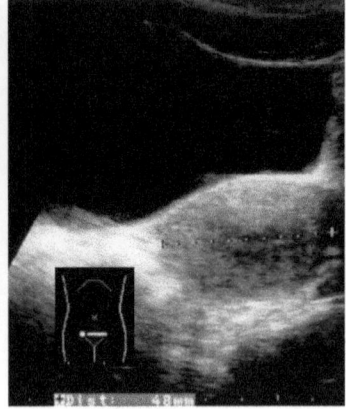

5.11b

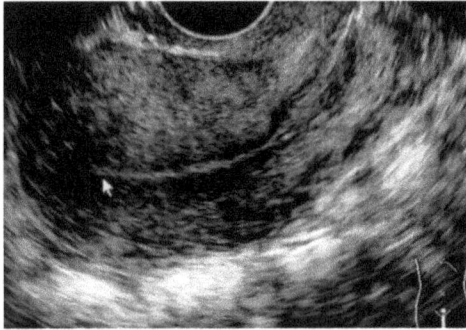

5.11c

UT – 81 x 48 x 34mm.

Note the very thin and echogenic endometrium (arrow head in 5.11c).

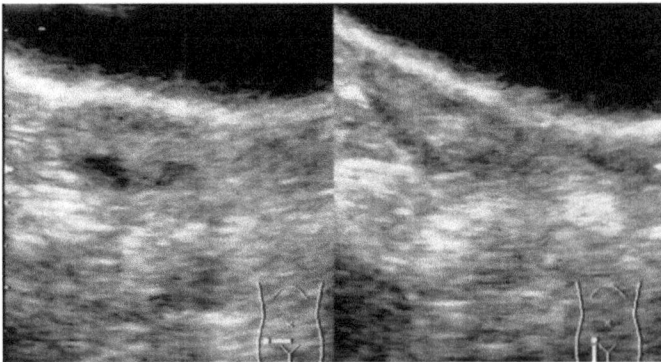

5.11d

RO – 30 x 12 x 20mm

Ultrasound Services in an Early Pregnancy and Acute Gynaecological Unit. Book 2

36

Right ovarian volume = 3.0 x 1.2 x 2.0 x 0.5233 = 3.77cc

LO – not visualized

Another patient on the Pill

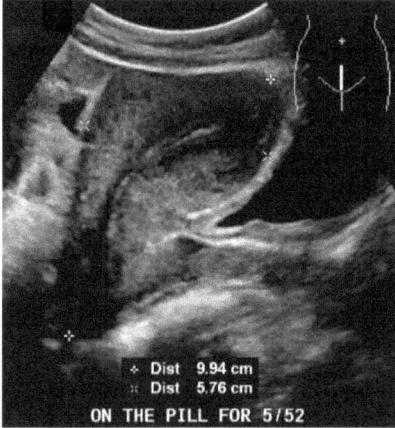 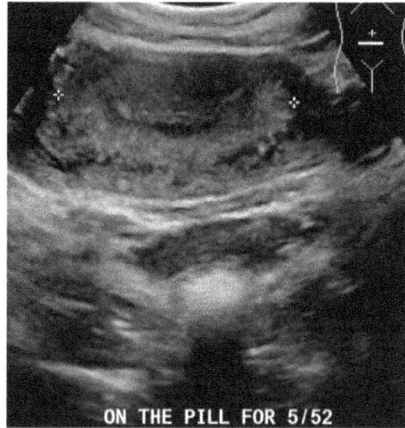

5.11e   **5.11f**

Uterine Abnormalities

The uterus develops in utero from the two mullerian ducts starting at 3-4/40 and continuing into the second trimester. Interruption of this process causes incomplete fusion which may not be apparent until the woman is post puberty. It is not unusual for any of the uterine abnormalities to be discovered during a gynaecology or early obstetric scan. A knowledge of the types of possible abnormalities and their effect is essential for the sonographer. It is believed that about 4-7% women have some form of uterine abnormality.

Bicornuate uterus

On ultrasound this is seen as two separate uterine cavities, with different thickness of the corresponding endometria but with only one cervix. It is not unusual that a woman with such a uterine deformity may be pregnant in one horn and be bleeding in the other horn. It is found in 20% of women with uterine abnormalities. The amniotic membranes of such a woman may break earlier than expected and cause preterm labour due to overstretching of the uterus. Ultrasound diagnosis of bicornuate uterus is easier on the TS view as two different or separate endometrial cavities will be seen and the TS diameter of the uterus is usually greater than 8cm.

Ultrasound Services in an Early Pregnancy and Acute Gynaecological Unit. Book 2

37

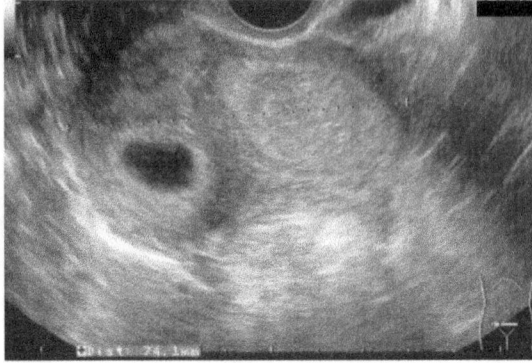

5.12 a

Differential diagnosis - uterus didelphys.

There is an IUGS in the right horn and thickened endometrium in the left horn.

A 15 year old girl presented on Day 1 of her menstrual cycle with a clinical indication of RIF pain and guarding for 7days radiating from the right flank to the pelvic rim. Below are the ultrasound findings:

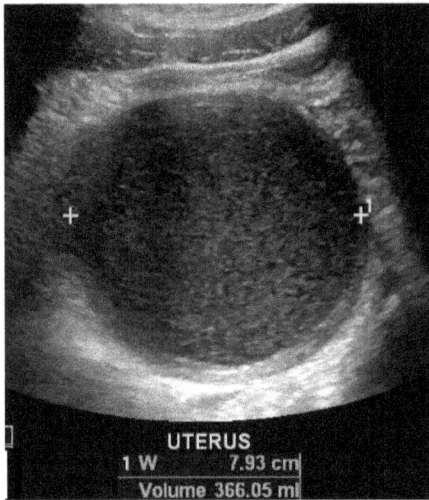

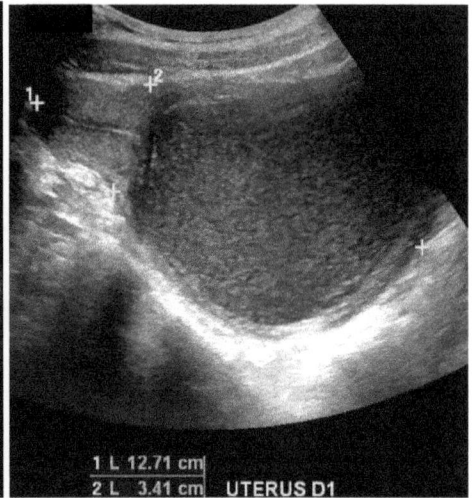

5.12aa   **5.12b**

Ultrasound Services in an Early Pregnancy and Acute Gynaecological Unit. Book 2

38

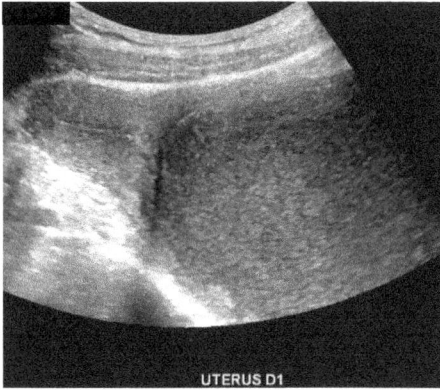

5.12c

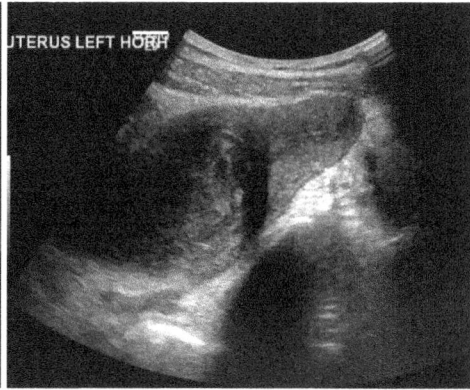

5.12d

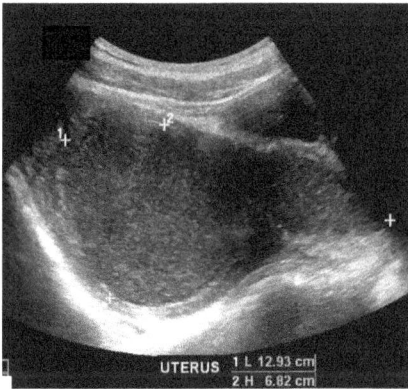

5.12e

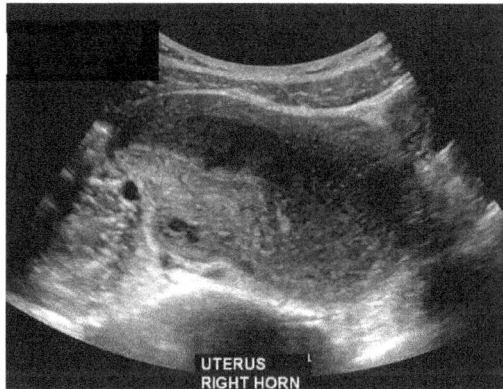

5.12f

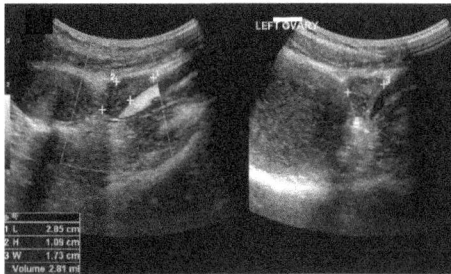

5.12g

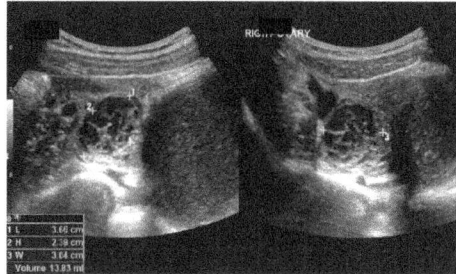

5.12h

Ultrasound Services in an Early Pregnancy and Acute Gynaecological Unit. Book 2

39

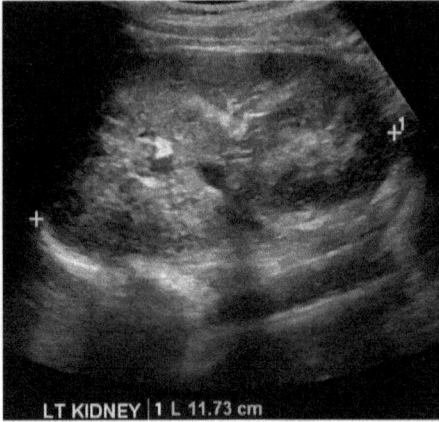
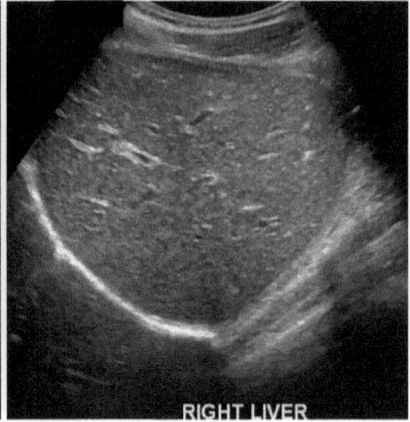

LT KIDNEY | 1 L 11.73 cm

RIGHT LIVER

5.12i

5.12j

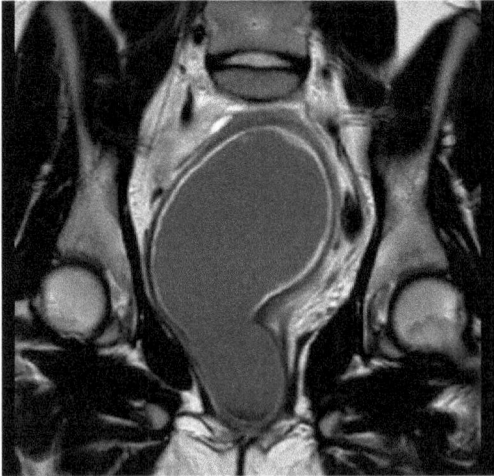
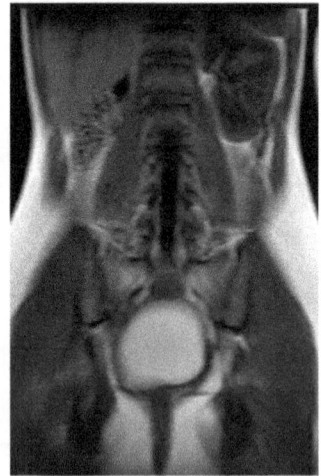

5.12k

5.12l

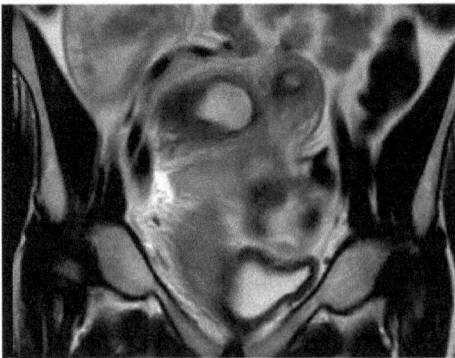
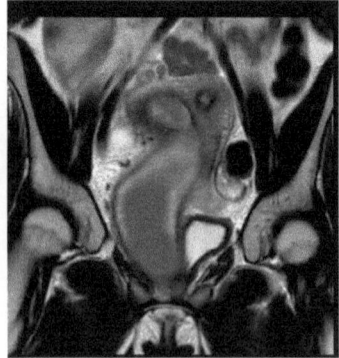

5.12m

5.12n

Ultrasound Services in an Early Pregnancy and Acute Gynaecological Unit. Book 2

40

Ultrasound and MRI findings

On both Ultrasound and MRI imaging, there was a bicornuate uterus with normal appearances of the left horn. (c. m-n). The right horn and cervical area are markedly distended and contain echogenic fluid, approximately 366mls. (a-b, e-f, k) . Both ovaries were clearly defined. There was a small hemorrhagic cyst on the right with a volume of 12mls. (h). The left ovary displays normal ultrasound appearances and has a volume of 3mls (g). Absent right kidney and single left kidney was noted. (i, j, l). No free fluid was present in the pelvis or abdomen. On MRI, a small amount of fluid was noted in the vagina.

** *This case has been included to show a paediatric bicornuate uterus with haematometra but patient was not scanned in the EPAGU*

Uterine didelphys

Ultrasound appearances is similar to that of bicornuate uterus but there will be two cervices. It is important that the patient should have a renal scan to rule out abnormalites such as renal agenesis. It comes as a result of no fusion of the uterine ducts in utero.

This patient was referred with a history of primary infertility. Below are the findings on Day 7.

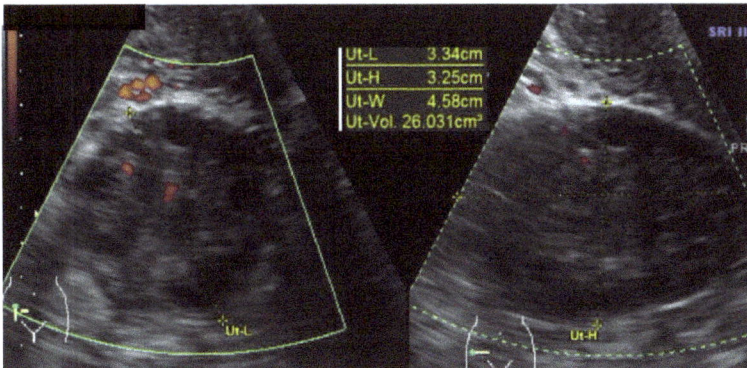

5.13 b

Ultrasound Services in an Early Pregnancy and Acute Gynaecological Unit. Book 2

41

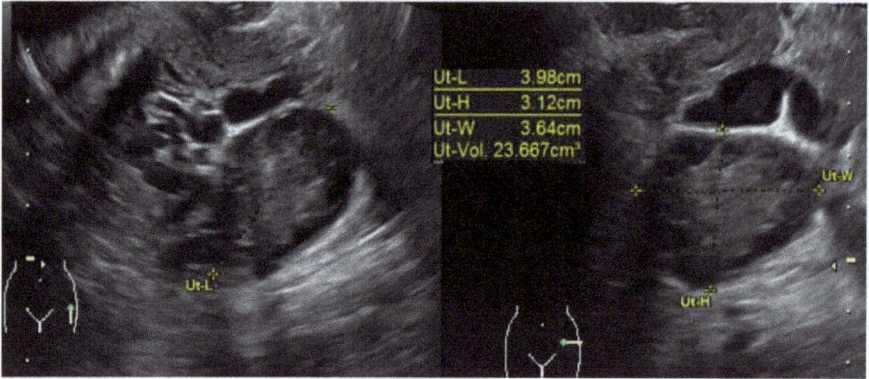

Ut-L   3.98cm
Ut-H   3.12cm
Ut-W   3.64cm
Ut-Vol. 23.667cm³

5.13c

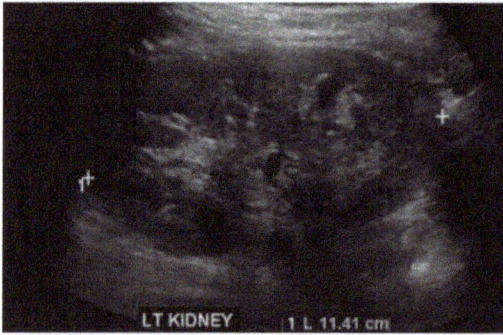

LT KIDNEY   1 L 11.41 cm

5.13d

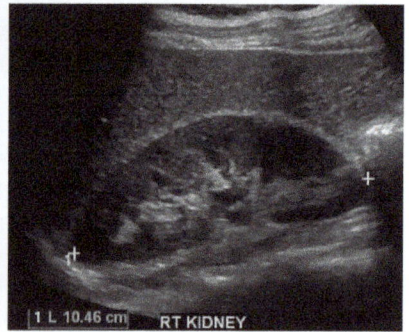

1 L 10.46 cm   RT KIDNEY

5.13e

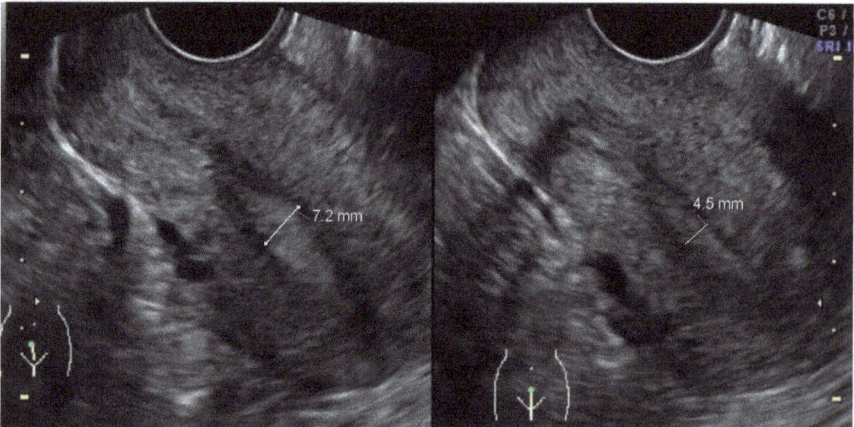

7.2 mm

4.5 mm

5.13f

Ultrasound Services in an Early Pregnancy and Acute Gynaecological Unit. Book 2

42

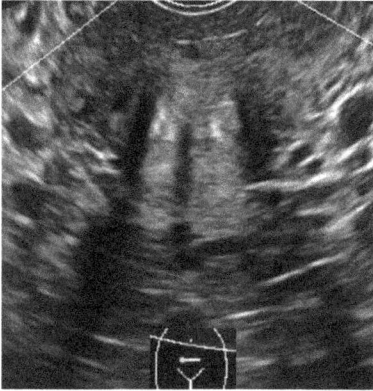

5.13g

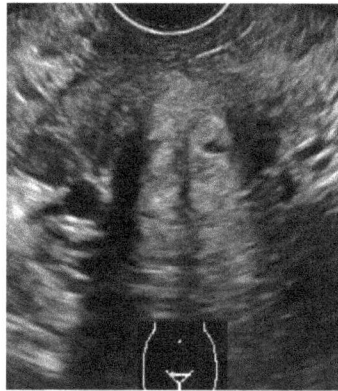

5.13h

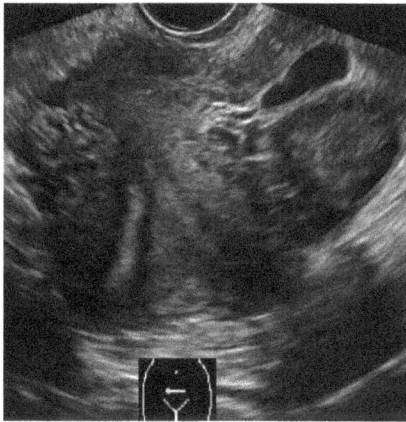

5.13i

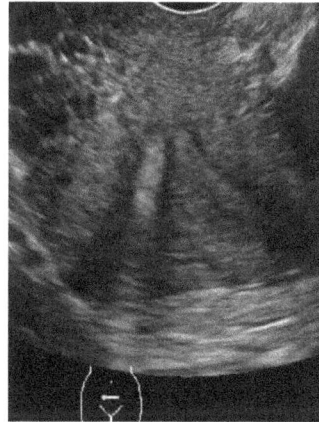

5.13j

MR Scan of the same patient:

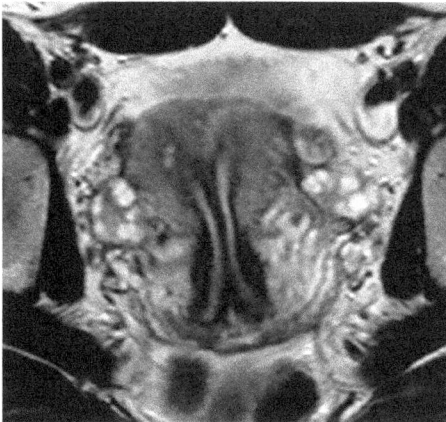

5.13k

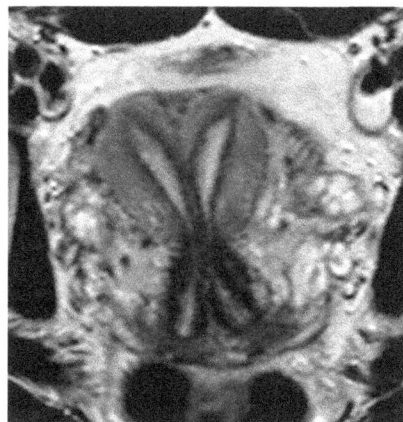

5.13l

Ultrasound Services in an Early Pregnancy and Acute Gynaecological Unit. Book 2

43

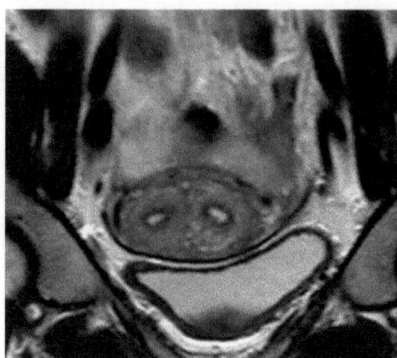 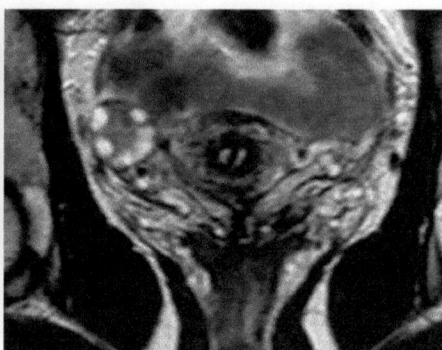

| 5.13m | 5.13n |

Ultrasound findings: The uterus have two endometrial cavities and two cervices (5.13f –j). It is normal in size and echo pattern. The endometrial thickness on the right measures 7.3mm and on the left 4.8mm (5.13f). Both ovaries are polycystic in appearance. ?left lydrosalpinx (5.13c & i). Right ovarian volume is 26cc and 23cc on the left (5.13b-c). Both kidneys appear normal in size and echo pattern (5.13d-e).

Impression: Uterine didelphys, ?septate or bicornuate uterus, bilateral PCO. Normal kidneys. ?left hydrosalpinx.

- MRI Report – Congenital uterine malformation with configuration of uterine didelphys. Two separate non communicating endometrial cavities and cervical canals. Bilateral PCO,
- Uterine didelphys may affect obstetric outcome including risk of preterm labour , IUGR
- *Hematometrocolpos and hematosalpinx if any of the cavities is non communicating.
- The vaginal septum may not be seen on ultrasound.
- This case is not from EPAGU but was included to demonstrate the uterine abnormality.

Septate uterus

May look similar to bicornuate uterus on ultrasound but the septate uterus is round at the top with a single cavity in the uterus whereas a bicornuate uterus 'dips' on the top forming a 'heart shape'. This uterus type is associated with the worst obstetric outcome as such patients are said to have a 90% rate of early

Ultrasound Services in an Early Pregnancy and Acute Gynaecological Unit. Book 2

44

miscarriage or premature birth.

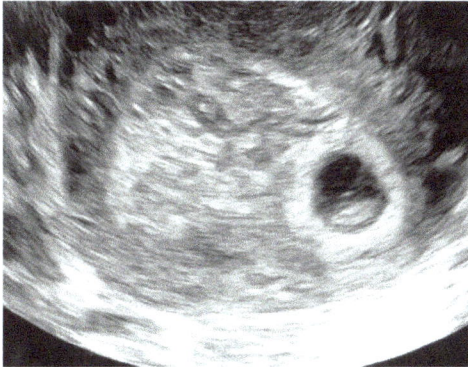

5.14 a There is an intrauterine pregnancy in the left horn.

* Differentials – Bicornuate uterus

Below is an MRI Image of a Septate uterus.

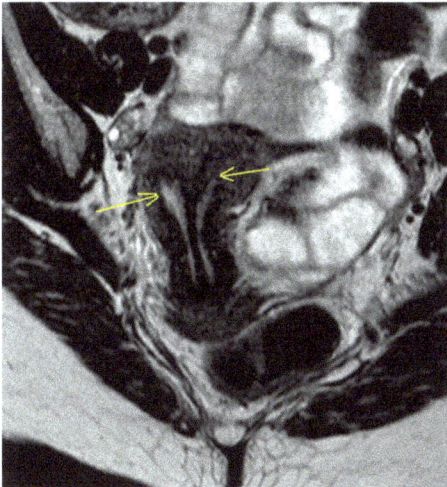

5.14b T2 axial complete septate

Complete Septate Uterus on T2 MRI with 2 endometrial channels (yellow arrows) separated by a fibrous septum which passes through to external cervical os.

Unicornuate uterus

- It has one horn that is connected to one fallopian tube. It has been described as half the size of a normal uterus. It may be difficult to identify on ultrasound. Both ovaries will be seen. It is a rare abnormality that is associated with a high incidence of pregnancy loss.

Ultrasound Services in an Early Pregnancy and Acute Gynaecological Unit. Book 2

45

- This type of uterus may be more laterally placed but normal in outline.
- There will be the absence of the normal rounded fundal contour.
- Where a rudimentary horn is present, it can be seen by its endometrium.
- A cystic mass (hematometra) may be seen where the endometrium is functional but the horn is obstructed.

Below is an MRI Image of a Unicornuate uterus.

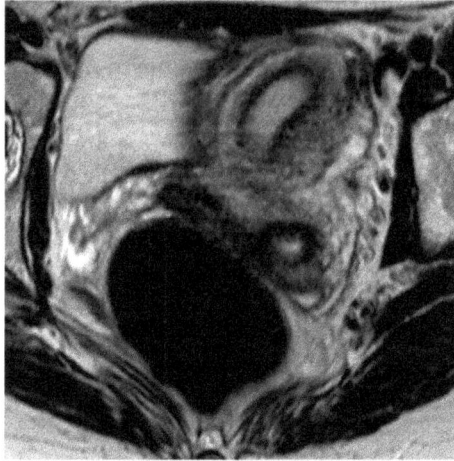

5.14c T2 Axial unicornual

Unicornuate Uterus – Single channel endometrial cavity with no right cornu – T2 angled axial image

HRT and the menstrual cycle

Menopause is one of the milestones in the life of a woman. (It is a time when she no longer experiences monthly periods and is considered naturally unable to be fertile). In the UK the average age for menopause is 52years. Vaginal bleeding post menopause is not normal. Such bleeding may cause anxiety to the patient.

All the types of HRT contain oestrogen that is meant to replace the oestrogen that the ovaries cease to make after menopause. This may cause the endometrial thickening. The risk of endometrial cancer is reduced when the oestrogen is combined with progestogen. Women on hormone replacement therapy can experience some bleeding which may be light or heavy.

The aim of the ultrasound examination of the pelvis is to

confirm or exclude the following conditions:

Ultrasound Services in an Early Pregnancy and Acute Gynaecological Unit. Book 2

46

- Endometritis
- Uterine fibroids
- Endometrial hyperplasia
- Endometrial or cervical polyps
- Endometrial or cervical cancer
- Cancer of the uterus including uterine sarcoma

Ovarian cysts

An ovarian cyst is a fluid filled sac in the ovary or cystic entity outside of the ovary but in the biological female pelvis. The cyst could be a functional cyst which is related to the woman's cycle or pathological cyst which is not menstrual cycle dependent. It may have a thin or thick wall, it may be well defined, with posterior enhancement or may not be well defined. To interpret a cystic appearance, the woman's age, LMP or approx. where she is in her menstrual cycle is essential. A cyst may contain clear echolucent fluid, low level echo fluid, it may contain echogenic debris, or solid lesion within it or in it's wall. It may have papillary projections from any side of it's wall, it may be small or big, unilateral or bilateral. It may be septated or not septated, it may be vascular or non vascular. It is essential to document the following once a cyst has been identified during a pelvic scan:

- The size of the cyst
- The location of the cyst
- Is it unilateral or bilateral?
- The wall of the cyst – is it thin or thick?
- Does it have any papillary projections?
- Cyst relationship with the ovary on that side
- Is there any associated ascites or free fluid in the pelvis or abdomen?
- The margins of the cyst – smooth or irregular, well or ill defined
- Is it septated or not and is there any flow in the septum or septa on Colour Doppler
- Any effect on the nearby pelvic organ, e.g. displacing the uterus or ovary etc.
- The content of the cyst – low leveled echoed or purely anechoic, mixed echo, heteregenous etc.
- Vascularity or otherwise around and within the cyst. Low resistant indices (RI) within the lesion raises the concern for suspicion of

Ultrasound Services in an Early Pregnancy and Acute Gynaecological Unit. Book 2

47

malignancy.

*The NICE guideline on ovarian cancer

B-rules	M- rules
Unilocular cysts	Irregular solid tumour
Presence of solid components where the largest solid component <7 mm	Ascites
Presence of acoustic shadowing	At least four papillary structures
Smooth multilocular tumour with a largest diameter <100 mm	Irregular multilocular solid tumour with largest diameter ^{3}100 mm
No blood flow	Very strong blood flow

Source: RCOG Green-top Guideline No. 62 © Royal College of Obstetricians and Gynaecologists

Corpus luteum cyst (CLC)

Always in the ovary, seen post ovulation in the luteal phase. There is vascularization around the cyst otherwise known as 'ring of fire' using Colour Doppler, may see some free fluid in the POD. Unlike the follicle, it tends to be irregular in outline, may be bigger, may contain some blood elements therefore becoming haemorrhagic, usually or often disappears with the next period. Where in doubt, a follow up scan six weeks later or in another menstrual phase usually shows it has disappeared or changed in size or appearance.

Multiple corpus luteum cysts may be seen e.g. if the woman releases two eggs in a normal menstrual cycle or post fertility treatment e.g. IVF. Here the ovaries may be enlarged, with multiple corpus luteum cysts and increased quantity of pelvic fluid.

Ultrasound Services in an Early Pregnancy and Acute Gynaecological Unit. Book 2

48

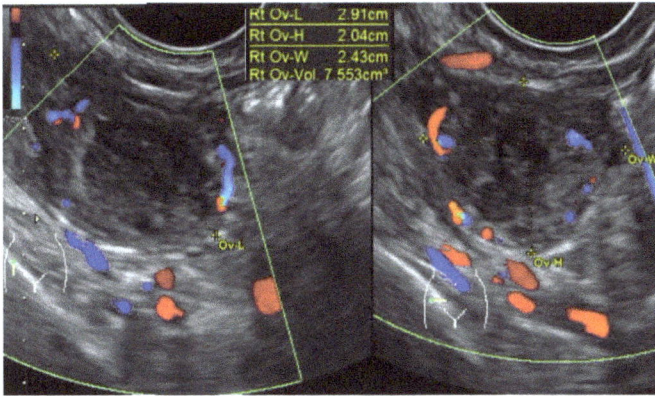

5.15a

Please note the ring of fire around the edges of the cyst.

A pelvic scan revealed this. Day 20 of a normal 28days cycle. The right ovary not shown here appeared sonographically normal. There was 9mm in depth fluid in the POD not shown here.

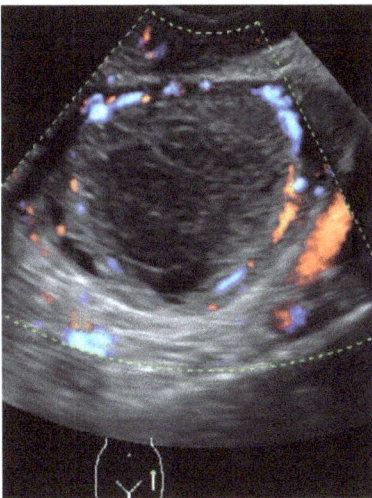
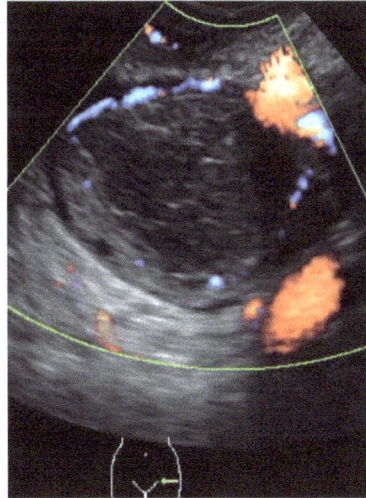

5.15b   **5.15c**

Ultrasound Services in an Early Pregnancy and Acute Gynaecological Unit. Book 2

49

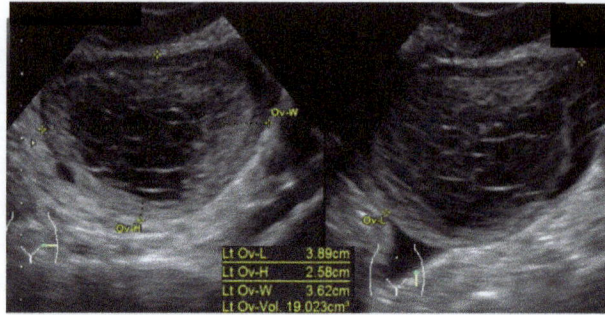

5.15d

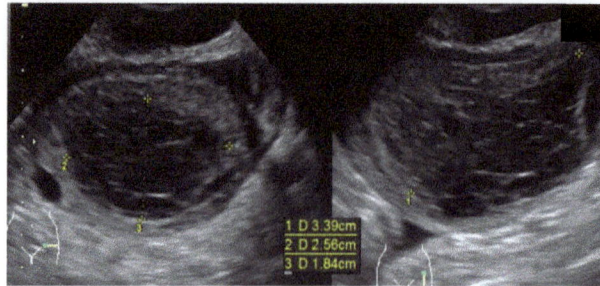

5.15e

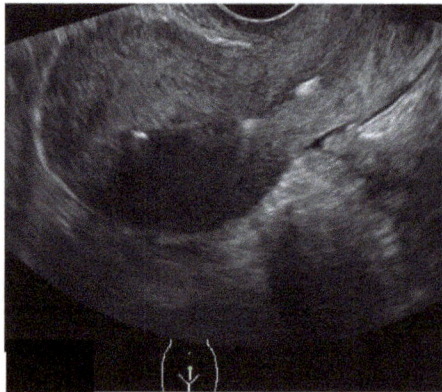

5.15f

Ultrasound findings: IUCD shaft is correctly positioned in endometrial cavity (5.15e). Haemorrhagic CLC in the left ovary (5.15a-d).

Follicular cyst

This is usually unilateral, enlarged, un ruptured big follicle that has not been released in ovulation. It is usually circular with no irregularity in its outline no internal echoes or debris. No vascularisation will be seen in or around this

Ultrasound Services in an Early Pregnancy and Acute Gynaecological Unit. Book 2

50

cyst. Usually this will be seen in conjunction with a thickened endometrium. It is a functional cyst. If it remains un released or un ruptured the patient will not have her next period and she will have a negative pregnancy test result. She may experience some pain in the area of the cyst. If she ovulates, the appearance will be different in another menstrual phase e.g. six weeks post the first scan.

Paraovarian cyst

Seen adjacent to the ovary not within it, lying on the broad ligament between the ovary and uterus. It is believed that it represent embryonic remnants and it is usually unilateral, accounting for 10% of pelvic masses. It is echo free and ovoid in shape. It is not a functional cyst. Usually very small, ranging from 2-20cm. Small sized cysts are of little or no clinical significance and the patient is likely to be asymptomatic, often found as an incidental finding during a pelvic scan. However large paraovarian cysts may cause pelvic pain and dyspareunia. May be mistakenly diagnosed as hydrosalpinx.

This patient was referred for a scan post miscarriage.

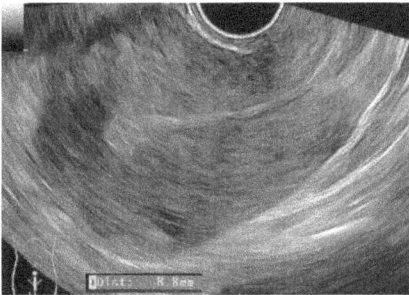

5.16a

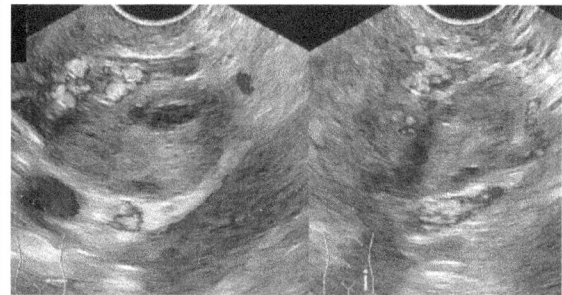

5.16b (31 x 34 x 21mm)

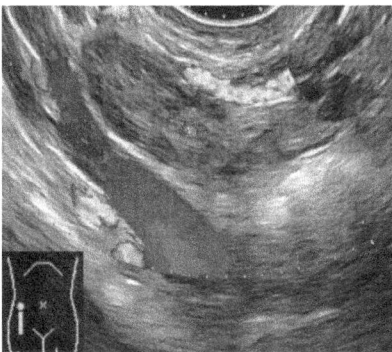

5.16c

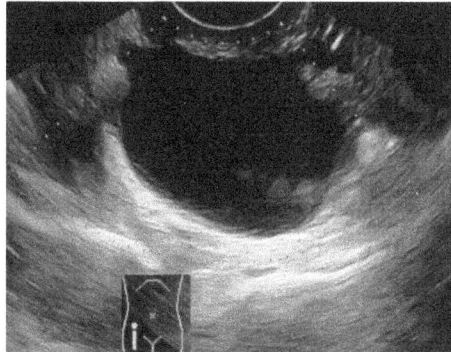

5.16d 26 x 28 x 15mm

Ultrasound Services in an Early Pregnancy and Acute Gynaecological Unit. Book 2

51

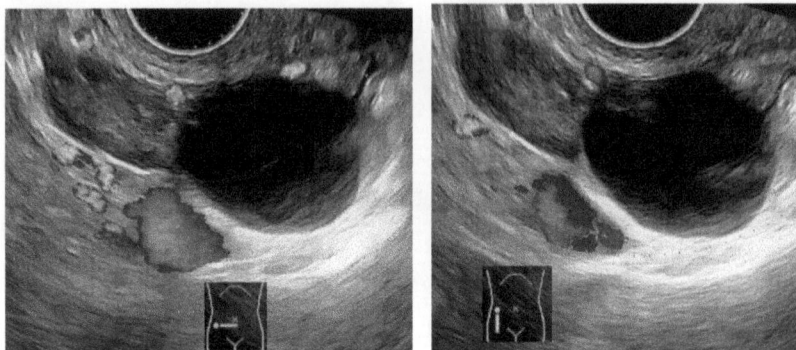

5.16e 30 x 27 x 28mm   **5.16f**

Ultrasound findings: An anteverted uterus with a 8.8mm endometrium. Left ovary – 31 x 34 x 21mm, volume = 11.5mls (5.16b). Right ovary – 26 x 28 x 15mm, volume = 5.7mls (5.16 c, e-f). Right paraovarian cyst – 30 x 27 x 28mm (5.16 d-f). No obvious free fluid is seen in the POD.

The above is an example of a right para ovarian cyst otherwise referred to as paratubal cyst or a hydatid cyst of Morgagni

- Hydrosalpinx will be tubular, 'sausage shaped' or coily. It will have double wall sign, occasionally possible to have a space between the ovary and the hydrosalpinx.
- Examining this structure from all the sides and observing its shape may be helpful in distinguishing this from a cyst.

Differentials - pelvic peritoneal inclusion cyst

Haemorrhagic cyst

It is a cyst that has fine inter digitating septations, giving it a fishnet weave or fine reticular appearance. It is a functional cyst. Scanning six weeks from the day of this scan or later in the cycle will demonstrate a different size and echo – pattern in a normal haemorrhagic cyst.

Ultrasound Services in an Early Pregnancy and Acute Gynaecological Unit. Book 2

52

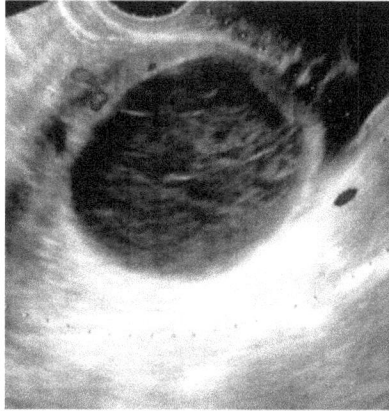

5.17a

Dermoid cyst

It is a benign neoplasm and is composed of tissue from at least two of the germ cell layers. The dermoid may contain hair, teeth etc. and this may make them show a wide range of ultrasonic appearances because of their variable composition. It may appear as hyperechoic or echogenic mass within the ovary. This is because it contains sebum and other fatty material. There may be attenuation seen posterior to the dermoid. Be aware of 'dirty' shadows from the bowel, that may try to cast hyperechoic shadows on the ovary. In most cases as the bowel churns, the overlying shadow from it also moves. They could also be cystic.

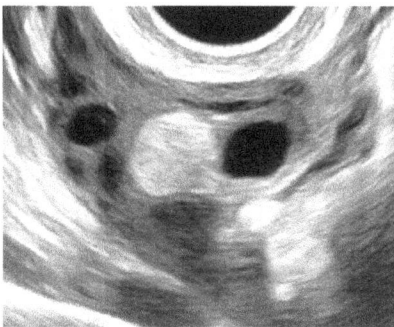 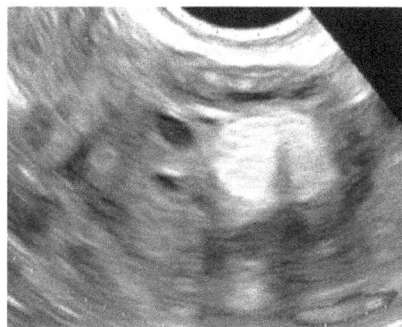

5.18a **5.18aa**

Above shows a dermoid cyst in an ovary

Ultrasound Services in an Early Pregnancy and Acute Gynaecological Unit. Book 2

53

Mature Cystic teratoma

It is seen on ultrasound as hypoechoic mass with some hyperechoic area in it. It is mostly unilateral, may demonstrate a fat-fluid level, may have 'tip of the iceberg' appearance which can be confused with overlying bowel gas, or hyperechoic lines which are by floating hair.

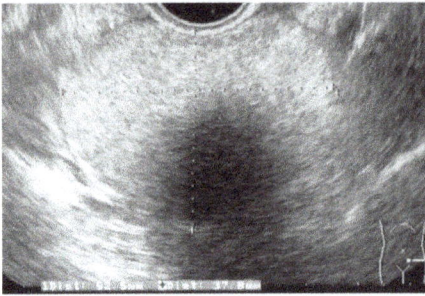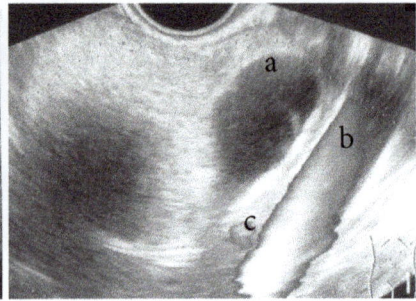

| 5.18b | 5.18c |

a. left teratoma, b- left iliac vein, c- left iliac artery.

Complications associated with teratomas include torsion, rupture, infection and rarely hemolytic anemia.

Another case of Ovarian Dermoid on MRI

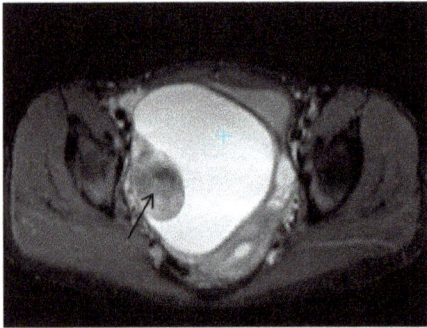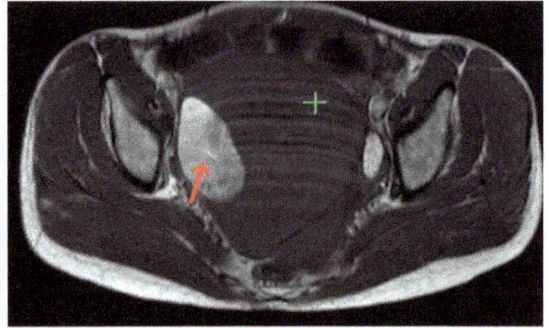

| 5.18c | 5.18d |
| T1 fatsat axial dermoid | T1 Axial dermoid |

Ultrasound Services in an Early Pregnancy and Acute Gynaecological Unit. Book 2

54

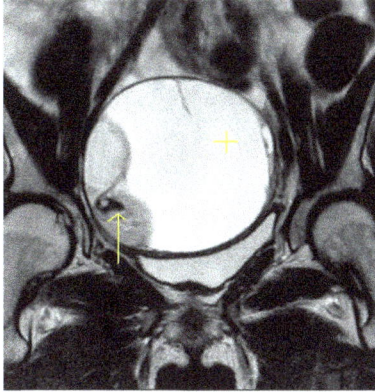

5.18e
T2 Coronal labeled

1. T1 Axial FATSAT image revealing low signal fat component (black arrow) and proteinaceous aqueous content (blue cross)
2. T1 Axial image showing large right ovarian dermoid (mature cystic teratoma) with fat content labelled with red arrow and majority low signal material labelled with green cross
3. Coronal T2 image revealing demoid plug with calcification (yellow arrow) and aqueous content (yellow cross)

Endometrioma

Otherwise known as 'chocolate cyst'. This shows homogeneous low level echoes within the ovary or outside the ovary. This is caused by bleeding from ectopic endometrial tissue within or outside the ovary. It has poor Doppler flow but thickened wall. They are of various sizes, unilateral or bilateral solid or homogeneous appearance. This may cause acute or chronic pelvic pain especially during normal menstruation, infertility, dyspareunia or dysmenorrhea. It will have posterior enhancement and may rupture therefore the need for follow up scans. Echogenic foci are seen in the wall in 30% of the cases. No fine strands will be seen coursing within the cyst, they lack septations and can be mistaken for a solid mass. MRI can be used to make the diagnosis.

Differentials are a} haemorrhagic cyst which will have fine strands coursing within the cyst and change in appearance in another menstrual phase or six weeks from the first scan and b} ovarian torsion

Ultrasound Services in an Early Pregnancy and Acute Gynaecological Unit. Book 2

55

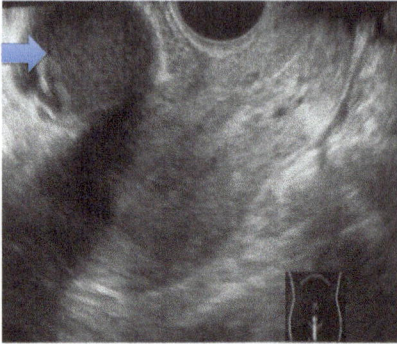 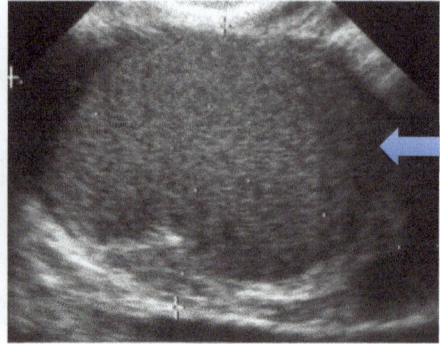

5.19a   **5.19b**

Arrows showing endometriomas in two different patients.

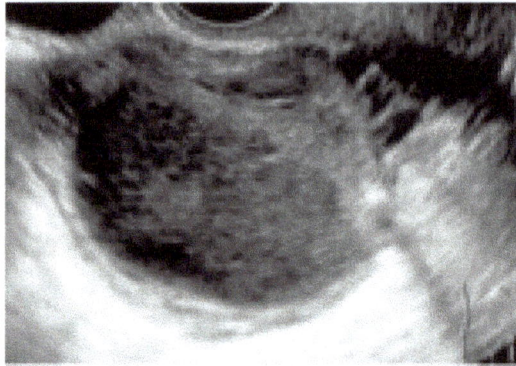

5.19c Above shows endometriomas in another patient

Another case of Endometriosis on MRI

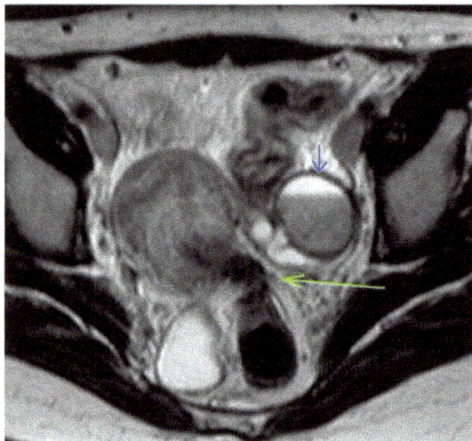

5.19d

T2 axial endometriosis

Ultrasound Services in an Early Pregnancy and Acute Gynaecological Unit. Book 2

56

Severe (Grade 4) Endometriosis on MRI with axial T2 image showing bilateral endometriomas (left labelled with blue arrow) and significant scarring at pouch of Douglas indrawing distal sigmoid colon (green arrow).

Multi cystic ovary

This is a common appearance of the ovary in girls just before their 1st menstrual period. The ovary is usually of normal size. The follicles are multiple, scattered all around the ovary, of various sizes, and small, less than 12mm in diameter. The affected ovary usually shows like a bunch of grapes or 'swiss cheese' or honeycomb appearance. After the first period it is seen when the patient has lost significant weight or where the patient is experiencing severe stress and anxiety. Often this is seen in young women who are in their teens or young adult life, had bulimia or anorexia nervosa but had recovered. The patient may have irregular or no periods. Egg or oocycte production is rare, therefore the woman could be infertile or experience sub-fertility.

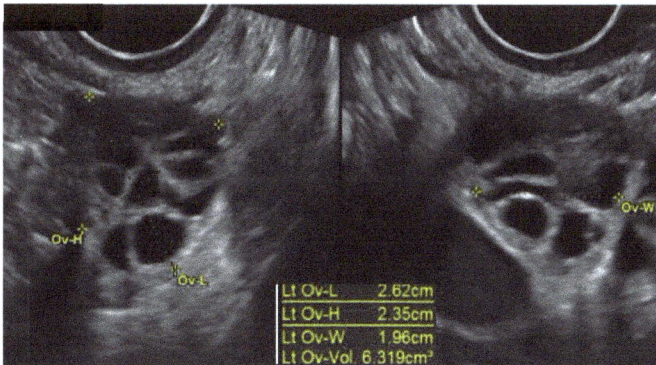

5.20a
An example of multicystic ovary

Polycystic ovary

Is seen in 20% of women of reproductive age. The affected ovary is enlarged, has a thick stroma, multiple follicles of no more than 10mm in diameter are seen neatly arranged around the periphery of the ovary referred to as the 'necklace sign' (at least 10 of them) and the follicles less than 10mm in diameter (average 4-5mm) or an ovary with an ovarian volume that is equal to or greater than 10mls in volume (without any cyst in it). It is possible to have one ovary with polycystic appearance

Ultrasound Services in an Early Pregnancy and Acute Gynaecological Unit. Book 2

57

and the other ovary with a normal appearance. It is possible to have PCO without having PCOS.

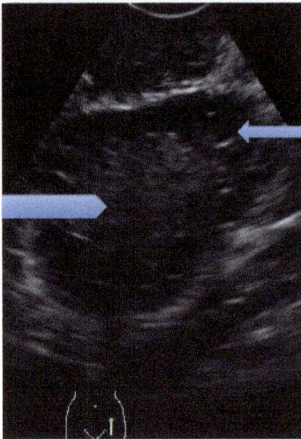 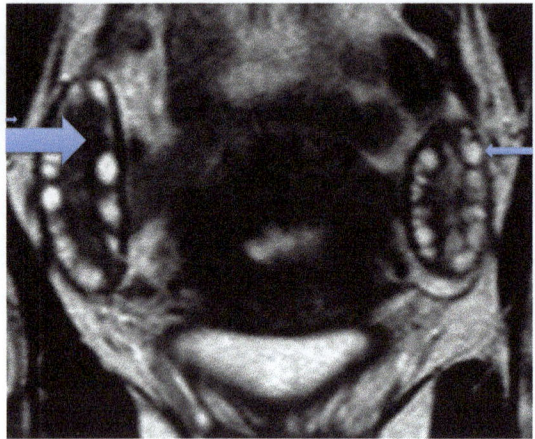

5.21 a   **5.21c**

Thin arrow –follicle, thicker arrow – thick stroma
PCO on ultrasound and on MRI

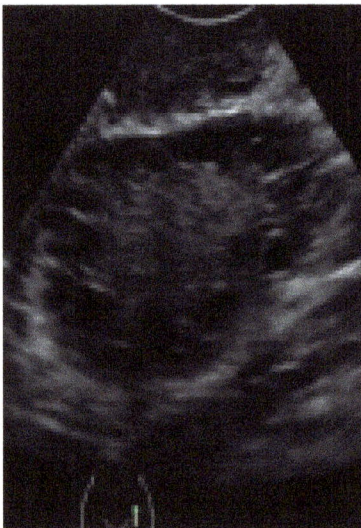 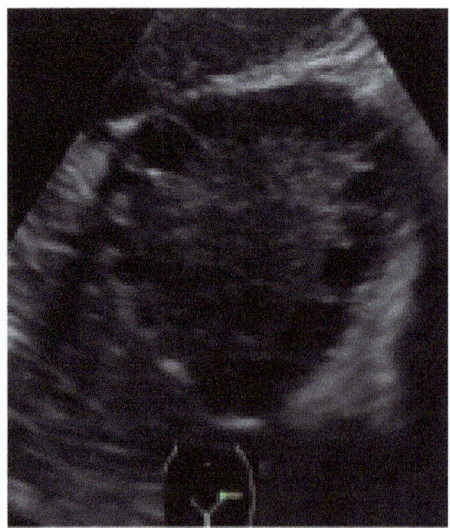

5.21a   **5.21b**

Note the peripheral follicles and the strong stoma. This is PCO

Ultrasound Services in an Early Pregnancy and Acute Gynaecological Unit. Book 2

58

Complex Cyst

This cyst is usually of complex composition often with cystic and solid components, could be regular or irregular in outline, could be unilateral or bilateral, could be small or big in size. May be septated or not septated. Use of Colour Dopplers to assess its vascularity is important. Finding a complex cyst should alert the sonographer to check the abdomen and pelvis for ascites, and mets in the liver and possibly assess the kidneys should obstruction be suspected. Where the sonographer has no training or qualification to perform abdominal ultrasound, the need for an ultrasound scan of the upper abdomen should be indicated in his report.

Ultrasound Services in an Early Pregnancy and Acute Gynaecological Unit. Book 2

59

Chapter Conclusion

Understanding the ultrasound appearance of the normal pelvic organs in a female and the various variants will help the Sonographer to identify abnormalities that may warrant further investigations or treatment.

Ultrasound Services in an Early Pregnancy and Acute Gynaecological Unit. Book 2

60

CHAPTER 6

In this chapter, we will consider some clinical indications that make women attend AGU or EPAGU for scan.

Clinical Indications for Ultrasound in AGU or EPAGU in no particular order:

- PMB
- Post TOP
- Missing IUCD
- Heavy bleeding
- Post miscarriage
- Abdominal bloating
- Sudden swollen legs
- Post op complications.
- Suspected ovarian cysts
- Post delivery complications
- Following fertility treatment
- Abnormal or irregular pv. bleeding
- Post cornual pregnancy treatment
- Post menopausal ovarian cysts or mass
- Sudden generalized or local pelvic pain
- No menstrual period and –ve pregnancy test result

The aim of scanning these ladies include:

- To assess the pelvis and identify any abnormality or cause for referral for the scan.
- It might become necessary to extend the examination to the abdomen e.g. in case of pelvic ascites, the upper abdomen needs to be scanned to

Ultrasound Services in an Early Pregnancy and Acute Gynaecological Unit. Book 2

61

assess the extent of the ascites or in case of large pelvic mass, the kidneys should be checked for hydronephrosis.

- All usual and other unusual findings must be documented and mentioned in the ultrasound report thereafter.

Technical challenges that the Sonographer may encounter

- High BMI
- Overlying bowel gas
- Shadows from fibroids
- Pain that limits the examination
- Very active or constipated bowel
- Patient refusing TVS when it is not contra indicated
- Lack of known anatomy landmark such as the uterus in post hysterectomy scans
- Heavy bleeding making the interpretation of the endometrium appearance difficult
- Presence of an IUCD in the endometrium which may make assessing the endometrium difficult
- Heavy abdominal bandaging or dressing following surgery thereby limiting the access to the area of interest

Examples of active bowel and overlying bowel gas seen during a TV Scan:

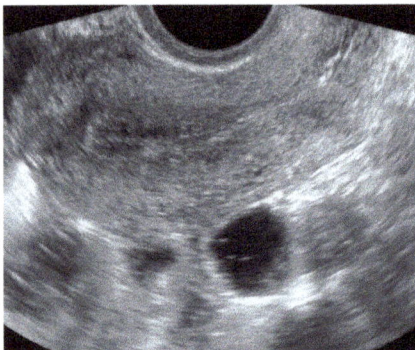

6.0a	6.0b
Active bowel and gas	Bowel gas in the RIF

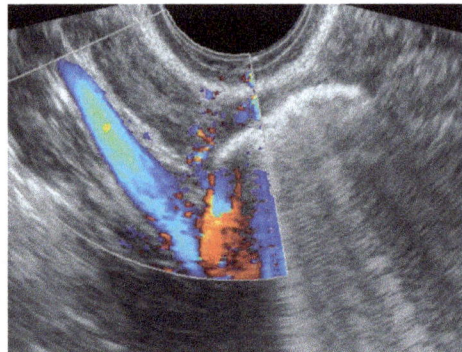

Right ovary lying superiorly to the right iliac vessel. White rings indicate shadows from bowel gas.

Ultrasound Services in an Early Pregnancy and Acute Gynaecological Unit. Book 2

62

Ultrasound Report

Immediately following the ultrasound examination an Ultrasound report should be generated specifying the following information:

- Hospital or and Departmental details
- Patient's details
- LMP when or where applicable
- Date of the Scan
- Reason for scan or Clinical History
- Any relevant Past medical history
- Answer to the scan reason or question
- Ultrasound Equipment used e.g. Aloka, Toshiba, GE, Siemens etc.
- Method of scanning TA or TVS or both
- Quality of views obtained - good, poor or restricted and why?
- Any other significant or relevant findings to or of the uterus ovaries or adnexa
- Name and designation about chaperone if present. If not this should ocumented and why
- Any problems encountered during the examination should be documented e.g. such that makes the examination limited either by the quality of the images or patient's discomfort or patients decline to TVS where it is not contraindicated
- Any need for follow up, referral or suggestion
- Sonographer's details

For medico-legal and clarity reasons amongst others, many hospitals in the UK tend to have a typed or word processed gynaecology ultrasound reporting system. In some departments, there are agreed templates with space for additional information which the Sonographer can use if and when necessary.

There are many obstetrics and Gynaecology reporting packages available including Viewpoint etc. It makes reporting easier, uniform whilst giving Sonographers the ability to add extra comments pertaining to each examination. It is important that the chosen reporting package be compatible with the hospital's reporting system and upgradable. The ultrasound report should be available for access by Clinicians

Ultrasound Services in an Early Pregnancy and Acute Gynaecological Unit. Book 2

63

who might need the report within the hospital. It should be easy to interprete by referring Clinicians including the GP's.

Which facilities may be required for a Gynaecology ultrasound Follow Up?

- Rapid access to Gynae. Clinic for referral and follow up where indicated
- Facilities for laboratory tests such as hormone tests, CA 125
- Other imaging modalities – CT, MRI
- Good theatre back up if and when need be
- Where the CA 125 is high, CT is used for staging
- Where the CA 125 is low, MRI is used to stage indeterminate masses
- MRI is usually used for staging and CT for assessment of disease spread in the body

WHAT TO LOOK FOR ON THE SCAN

Ideally every effort should be made to identify and assess the uterus, ovaries and adnexae. Choice of scanning method will depend on many factors. Where and when the patient can drink and it's her first gynecology ultrasound scan, it is prudent to do both a TAS and TVS, provided TVS is not contra indicated. With both approaches, a full pelvic view and assessment can be done. This can provide the baseline information that can be used to monitor any future growth or echo pattern changes or response to any treatment.

It is however essential that the Sonographer be familiar with normal ultrasound patterns of the uterus, ovaries and adnexae over a normal menstrual cycle both with TAS or TVS approach.

Before embarking on any non pregnant pelvic scan, it is important to find out from the patient her LMP, how often she has a menstrual period, if she is on the pill or not, if she has had any pelvic surgery before and for the peri or post menopausal if she is on HRT. This will help in the interpretation of the obtained images of the uterus, ovaries and POD. It is also important that the Sonographer asks and verifies that TVS is not contra indicated in the patient. It must not be assumed that every patient requiring gynaecological examination is suitable to have a TVS irrespective of her age.

Ultrasound Services in an Early Pregnancy and Acute Gynaecological Unit. Book 2

64

For patients who are menopausal, she should be asked approximately the date of her menopause. For the normal postmenopausal woman, the longer it has been that or when she became menopausal, the smaller the ovaries should be and the less chances it may be of seeing them on ultrasound especially when there is a lot of bowel activity or overlying bowel gas.

Post Menopausal bleeding (PMB)

Menopause is defined by the World Health Organization as the permanent cessation of menstruation resulting from the loss of ovarian follicular activity.

PMB is vaginal bleeding occurring twelve months post amenorrhea in a woman:

- Of the age where the menopause can be expected or
- Who has had an early or premature menopause or premature ovarian failure.

Predisposing factors for PMB include:

- It is likely to occur if exogenous oestrogens are taken
- Tamoxifen has an anti-oestrogen effect on the breast, but a pro-oestrogen effect on the uterus and bones
- Polycystic ovarian disease increases risk
- Hereditary non-polyposis colorectal carcinoma
- Obesity combined with diabetes

PMB is a common reason for postmenopausal women needing a gynaecological scan. It affects 1 in 10 women aged 55 years old and above. Women with PMB often attend with some anxiety, as PMB is a common symptom for both benign and malignant conditions.

PMB could be due to:

- Vaginal atrophy
- Endometrial carcinoma
- Carcinoma of cervix or cervix
- Trauma or bleeding disorder
- Endometrial or cervical polyps
- Use of hormone replacement therapy (HRT)
- Endometrial hyperplasia; simple, complex, and atypical

Whilst the focus is primarily on the integrity, thickness and appearance of the

Ultrasound Services in an Early Pregnancy and Acute Gynaecological Unit. Book 2

65

endometrium and cervix in particular, it is not unusual to find pathologies in the ovary (ies) or urinary bladder or adnexae.

- TAS should be performed first to exclude any urinary bladder pathology, pelvic mass (es) or fibroids. TAS is not sufficient enough due to the need for good resolution of the uterus (especially the endometrium) therefore making a TVS mandatory in these women (unless contra indicated or patient decline). The sonographer should confirm that TVS is not contra-indicated in the patient, verify patient's allergy to latex and need to obtain the patient's consent. The sonographer should apply more gel on the probe cover and be very gentle in scanning technique and comply with protocol for chaperoning.
- TVS is painless and well tolerated by most women.

What are we looking for when scanning women with PMB?:
- Ultrasound appearances of the urinary bladder, uterus, ovaries and the adnexae.
- Endometrial lining – is it thin or thick? Measure it in the LS view.
- Is the outline smooth or irregular, homogenous or heterogeneous?
- Does it have any space occupying lesion (SOL)?
- Is it eroding it's neighbouring myometrium?
- Is it vascular or non vascular – using Dopplers?
- Is it fluid filled? If yes what is the nature of the fluid?
- The cervix and its integrity.
- The thickness of endometrium should be measured as the AP diameter in the LS section excluding any fluid measurement. An endometrium of 5mm or less in a postmenopausal woman is considered normal. The integrity or smoothness or otherwise of the endometrium should be assessed and documented plus the presence of any ultrasound identifiable pathology including sub mucous fibroid, endometrial hyperplasia, polyp and cancer. There may be need to extend the scan to the upper abdomen e.g. when there is a big mass – to exclude hydronephrosis or assess abdominal ascites. Occasionally there may be the need for other imaging modalities such as CT or MRI.

Ultrasound Services in an Early Pregnancy and Acute Gynaecological Unit. Book 2

66

A saline infusion ultrasound (Sonohysterography) can help assess the endometrium better when an endometrial pathology is suspected. Shadows from intra mural fibroids may impede the visualisation of the endometrium. It is not uncommon not to find any ultrasound identifiable cause for the bleeding. Ultrasound findings of the ovaries and adnexae should be documented.

This woman was referred for a pelvic scan with a clinical history of PMB.

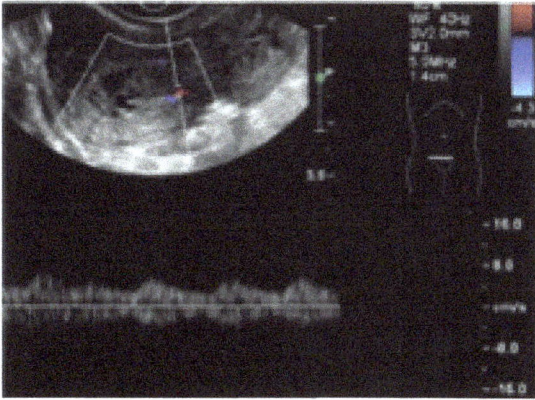

6.1a

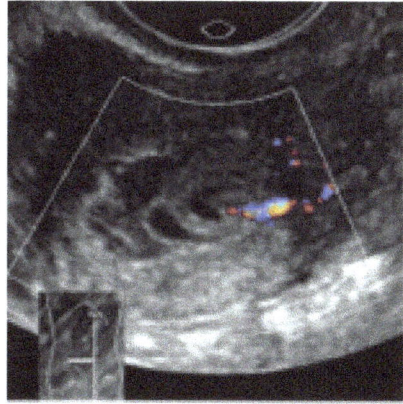

6.1b

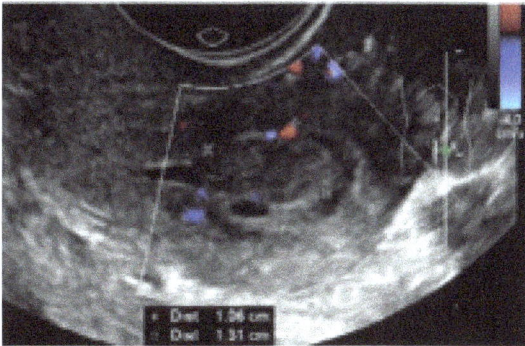

6.1c

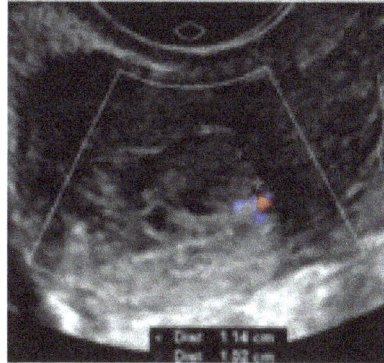

6.1d

Ultrasound findings: The endometrial thickness is 11mm (6.1d). Within the thickened endometrium is a 13 x 11 x 10mm predominantly hyper echoic structure that also had some cystic entity(6.1a-d). There is a feeding stalk on Doppler's (6.1b-d x in 6.1b).

Impression: Endometrial polyp but other endometrial pathology cannot be excluded such as endometrial adenocarcinoma or hyperplasia.

Ultrasound Services in an Early Pregnancy and Acute Gynaecological Unit. Book 2

67

This woman was referred for a scan with a clinical history of PMB on long term HRT. The left ovary not shown here appeared sonographically normal.

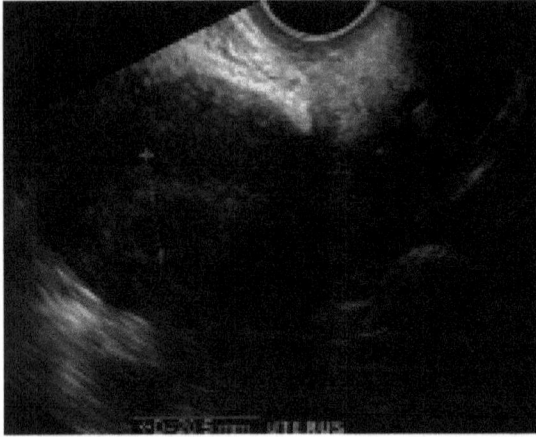

6.2a

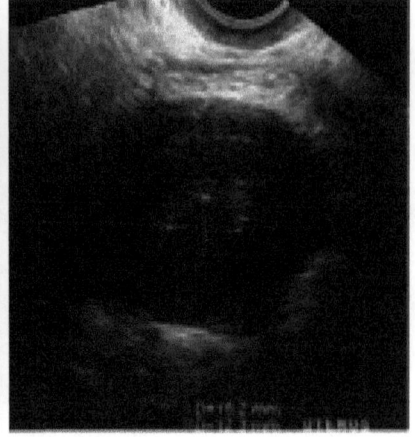

6.2b

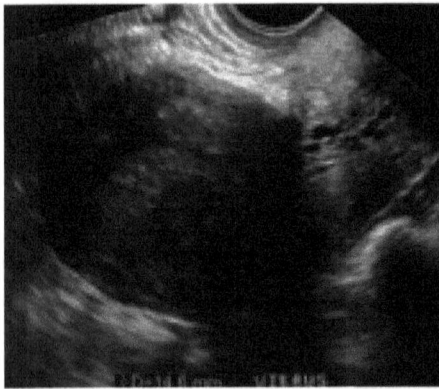

6.2c

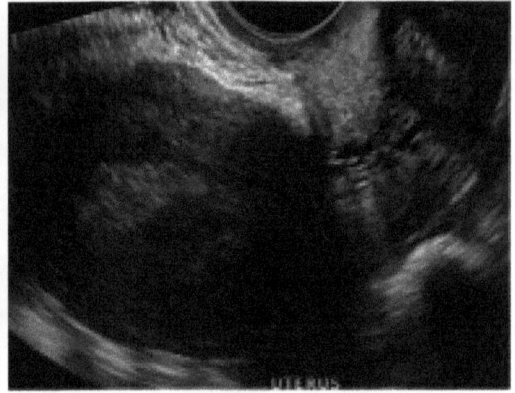

6.2d

Ultrasound Services in an Early Pregnancy and Acute Gynaecological Unit. Book 2

68

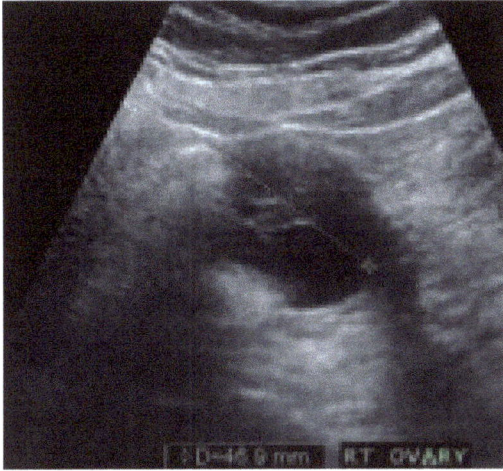
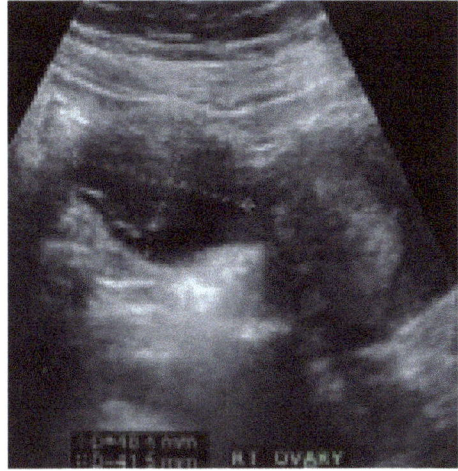

6.2e   **6.2f**

Ultrasound findings: An anteverted uterus with an endometrium that is irregular and markedly thickened measuring 21mm at the fundus (6.a). There appear to be small cystic areas within the endometrium. ? Cystic hyperplasia but other pathology cannot be excluded (6.2a,c-d). There is a hypoechoic area within the endometrium measuring approximately 16 x12 x15mm ?fibroid ?atypical polyp (6.2a-d)

The right ovary measures 48 x 42x 47mm and contains a complex cyst with thickened septae (6.2e-f). No free fluid is demonstrated in the POD.

Impression: Thickened and irregular in outline endometrium with a hypoechoic structure in it. Endometrial pathology cannot be excluded.

Complex cyst in the right ovary.

*Where and when available, performing a Sonohysterography will help in reaching the diagnosis of the endometrial entity as better views will be obtained.

This postmenopausal woman was referred with a history of 1/7 pv bleeding. Nulliparous, never been on HRT or Tamoxifen. TVS declined. Menopause over 20years before the scan. Both ovaries were not identified.

Ultrasound Services in an Early Pregnancy and Acute Gynaecological Unit. Book 2

69

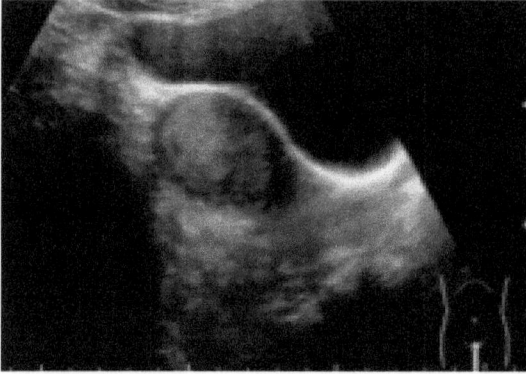

6.3a

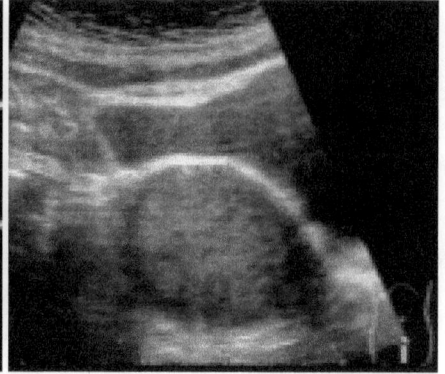

6.3b

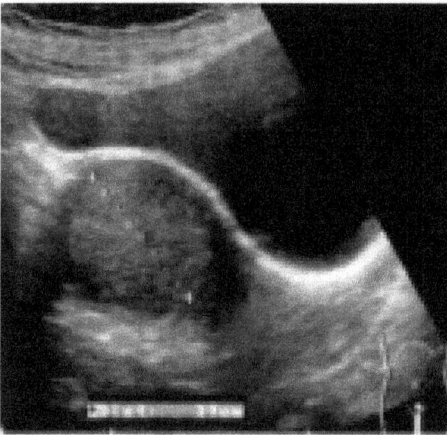

6.3c

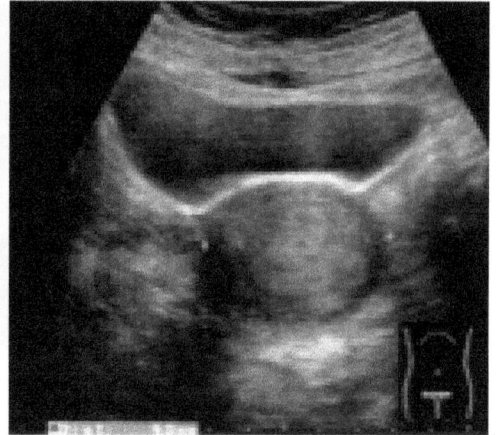

6.3d

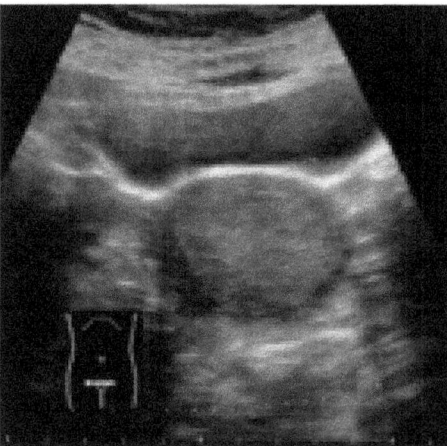

6.3e

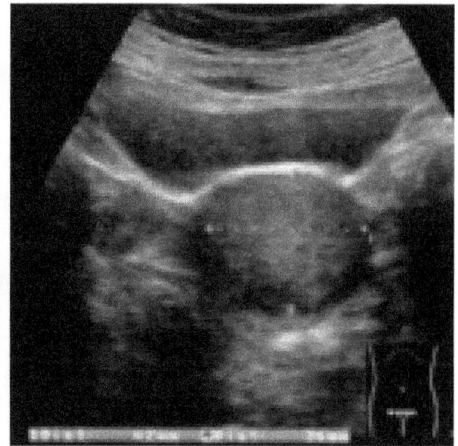

6.3f

Ultrasound Services in an Early Pregnancy and Acute Gynaecological Unit. Book 2

70

Ultrasound findings: Completely filling the endometrium is an approx. 42 x 42 x 36mm predominantly echogenic area that did not show any flow on Dopplers. (6.c-f). The myometrium is very thin (6.3a-c)

Impression:?cystic endometrial hyperplasia, ?Endometrial Ca. ?other pathology.
* Follow up histology report: hysterectomy specimen showed Grade 2 endometrial adenocarcinoma

This post menopausal woman was referred with a history of brownish discharge. ?PMB. TVS was declined. Below are the images.

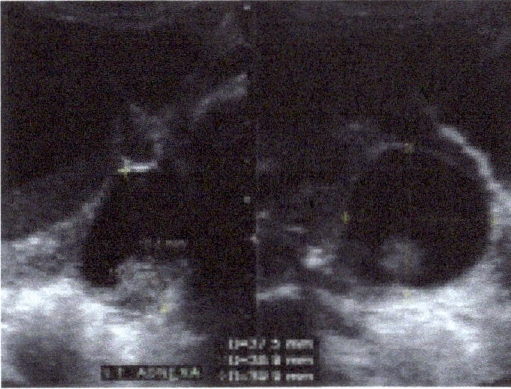

6.4a

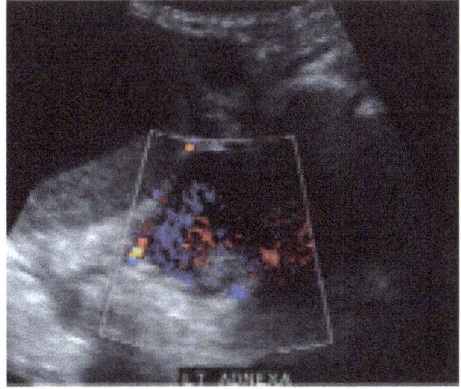

6.4b

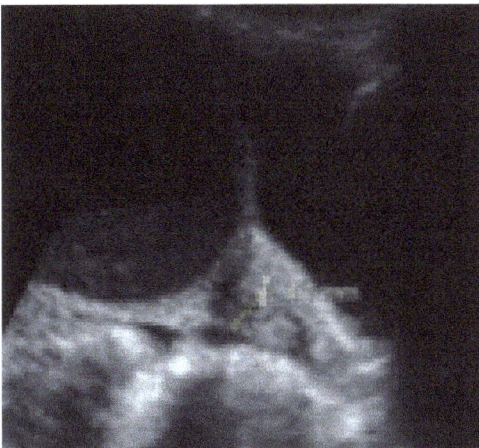

6.4c

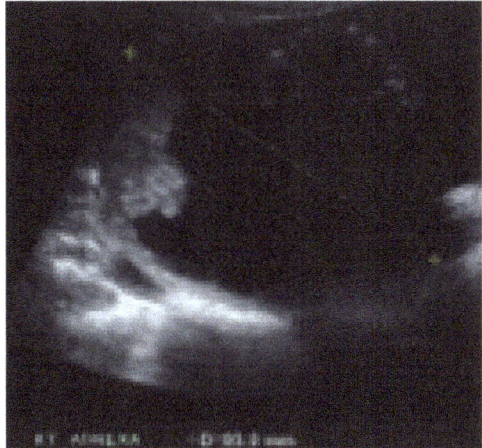

6.4d

Ultrasound Services in an Early Pregnancy and Acute Gynaecological Unit. Book 2

71

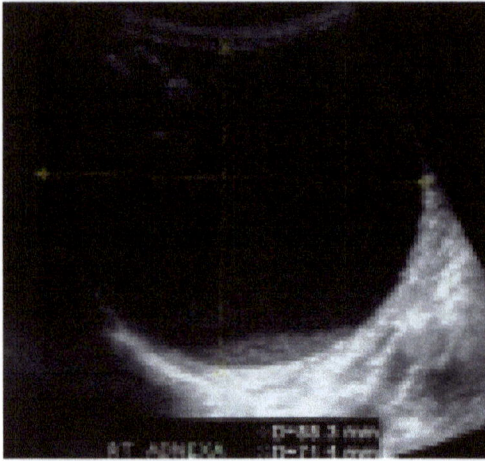
6.4e

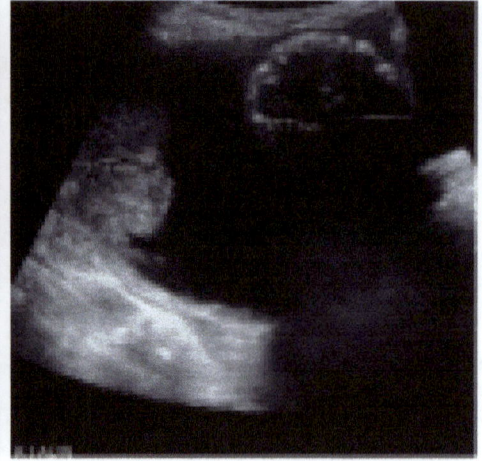
6.4f

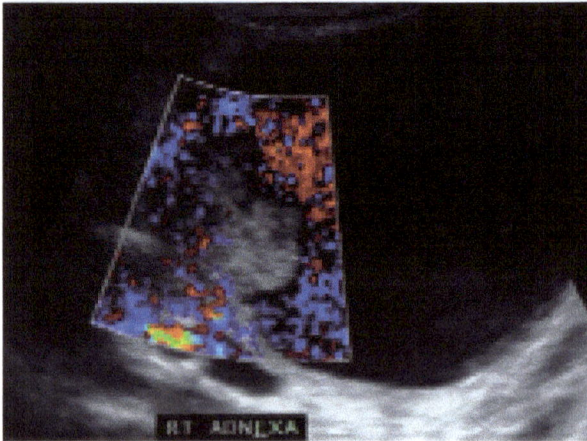
6.4g

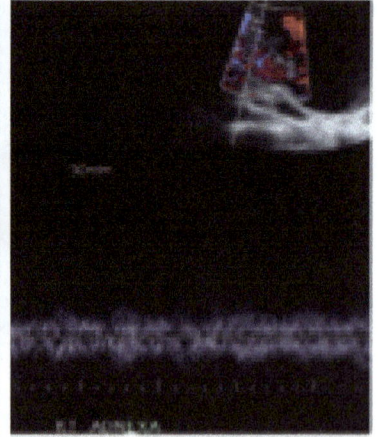
6.4h

Ultrasound findings: Normal size uterus (appropriate for post menopausal woman) with a 4.7mm endometrium (6.4c). In the right adnexal is a complex predominantly low level echoed cyst that had sedimentations at it's base. There is an irregular papillary projection arising from it's wall and superiorly within the cyst is a ?calcified papilla. There is blood flow to the papillas (6.4d-h). Inferior to the uterus and ? in the left adnexa is another cystic entity with irregular in outline ?papillas (6.4a –b). Both ovaries were not seen separate from these complex entities.

Impression: Bilateral complex masses. Bilateral ovarian malignancy could not be excluded.

Ultrasound Services in an Early Pregnancy and Acute Gynaecological Unit. Book 2

72

The woman later had a CT scan in view of the ultrasound findings.

* CT was able to identify a right ovary, identify a heterogenous multi loculated mass in the left adnexal region with an irregular lobulated soft tissue area superiorly within the cystic area. Left ovary was not seen separate from the mass. Rounded soft tissue mass was seen in the retro uterine pouch suspicious of peritoneal deposit. CT concluded that there is complex left adnexal cyst likely to represent primary ovarian malignancy with associated ascites and peritoneal deposits.

*This case demonstrates that not all post menopausal patients with ?discharge or pv bleeding is as a result of or from endometrial pathology.

This woman in her fifties was referred with a history of RIF mass, PMB and previous gastric cancer. Both ovaries were not identified and both kidneys had normal sonographic appearances with no evidence of hydronephrosis.

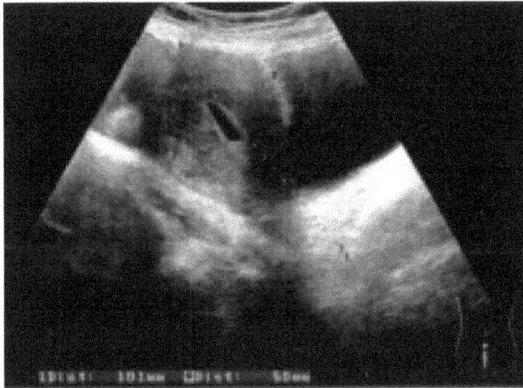

6.5a

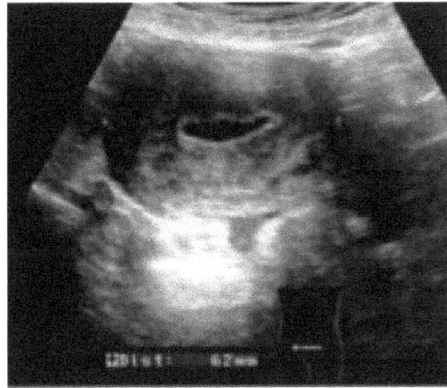

6.5b

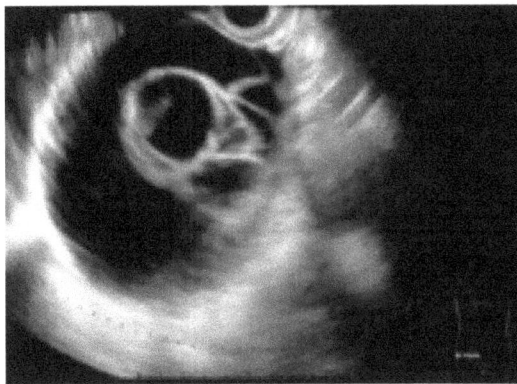

6.5c

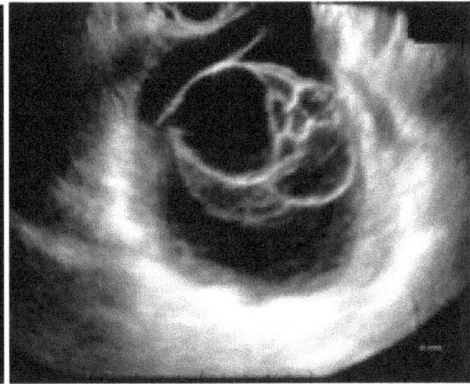

6.5d

Ultrasound Services in an Early Pregnancy and Acute Gynaecological Unit. Book 2

73

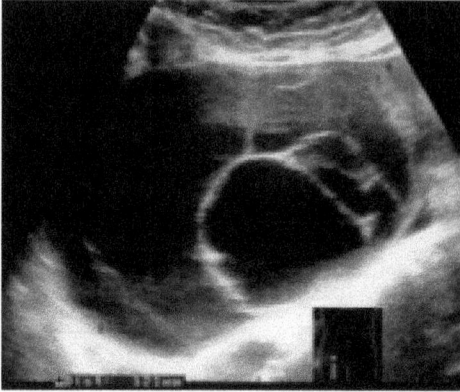

6.5e

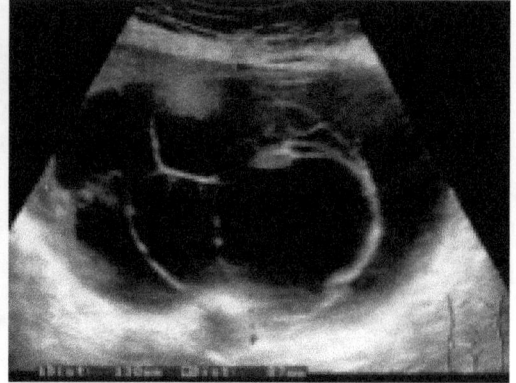

6.5f

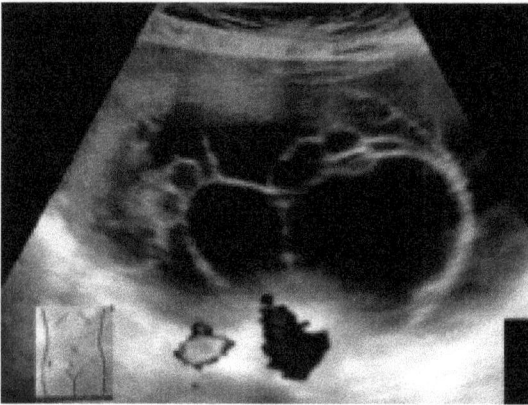

6.5g

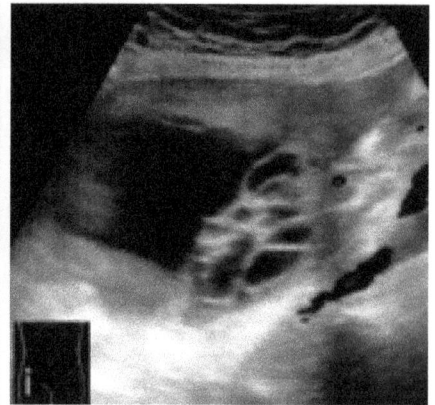

6.5h

Ultrasound findings: An anteverted uterus measuring approx. 101 x 50 x 62mm (6.5a-b). There is some fluid and some echogenic structure slightly irregular in outline measuring approx. 28 x 9mm in the endometrium. Predominantly in the RIF and towards the midline is an approx. 131 x 132 x 133mm multi septated cyst that does not demonstrate any flow on Dopplers. Both ovaries have not been identified. 6.5c -h)

Impression: Cystadenoma although other pathology cannot be excluded.
CT/ MRI is suggested.

- MRI report confirmed a large right adnexal 13cm mass with appearances that are consistent with tumour.
- CT reported significant enlargement of Krukenberg type tumour of the right ovary.

Ultrasound Services in an Early Pregnancy and Acute Gynaecological Unit. Book 2

74

Krukenberg tumors - Experts claim that:

- They are uncommon, that it accounts for 1-2% (in some literature) or 5 -6% in other literature of all ovarian tumors..
- It is a type of ovarian tumor which starts in another area of the body and migrates to the ovaries.
- They tend to originate from cancer of the GIT system and less commonly from breast, colon, pancreas, appendix cancer.
- Patients typically present with this problem in their fourth or fifth decade of life. The common presenting symptoms are related to the ovary and include abdominal pain and distension due to the bilateral, often large ovarian masses.
- They often have poor prognosis.

This woman was referred with a history of PMB for 5/52. Both ovaries were not identified.

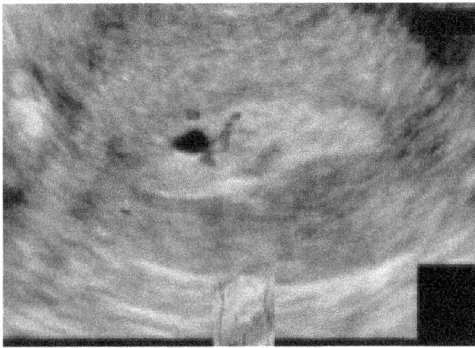

6.6a

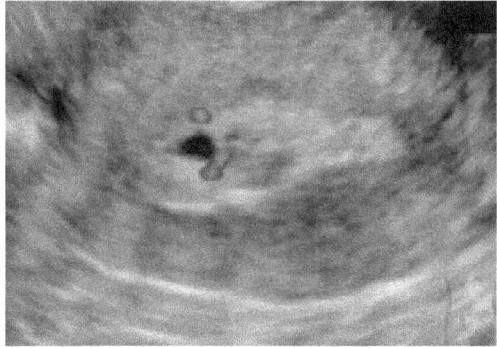

6.6b

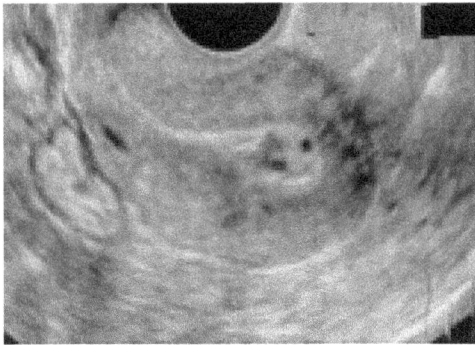

6.6c

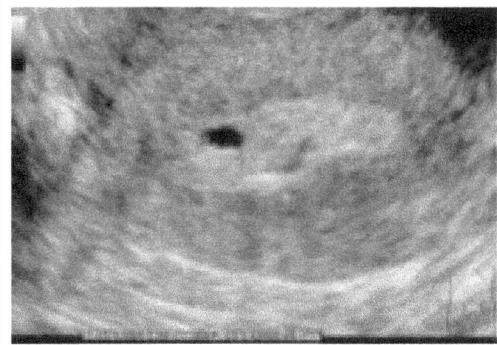

6.6d

Ultrasound Services in an Early Pregnancy and Acute Gynaecological Unit. Book 2

75

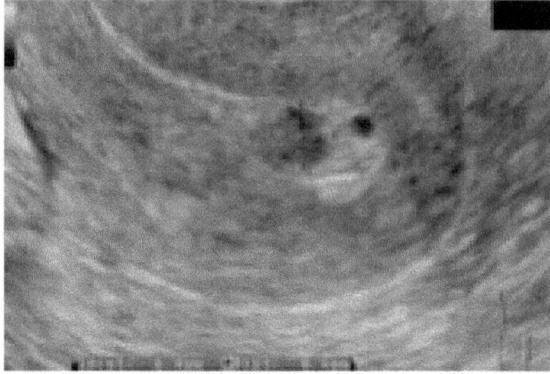

6.6e

Ultrasound findings: Retroverted uterus – measurements not included. There are three hypoechoic areas, the biggest being approx. 6 x 6 x 8mm and irregular in outline(6.6e). There is an approx. 14 x 8mm hyperechoic area in the endometrium that show some flow on Dopplers (6.6a-b).

Impression: ?Polyp, ? hyperplasia but other endometrial pathology cannot be excluded.

This Post Menopausal woman was referred for PMB, both ovaries were not identified.

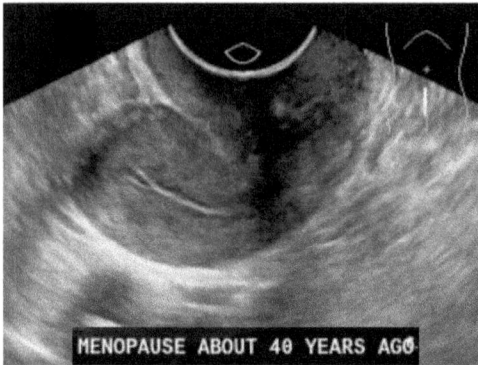

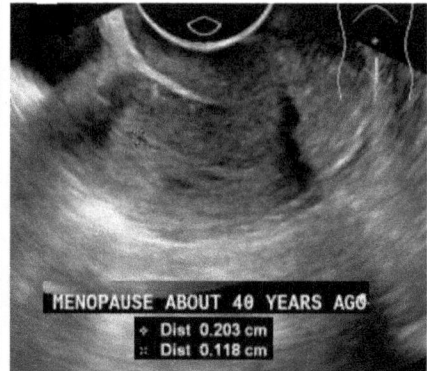

6.6f   **6.6g**

Uterine measurements above is 53 x 29 x 22mm

Note the tiny fluid in the endometrium. The endometrium is smooth and thin.

Endometrial thickness in this case is 2.03mm – 1.18 = 0.85mm.

Ultrasound Services in an Early Pregnancy and Acute Gynaecological Unit. Book 2

76

Post Termination of Pregnancy (TOP)

Women terminate pregnancies for social or medical reasons and at various gestational ages. Some women will have medical termination whilst others will have surgical termination. For women who are referred for a post TOP scan it is important to confirm or exclude intrauterine gestational sac or RPOC primarily. The aim is to confirm or refute RPOC which if left in the uterus can cause bleeding, infection, abdominal pain, delay in the return of normal menstrual period and other complications.

This woman was referred with a history of vomiting post TOP. Both ovaries not shown here appeared sonographically normal.

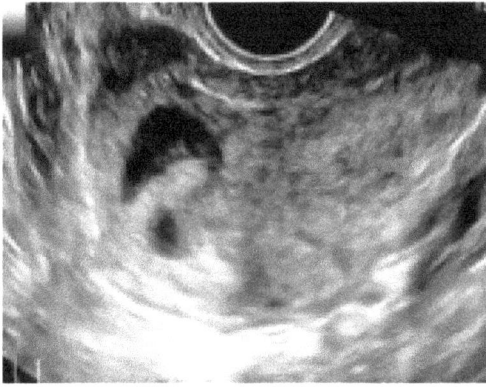 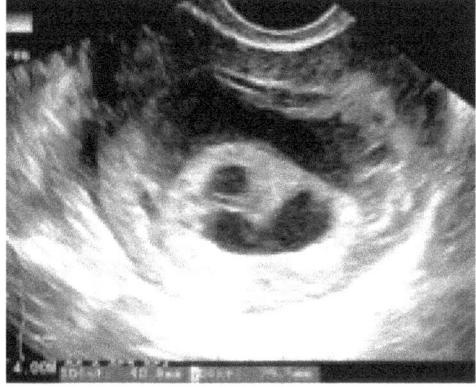

| 6.7a | 6.7b |

Ultrasound findings: An anteverted uterus with a fluid filled endometrium as well as echogenic structures. TS measurement of the endometrial cavity = 41 x 30mm. **Impression:** RPOC.

This woman was referred for a scan with a history of ?RPOC at 4/52 and 8/52 post TOP. Both ovaries not shown here appear normal.
Below are the ultrasound findings at 4/52

Ultrasound Services in an Early Pregnancy and Acute Gynaecological Unit. Book 2

77

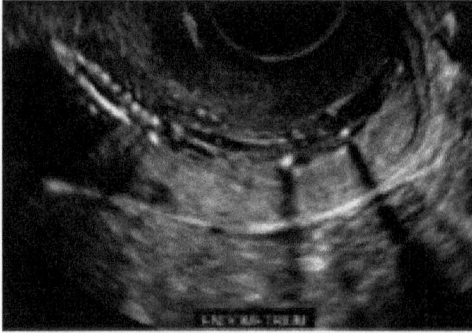
6.8a

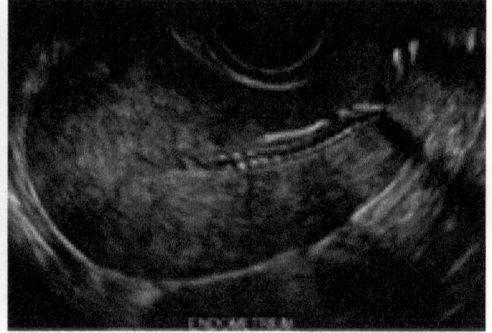
6.8b

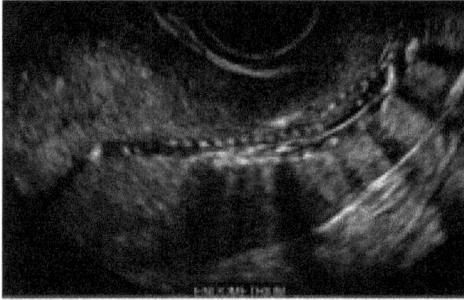
6.8c

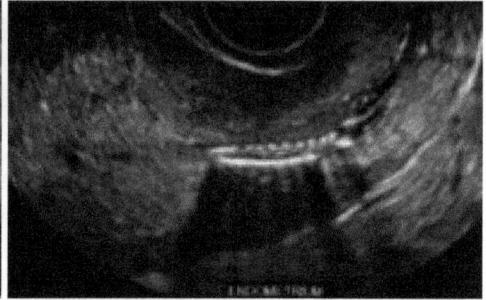
6.8d

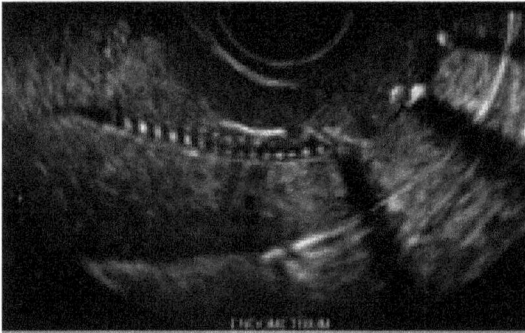
6.8e

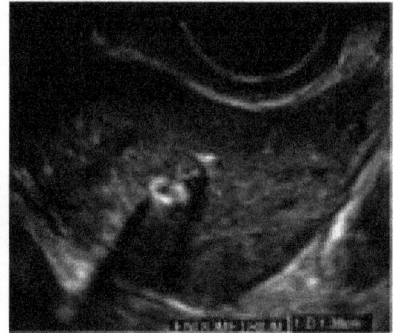
6.8e

***Ultrasound findings* at 4/52:**

- In the fundal portion of the cavity, the endometrium is expanded up to 18mm with blood clot. Along the entire length of the endometrial cavity, there are evenly spaced echogenic foci with the appearance of a fetal spine, however a foreign body cannot be excluded.

No abnormal adnexal masses or free fluid seen. Both ovaries not shown here appear normal.

Ultrasound Services in an Early Pregnancy and Acute Gynaecological Unit. Book 2

78

Impression: RPOC.

At 8/52

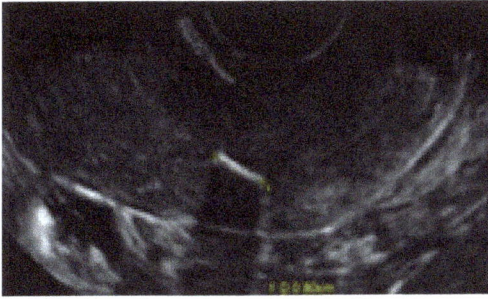

6.9a +3mm+

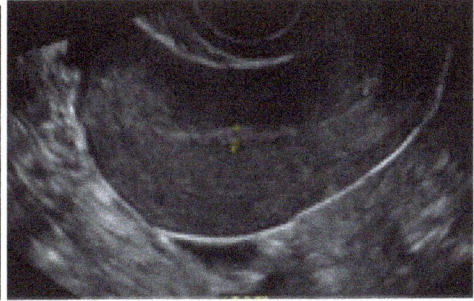

6.9b

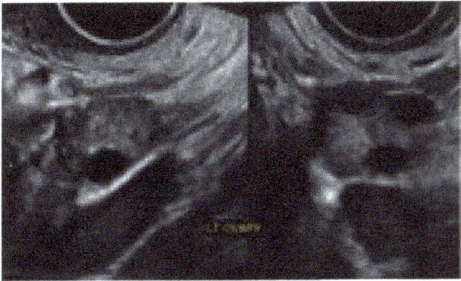

6.9c

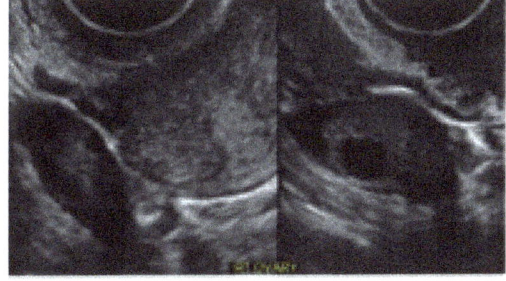

6.9d

Ultrasound findings at 8/52: The fundal endometrium appears thin and regular with a 3mm thickness. (6.9b) There are 2 echogenic, shadowing linear structures within the cavity at the level of the lower uterine segment (only one shown above 6.9a). These measure 8mm and 10mm and have the appearance of fetal long bones, which were present at the previous scan however as mentioned foreign body cannot be ruled out. Both ovaries appear normal (6.9c-d). No adnexal masses or free fluid seen.

Impression: RPOC

This woman was referred with a history of ?RPOC, Post TOP.

Ultrasound Services in an Early Pregnancy and Acute Gynaecological Unit. Book 2

79

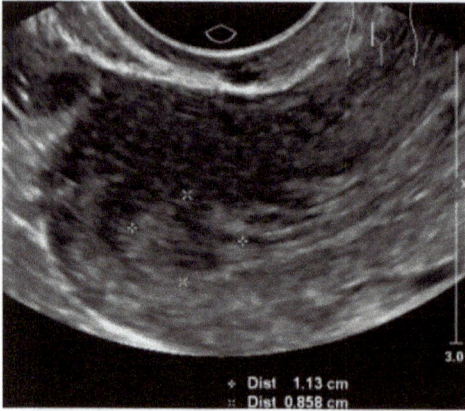

6.10a

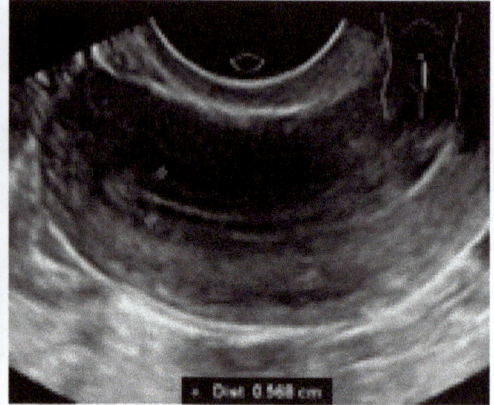

6.10b

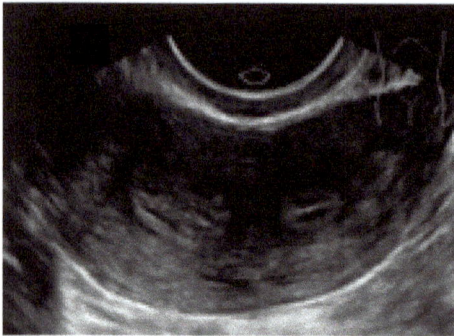

6.10c

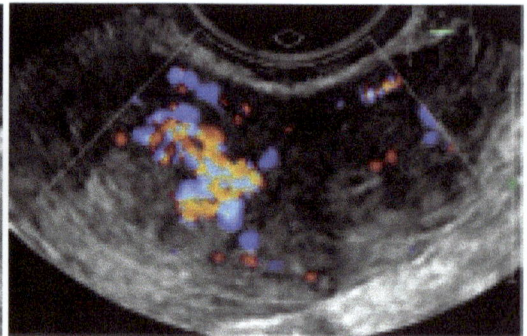

6.10d

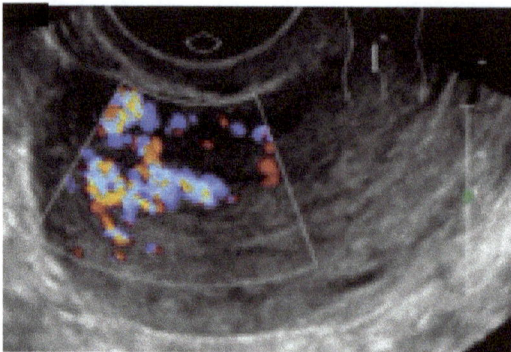

6.10e

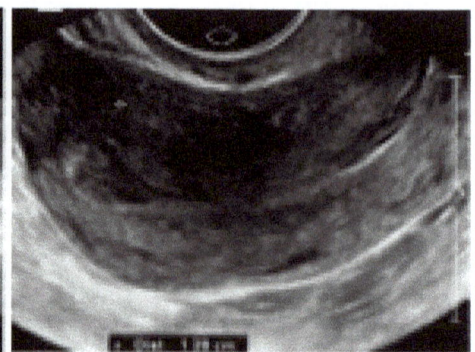

6.10f

Ultrasound findings: An anterverted uterus with two endometrial cavities possibly bi-cornuate or septated uterus with normal echo pattern of the myeometrium(6.10a –d). The endometrial cavity on the right is filled with

Ultrasound Services in an Early Pregnancy and Acute Gynaecological Unit. Book 2

80

predominantly vascular echogenic material the largest being approx. 9 x 11mm (6.10a, d-e). The endometrial thickness on the right is 12.8mm (6.10f). The left endometrium is triple lined in appearance and is 5.7mm in thickness (6.10b-c).

Impression: -Bi-cornuate or septated uterus with RPOC in the right horn. Triple line endometrium is noted on the left.

Missing Intrauterine Contraceptive Device (IUCD)

When an IUCD is gone missing or the string cannot be felt, the 1st diagnostic imaging examination used is ultrasound. The aim is to confirm or otherwise that the IUCD is in the uterus and where it is in the uterus - in the endometrium or in the cervix, in the endometrium or in the myometrium? Women also get referred for pelvic ultrasound post IUCD insertion for any of the following reasons with regards to IUCD:

- PID
- ?Lost string
- ? Lost IUCD
- Pelvic pain
- Abnormal bleeding
- ? Perforated uterus or mal position of IUCD in the uterus.

IUCD that is not correctly positioned in the endometrium is the cause of many pregnancies whilst in situ.

There are various types of IUCD and it is always good for the sonographer to establish from the patient, which she has been given. The older types including Copper T are easier to visualize on ultrasound because it has copper wire around it whilst mirena coil is more difficult to visualize on ultrasound because there is no metal in or around it. The IUCD should be in the fundus of the endometrium if it is to have the maximum effect. Where 3D ultrasound is available and the sonographer is familiar with obtaining the image and interpreting it, it should be used especially in the locating and monitoring of IUCD. The reason being that whilst with the 2D ultrasound the shaft of the IUCD can be seen clearly only with the 3D can the arms of the IUCD be accurately determined.

This woman was referred with a history of not feeling the string of the IUCD. Both ovaries not shown here appear sonographically normal.

Ultrasound Services in an Early Pregnancy and Acute Gynaecological Unit. Book 2

81

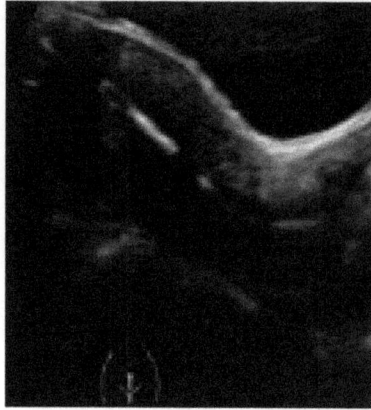

6.11a
LS view TAS

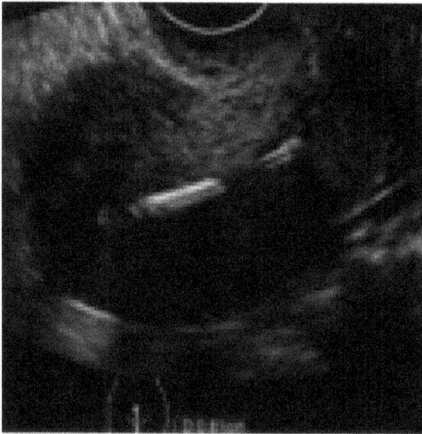

6.11b

LS view

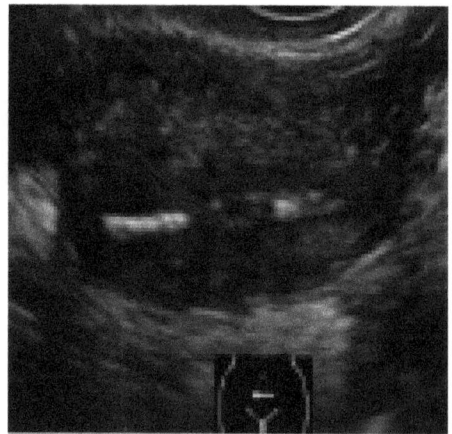

6.11c

TS view

Ultrasound findings: The IUCD shaft is correctly positioned in the endometrium approx. 6mm from the fundus (6.11b). The string is seen in the cervical canal (c in 6.11a-b)

Impression; Correctly positioned IUCD shaft in the endometrium.

Not being able to feel the IUCD string may be due to any of the following:

- That the IUCD is in the uterus in a normal or abnormal position. It is important that the myometrium be examined in relation to the position of the IUCD so that a perforation can be excluded.
- That the IUCD has been mistakenly expelled and it is no longer in the uterus.

Ultrasound Services in an Early Pregnancy and Acute Gynaecological Unit. Book 2

82

- The IUCD may still be in the uterus but the string might have been broken or displaced.

*It has been observed that women who have their IUCD fitted in the immediate post partum period after a vaginal delivery have the highest rate of expelling IUCD.

This woman was referred with a history of RIF pain. Left ovary not shown appears sonographically normal

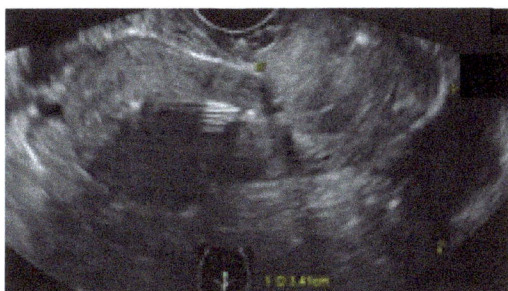

6.12a

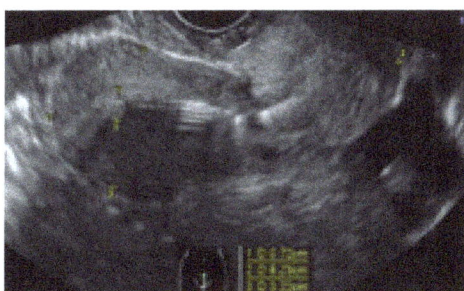

6.12b

// - previous C/S scar

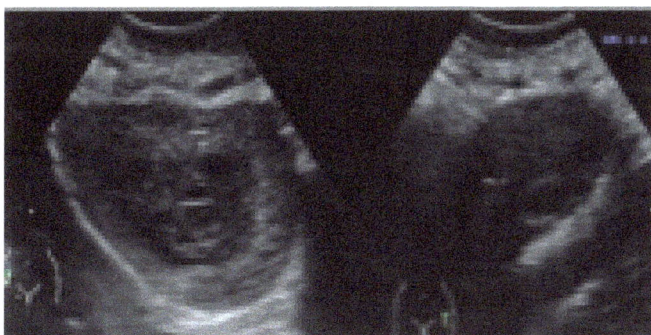

6.12c

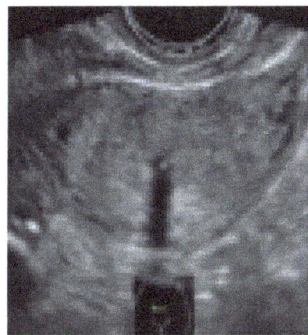

6.12d

Ultrasound findings: There is a mirena coil shaft correctly positioned in the endometrium. The endometrium is 7.2mm thick (6.12a-b & d_. There is some free fluid in the POD up to 34mm in depth. There is a hemorrhagic cyst in the right ovary (area of patient's pain 6.12c).

Impression: Normal mid cycle appearances with Mirena coil in situ. Appendicitis has not been excluded in this scan.

Ultrasound Services in an Early Pregnancy and Acute Gynaecological Unit. Book 2

83

This woman was referred with a history of heavy pv bleeding: Both ovaries not shown appeared polycystic. Ultrasound findings on Day 12 of her cycle.

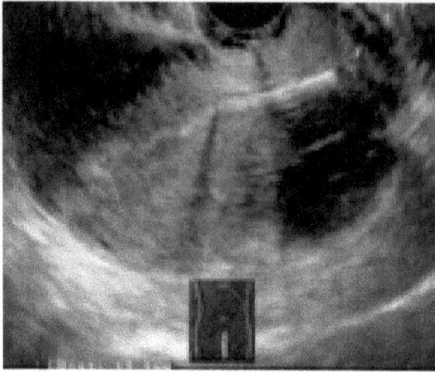

6.13a

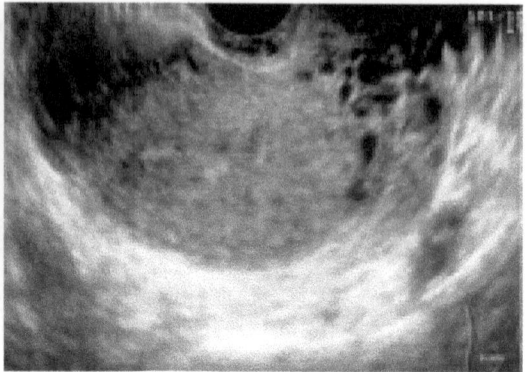

6.13b

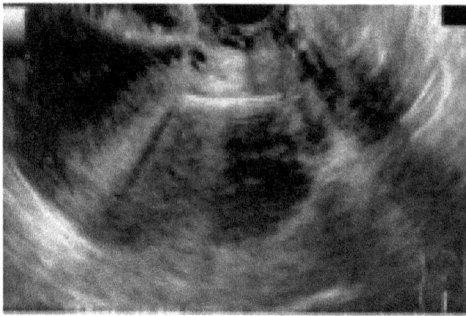

6.13c

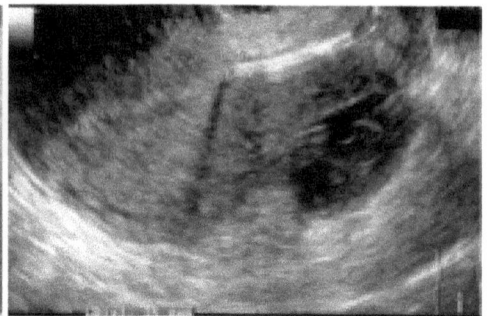

6.13d

Ultrasound findings: There is an IUCD shaft in the cervical canal that is approx. 35mm from the fundus and 12.5mm from the os (6.13 a, c-d). The endometrial thickness is 13mm (6.13a). Endometrial structure and thickness is appropriate for menstruation.

Impression: IUCD shaft in the cervical canal.

- In the absence of no other ultrasound identifiable findings, this woman's heavy pv bleed is likely to be due to the wrong positioning of the IUCD.
- The IUCD is currently not providing any protection against any on coming pregnancy.

This woman was referred with a history of heavy continous pv bleeding for five weeks. Both ovaries not shown appear sonographically normal.

Ultrasound Services in an Early Pregnancy and Acute Gynaecological Unit. Book 2

84

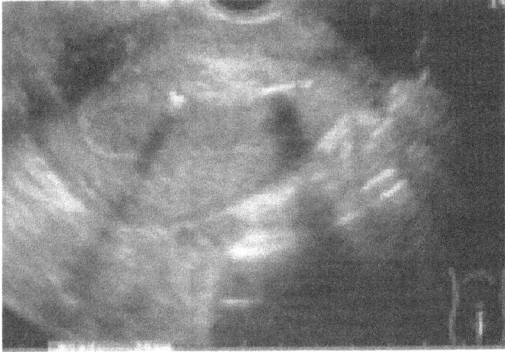

6.14a

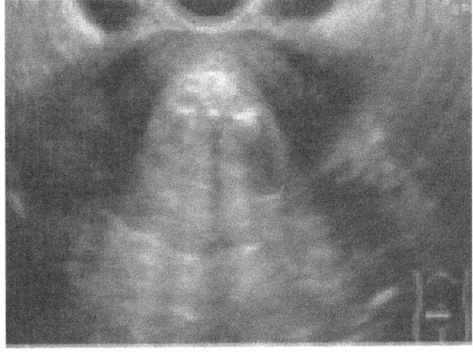

6.14b

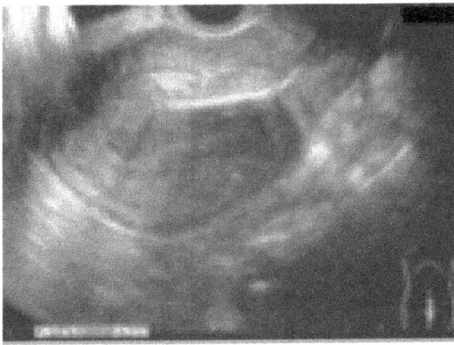

6.14c

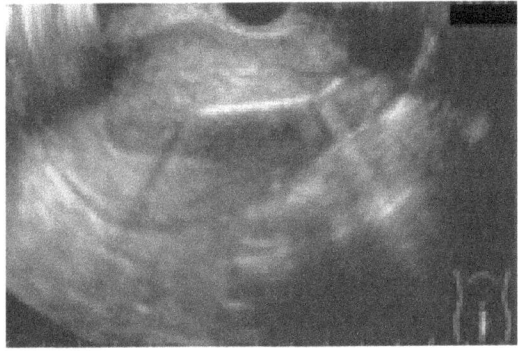

6.14d

Ultrasound findings: There is a Copper T shaft in the endometrium and approx. 25mm from the uterine fundus (6.14a). The endometrium is filled with low level echoed fluid. Blood cannot be excluded.

Impression: Copper T IUCD shaft in a low level echo fluid filled endometrial cavity. The IUCD is 25mm away from the fundus.

A pelvic scan revealed this on day 54 of the cycle. The woman was referred with a history of pelvic pain.

Ultrasound Services in an Early Pregnancy and Acute Gynaecological Unit. Book 2

85

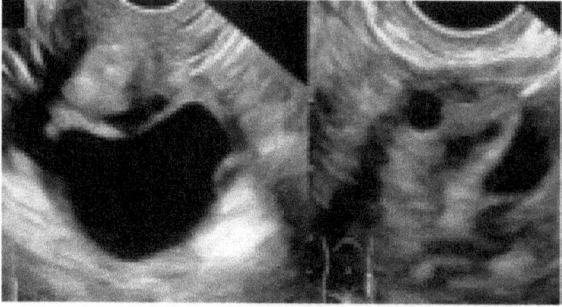

6.15a

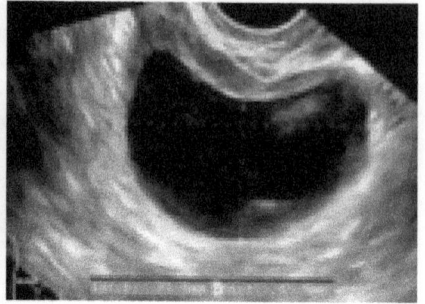

6.15b

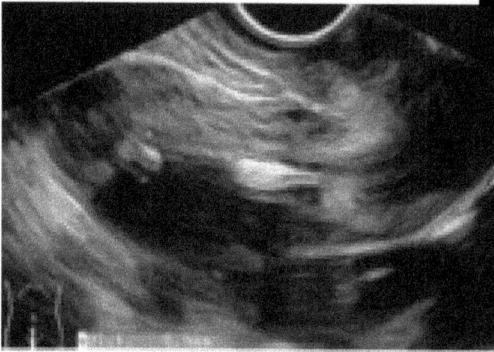

6.15c

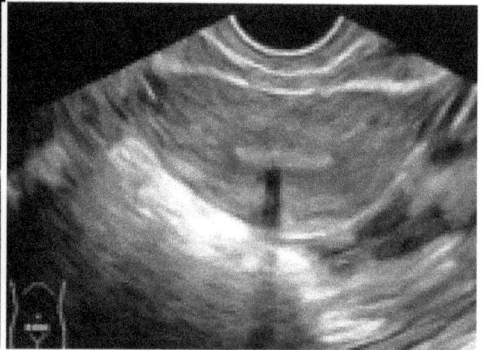

6.15d

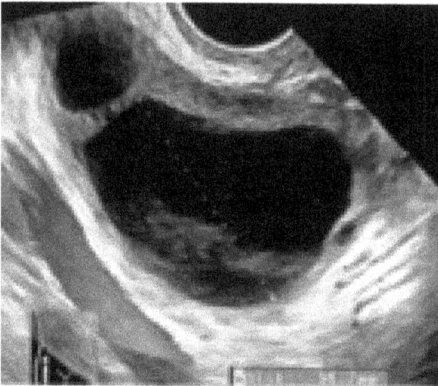

6.15e

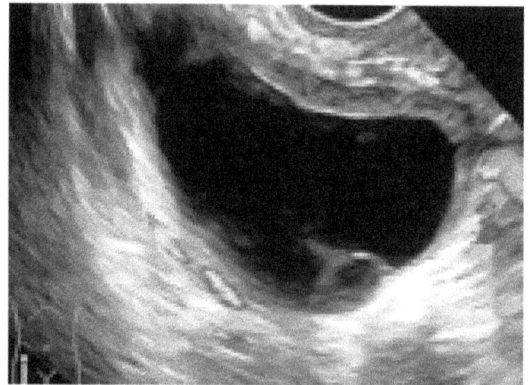

6.15f

Ultrasound Services in an Early Pregnancy and Acute Gynaecological Unit. Book 2

86

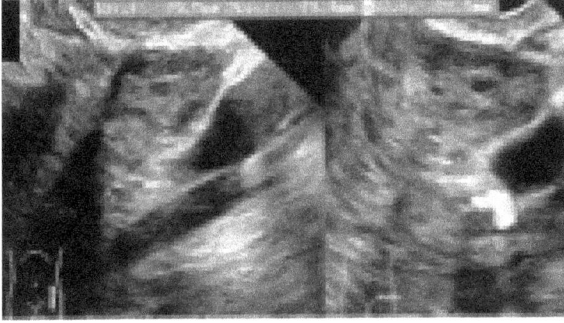

6.15g

Ultrasound findings: There is an IUCD shaft (mirena coil) correctly positioned in endometrial cavity (6.15b-c). Endometrial thickness is 6.9mm. There is a cyst with 'daughter cyst' in the right adnexal measuring 35 x 26 x 46mm (6.15a – b & e-f). Normal sonographically appearing left ovary measuring 29 x 19 x 22mm (6.15g). No free fluid in the POD.

- Whilst levonorgestrel released from Mirena coil is meant to prevent ovulation it does not always happen. Some may still ovulate and develop hemorrhagic cyst subsequently.
- Copper T IUCD, contains copper, which is slowly released into the uterine cavity. The copper stops the sperm from getting through the vagina and uterus to reach the egg, thus preventing fertilization.
- A mirena coil must be replaced every five years.

Experts claim that IUCD may:

- Increase menstrual cramps and bleeding. A reason for removal in 5-15% of patients.
- Prevents sperm transport through the uterine cavity, mechanism of action is not mainly by inhibition of implantation.
- Mobilize white blood cells and release of endotoxin, which prevents fertilization.
- Copper modifies cervical mucus inhibiting sperm transport.
- Uterine perforation is quoted to be in 1-3/1000 women, most cases of perforation occur often at the time of insertion.

Ultrasound Services in an Early Pregnancy and Acute Gynaecological Unit. Book 2

87

Both patients below were referred for IUCD location

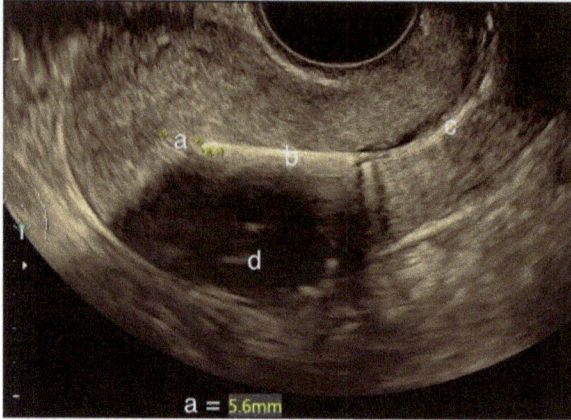

6.15h

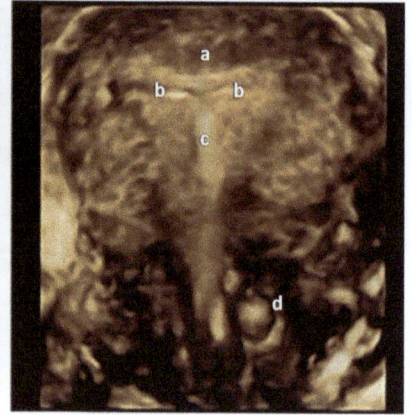

6.15i

6.15h *A-distance between IUCD and uterine fundus, b-IUCD shaft, c- IUCD string, d-posterior acoustic shadows from the shaft*

6.15i *a- uterine fundus, b -arm of the IUCD, c- IUCD shaft, d-nabothian cyst in the cervix*

Untrasound finding: *Correctly postioned shaft and arm of coil in endometrium. Note d is a nabotian cyst in the cervix*

Another patient:

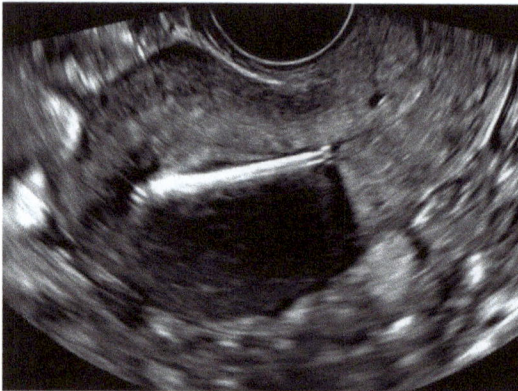

6.15j

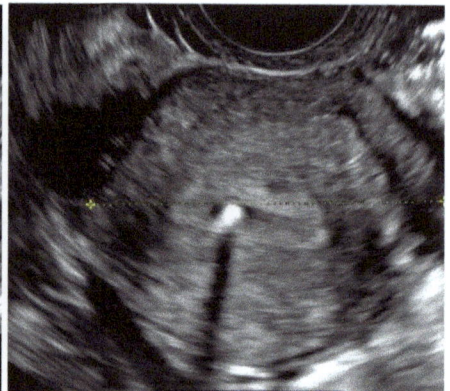

6.15k

Ultrasound Services in an Early Pregnancy and Acute Gynaecological Unit. Book 2

88

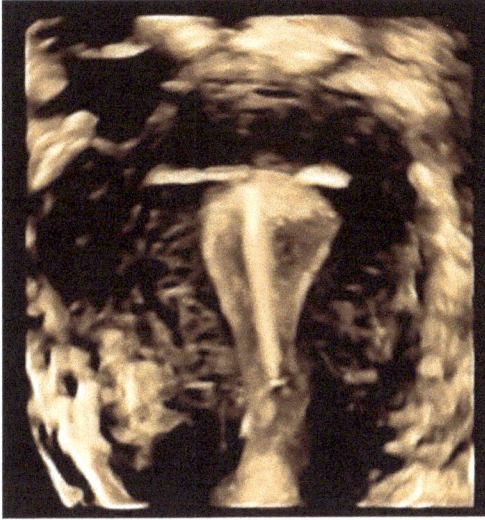

6.15l

The IUCD arms are incorectly positioned and in the myometrium

Ultrasound findings: whilst the shaft of the IUCD above is correctly postioned, the arms are not.

Heavy or Prolonged bleeding

Assess the uterus to confirm or exclude fibroids especially in the endometrium (sub mucousal) or indenting the endometrium or adenomyosis. Fibroid location and size should be documented. Where the uterus is now being enlarged due to the size or number of fibroids, the kidneys should be assessed to exclude or confirm hydronephrosis. Heavy or prolonged bleeding may also occur in patients with known IUCD in situ. IUCD presence and position should be assessed and documented.

This woman was referred with a history of painful periods. ?cause
Below are the ultrasound findings on Day 10

Ultrasound Services in an Early Pregnancy and Acute Gynaecological Unit. Book 2

89

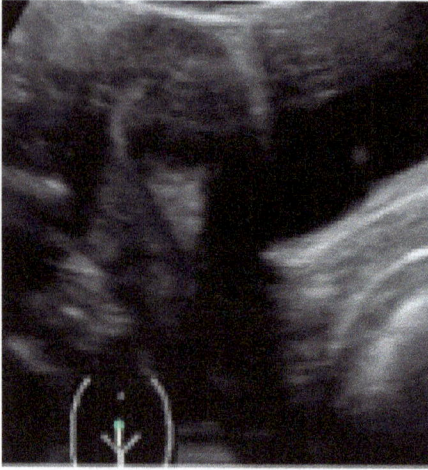
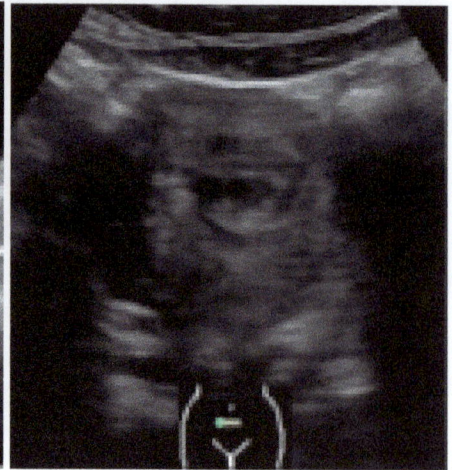

6.16a   **6.16b**

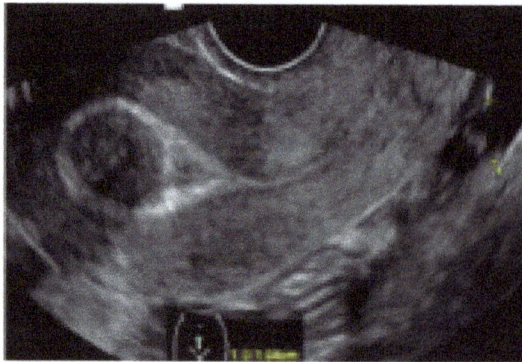
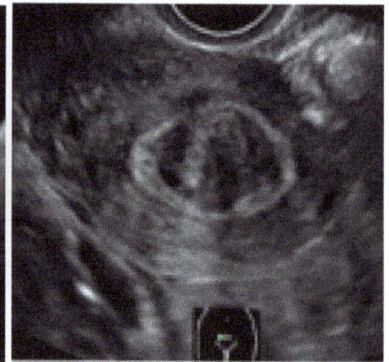

6.16c   **6.16d**

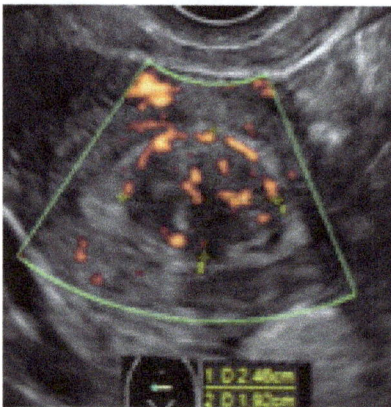
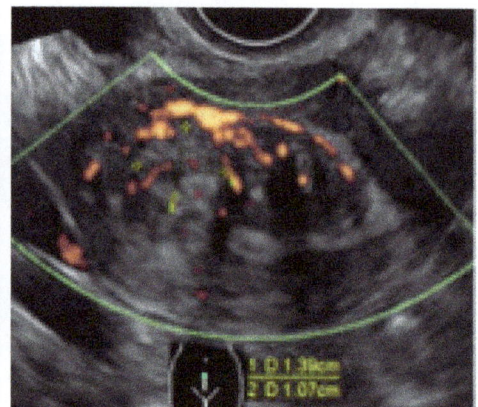

6.16e   **6.16f**

Ultrasound Services in an Early Pregnancy and Acute Gynaecological Unit. Book 2

90

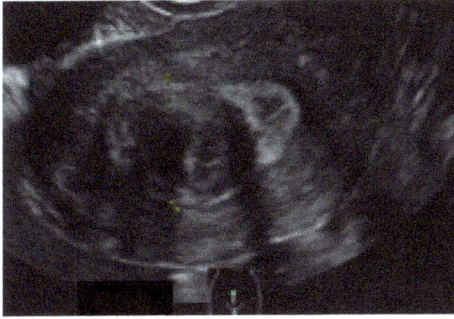 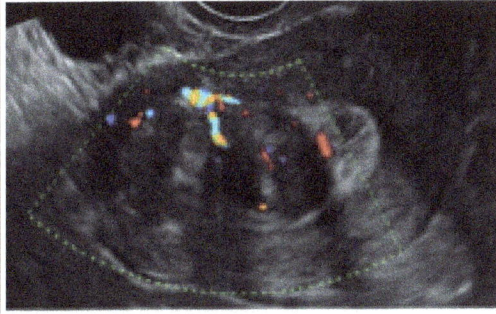

6.16g ++ 22mm   **6.16h**

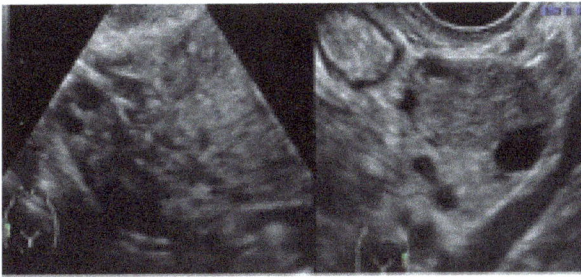

6.16i

Ultrasound findings: An anteverted uterus with a 22mm endometrium (6.16g). Within the endometrial cavity are two predominantly hypoechoic areas that has some posterior acoustic shadowing, the bigger one being approx. 19 x 25mm and an approx. 14 x 11mm echogenic or hyperechoic structure with a feeding stalk (6.16 e-h & a-d) . The right ovary appears sonographically normal and there is a corpus luteal cyst in the left ovary (6.16i). (There is some fluid in the POD up to 10mm in depth not shown here).

Impression: Fibroids and polyp in the endometrial cavity.

Fibroids otherwise called leiomyomas

Experts claim that fibroids:

- Can sometimes run in the family.
- Affects 1 in 5 of women at sometime in their life.
- Are a benign tumour of the smooth muscle of the uterus.
- More common in African –Caribbean's than in Caucasian women.
- May or may not be symptomatic depending on size and its location.

Ultrasound Services in an Early Pregnancy and Acute Gynaecological Unit. Book 2

91

- Can be of any size – small or big, can be single or multiple in a woman.
- Are very common in 20% of women in their 20's and 40% of women in their forties.
- Obese and overweight women are more at risk of developing fibroids than normal sized women.
- Large fibroids can cause urinary problems such as constant or regular visit to the toilet to urinate or inability to hold the urine.
- Can cause painful periods, excessive bleeding leading to anemia, clots during menstruation, bloating, infertility, miscarriage, preterm labour, or painful sexual intercourse especially posterior wall or posterior pedunculated fibroids.
- Fibroids can be in the endometrium – intracavity or submucosal, in the myometrium but putting pressure on the endometrium – submucosal which can cause excessive menstrual bleeding and infertility. In the myometrium - (intramural), close to the wall of the uterus – (subserosal} or outside the uterus and connected to it with a stalk – (pedunculated) which is prone to torsion. Fibroids can be anywhere in the endometrium or myometrium – they can be fundal, anterior, posterior or cervical as shown below:

Figure 6.a Possible location of uterine fibroid.

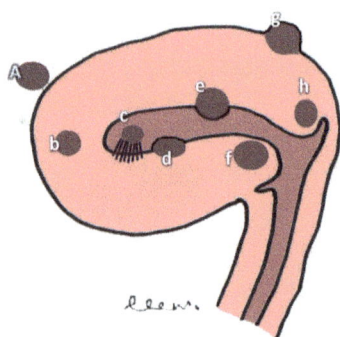
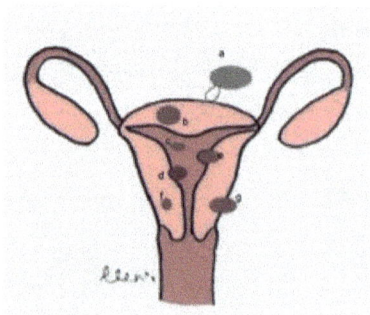

6.a   **6.b**

Ultrasound Services in an Early Pregnancy and Acute Gynaecological Unit. Book 2

92

6.a . - Sagittal view

a- pedunculated fundal fibroid

b- fundal intramural fibroid

c- intracavitary fibroid

d- posterior submucosal fibroid

e- anterior submucosal fibroid

f - posterior cervical intramural fibroid

g- anterior subserosal fibroid

h- anterior cervical intramural fibroid

6.b - Coronal View

a- pedunculated fundal fibroid

b- fundal intramural fibroid

c- intracavitary fibroid

d- submucosal fibroid

e- submucosal fibroid

f - cervical intramural fibroid

g- subserosal fibroid

The location and size of fibroids should be always be documented so that comparison can be made over time. Fibroids can be hypoechoic, heterogeneous, calcified completely or have areas of calcifications within or have echogenic rim. A uterus with fibroids may be difficult to assess because of shadows from it. The fibroids can be discrete as above or non discrete and this may be difficult to differentiate on ultrasound between this generalized fibroidy appearance and adenomyosis. Sometimes there is an echopoor area within the fibroid, referred to as degeneration. In a non pregnant patient, it does not cause pain but in a pregnant patient, it is called 'red degeneration' and causes pain.

Some reporting packages are able to plot the graphs of the fibroids each time so each fibroid can be reassessed and monitored over time.

Ultrasound Services in an Early Pregnancy and Acute Gynaecological Unit. Book 2

93

Uterine Fibroids Locations
MRI Image of locations of fibroids:

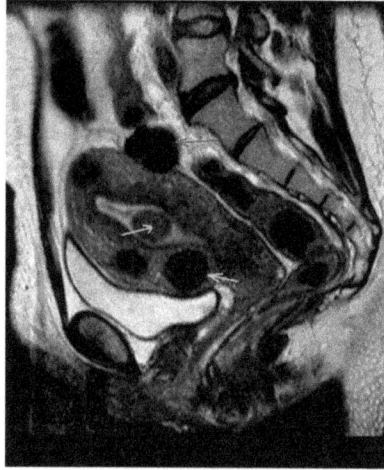

6.16j

Sagital T2 MRI:

The three main locations of uterine fibroids: Intramural (turquoise arrow), Subserosal (pink), and Sub- mucosal(green).

Examples of fibroid location on Ultrasound

- An ultrasound image of a subserosal fibroid:

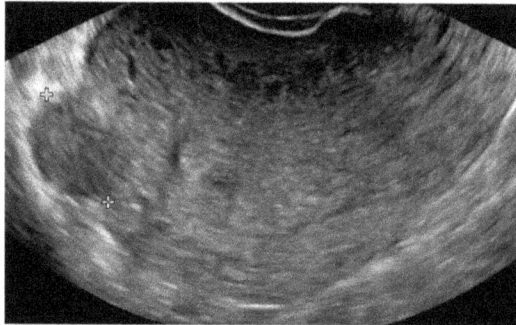

6.16k

The above is a fundal sub serousal fibroid.

Ultrasound Services in an Early Pregnancy and Acute Gynaecological Unit. Book 2

94

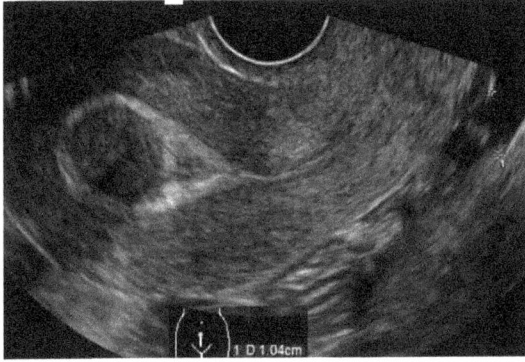

6.16l

Ultrasound image of a sub mucosal fibroid (arrow). Note the posterior acoustic shadow.

This woman was referred with a history of lost IUCD. LMP –About 2 weeks before the scan. Both ovaries were not identified during the examination.

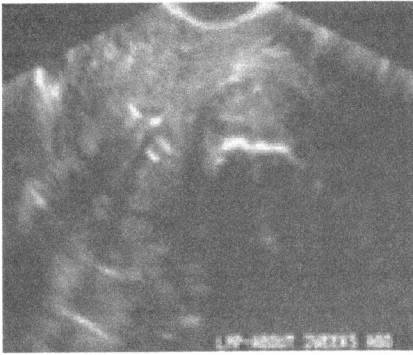

6.17a

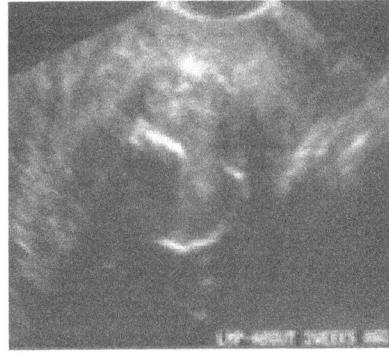

6.17b

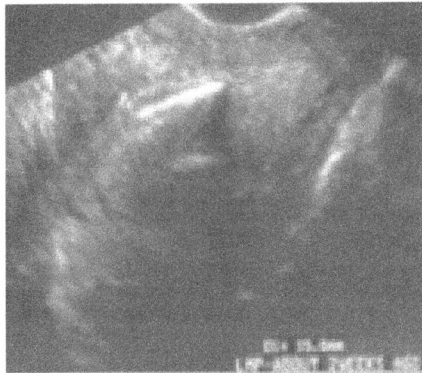

6.17c

Ultrasound Services in an Early Pregnancy and Acute Gynaecological Unit. Book 2

95

Ultrasound findings: An anteverted uterus that is heterogenous in echotexture. There is an IUCD shaft that is correctly positioned in the endometrial cavity (6.17c). The endometrial thickness is 15.6mm. There is a posterior intramural fibroid that has some calcifications in it and around it. (6.17a-b) measurements not included).

Post single or recurrent miscarriage

The aim is to confirm or refute RPOC which if left in the uterus can cause infection and bleeding. Informing women who would like to become pregnant after the miscarriage that the endometrium is normal is important. The ovaries should be assessed for cysts and PCO. It is not unusual for the patient not to have a LMP if the miscarriage is close to the time of the ultrasound examination.

The RCOG guideline stipulates that a woman who has experienced first trimester recurrent miscarriages or women with one or more second-trimester miscarriages should have a pelvic scan. (It is important that the ultrasonographer confirms or excludes uterine or ovarian abnormality that may be responsible for such). Where a uterine anomaly is suspected, a three – dimensional ultrasound scanning may be able to provide definitive diagnosis for that.

This woman was referred with a history of follow up post recent miscarriage. She does not remember her LMP. Her right ovary was not visualized at the time of the scan.

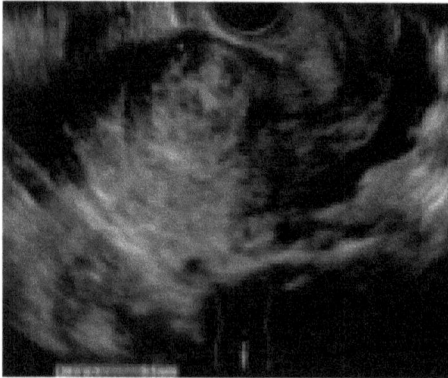 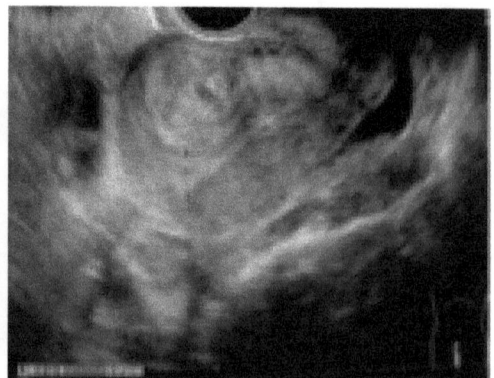

6.18a	**6.18b**

Ultrasound Services in an Early Pregnancy and Acute Gynaecological Unit. Book 2

96

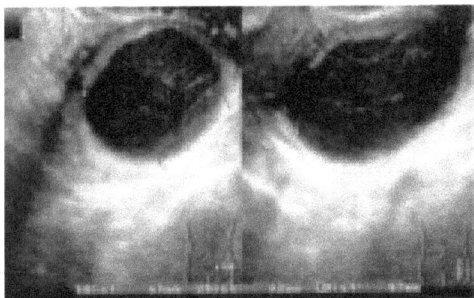

6.18c

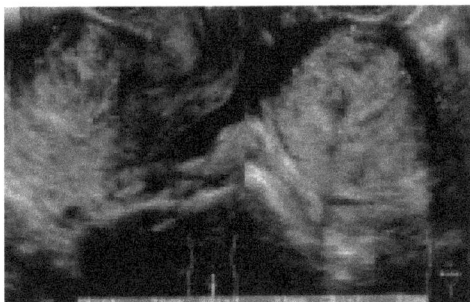

6.18d

Ultrasound findings: . LMP – Unknown. An anteverted uterus with a 12mm endometrium (6.18b) There is an approx. 34 x 33 x 31mm anterior submucosal fibroid that is displacing the endometrium posteriorly (6.18 a & d). There is an approx. 51 x 43 x 23mm ?endometrioma, ?haemorhagic cyst in the left adnexae. (6.18c). No separate left ovary is seen. There is some fluid in the POD (6.18 a-b)

Impression:

1. Anterior submucosal fibroid that is displacing the endometrium posteriorly.

2. There is no ultrasound evidence of RPOC.

3. Ultrasound appearance is suggestive of a recent ovulation.

This patient was referred with a history of miscarriage at 14/40. She had a normal 12/40 scan. Both ovaries were not identified during the ultrasound examination.

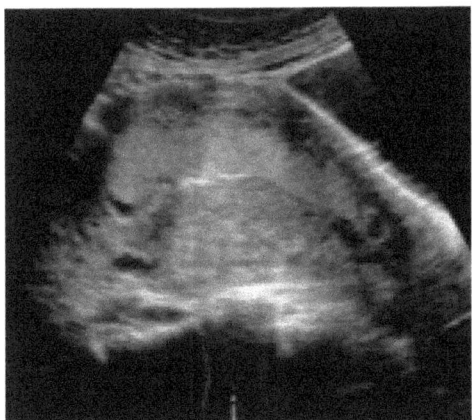

6.19a

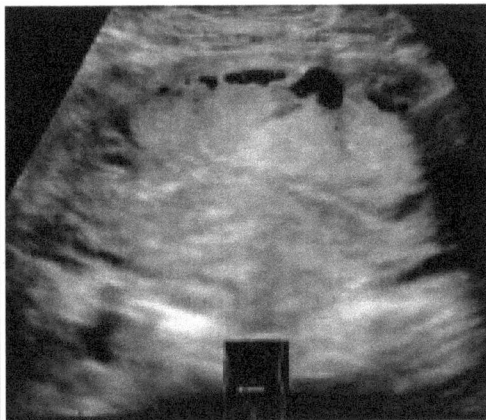

6.19b

Ultrasound Services in an Early Pregnancy and Acute Gynaecological Unit. Book 2

97

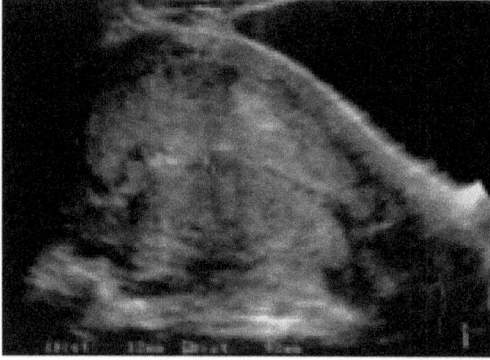
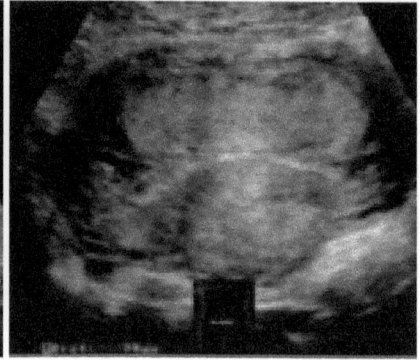

6.19c   **6.19d**

Ultrasound findings: Bulky uterus with no IUGS or fetus, there is an approx. 92 x 79 x 32mm hyperechoic structure within the uterus in the anterior aspect. (6.19a-d) This is probably the placenta.

Impression: Bulky uterus with RPOC.

This woman was referred for a follow up post recent miscarriage. LMP unknown.

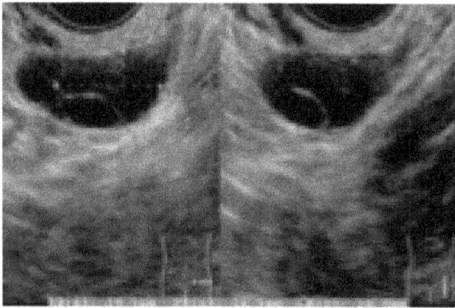
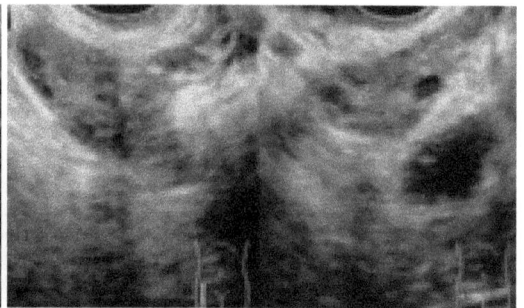

6.20 a   **6.20b**

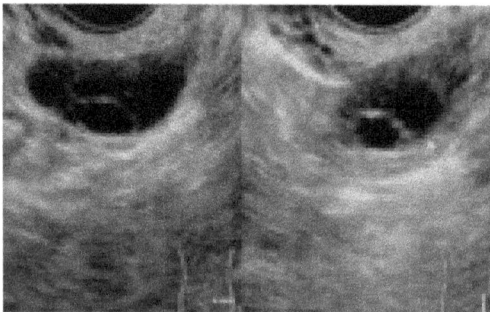
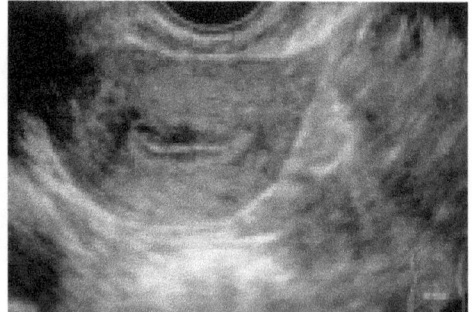

6.20c   **6.20d**

Ultrasound Services in an Early Pregnancy and Acute Gynaecological Unit. Book 2

98

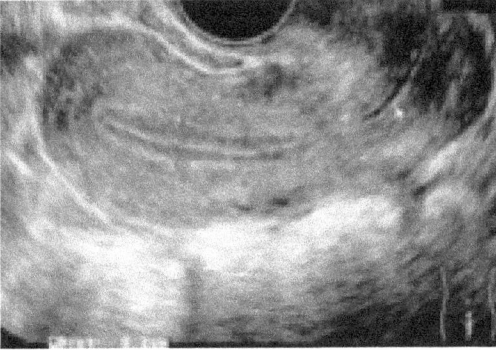
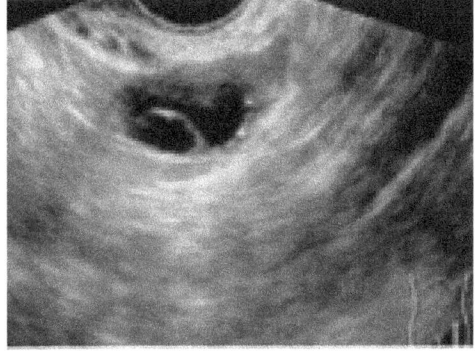

6.20e   6.20f

Ultrasound findings: Normal sized anteverted uterus with a triple line endometrium measuring 8.2mm.(images 6.20d & e) There is small quantity of fluid in the cervical canal (6.20e arrow). Both ovaries appear sonographically normal and there is a cyst and 'daughter cyst' (images 6.20a, c & f) in the left ovary. No obvious free fluid is demonstrated in the POD.

Impression: No obvious RPOC, normal mid cycle appearances.

This woman in her forties was referred with a history of miscarriage 1/52 ago. Previous 3 miscarriages.

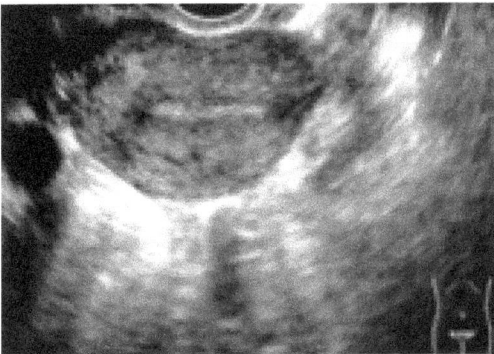
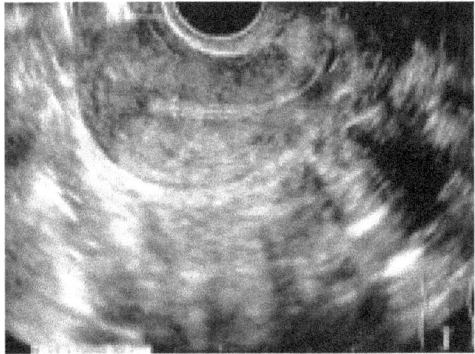

6.21a   6.21 b

Ultrasound Services in an Early Pregnancy and Acute Gynaecological Unit. Book 2

99

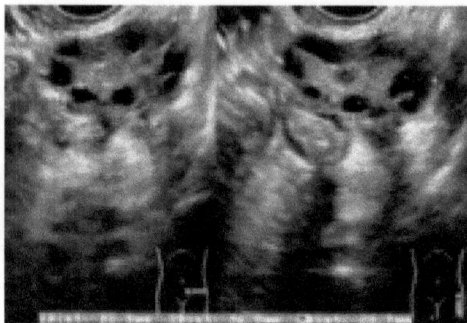

6.21c

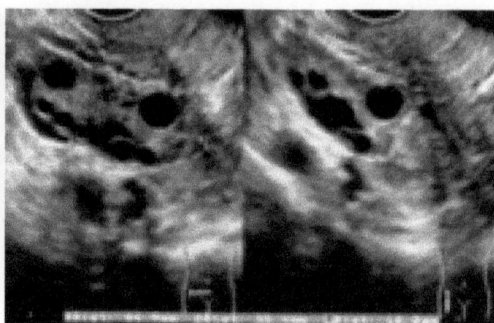

6.21d

Ultrasound findings: Normal sized anteverted uterus with a triple line endometrium measuring 3.7mm.(images 6.21a & b) The right ovarian volume is 17mls and the left ovarian volume is 13.1mls. Both ovaries appear sonographically polycystic. (images 6.21a & d)

No obvious free fluid is demonstrated in the POD.

Impression: No obvious RPOC, thin endometrium, bilateral PCO.

This woman was referred with a history of recent miscarriage.

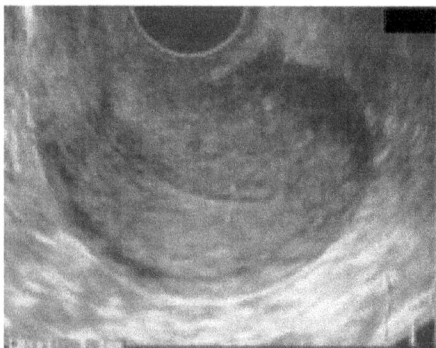

6.22a

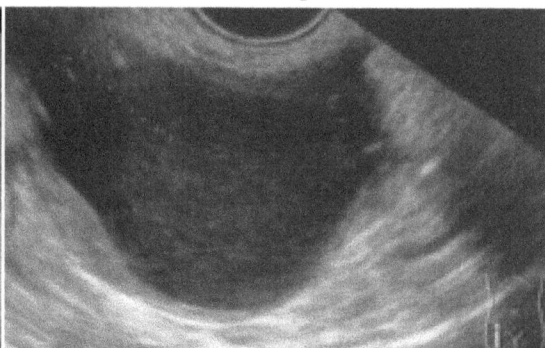

6.22 b

Ultrasound Services in an Early Pregnancy and Acute Gynaecological Unit. Book 2

100

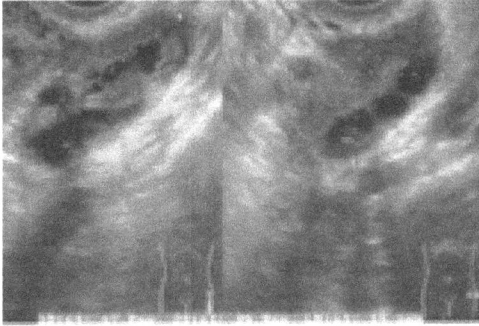 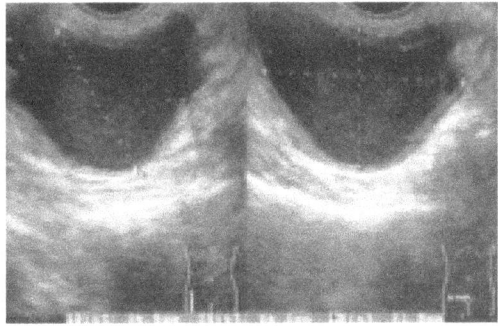

| 6.22c | 6.22d |

Ultrasound findings: Normal sized retroverted uterus with an endometrium measuring 5.3mm (6.22a). There is an approx. a 37 x 46 x 32mm low level echoed irregular in outline predominantly cystic area in the right adnexa with some ovarian tissue in its rim (6.22b & d}. The right ovary is not seen separately from this entity. The left ovarian volume is 22.2mls and in it there is a corpus luteum – measurement not included. (6.22c)

Impression: No obvious RPOC, ?endometrioma in the right ovary.

Differentials : ?haemorrhagic cyst.

Suggest a follow up scan in six weeks from this examination or in another menstrual phase to re-assess the ovaries

This woman was referred with a history of previous miscarriage. Known 40 days cycle.

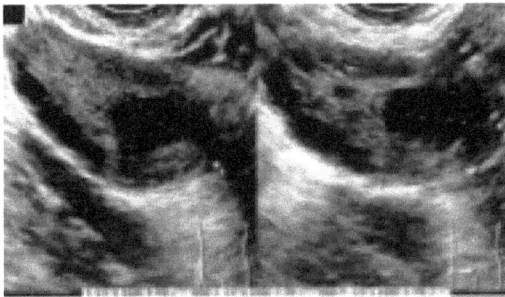 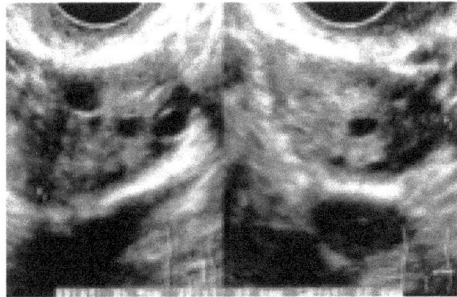

| 6.23a | 6.23b |

Ultrasound Services in an Early Pregnancy and Acute Gynaecological Unit. Book 2

101

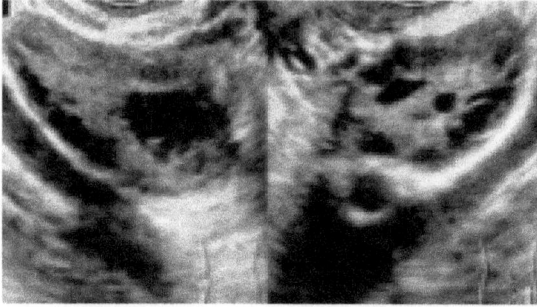

6.23c

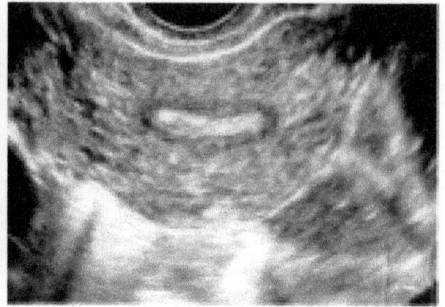

6.23d

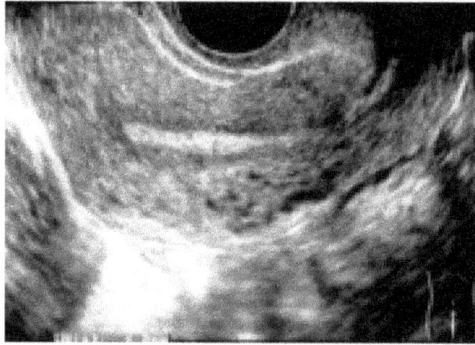

6.23e

Ultrasound findings: Normal sized anteverted uterus with an endometrium measuring 4mm (6.23d &e). The right ovarian volume is 21.7mls (6.23a &c) and the left ovarian volume is 13.3mls (6.23b & c). There is a corpus luteum in the right ovary (measurements are not included.) Both ovaries appear sonographically polycystic. (images 6.23a - c)

No obvious free fluid is demonstrated in the POD.

Impression: No obvious RPOC, thin endometrium and bilateral PCO.

*Though the same clinical indication, the above shows diverse ultrasound findings in various patients.

Irregular bleeding or abnormal pv. bleeding

It is important to assess the uterus especially the endometrial and cervical cavity for fibroids, endometrial or cervical polyps or any other endometrial pathology. The ovaries should be assessed for size and echo pattern. They should be measured.

Ultrasound Services in an Early Pregnancy and Acute Gynaecological Unit. Book 2

102

This woman was referred with a history of irregular bleeding.

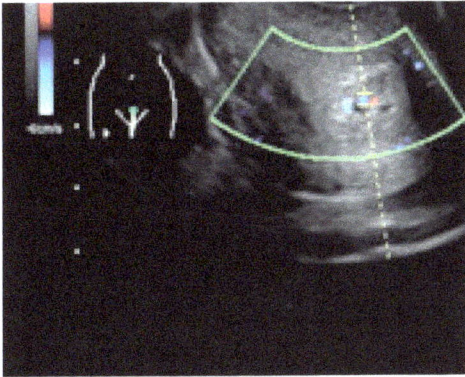 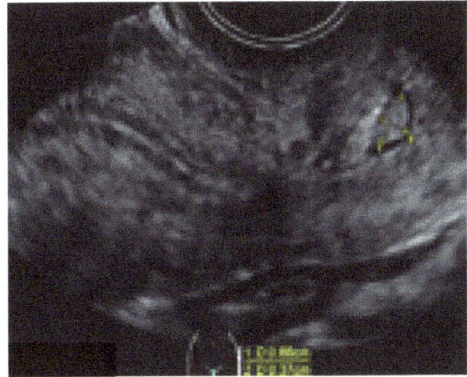

6.24a   **6.24b**

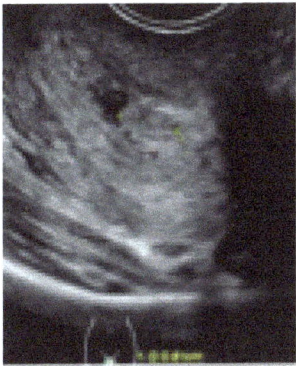 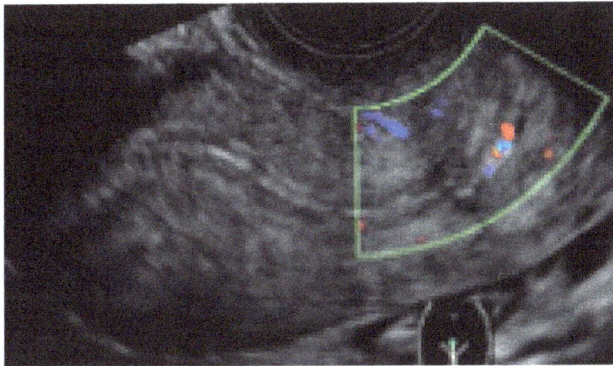

6.24c   6.24d

Ultrasound findings: An anteverted uterus with a triple line endometrium (6.24b & d measurements not included). There is an approx. 8 x 7 x 4mm hyperechoic structure in the cervical canal with a feeding stalk on Dopplers - arrow(6.24a –d).
Impression: Cervical polyp.

Abdominal bloating

This can be as a result of bowel distension, ascites or ovarian pathologies. When ascites is found, its location and depth in the pelvis should be documented. The upper abdomen should be scanned at the same time for ascites in the Morrison's pouch, around the liver etc. A normal pelvic ultrasound scan cannot exclude GIT problems.

Ultrasound Services in an Early Pregnancy and Acute Gynaecological Unit. Book 2

103

This woman was referred with a history of sepsis and abdominal bloating. LMP – Unsure. The scan was extended to the upper abdomen where other pathologies and more ascites were discovered.(not shown here) Ultrasound may be used to guide the draining of the ascites and to monitor the improvement or otherwise of the ascites.

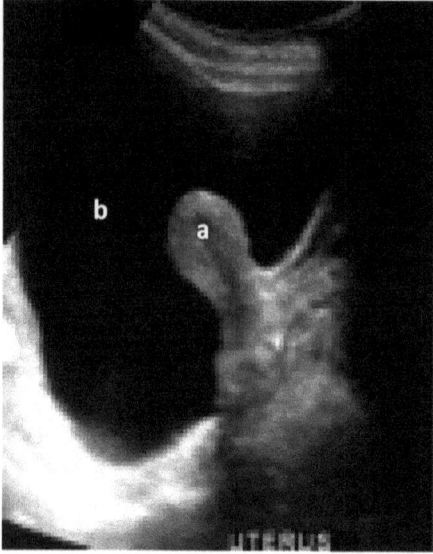

6.25a

a- uterus, b-ascites

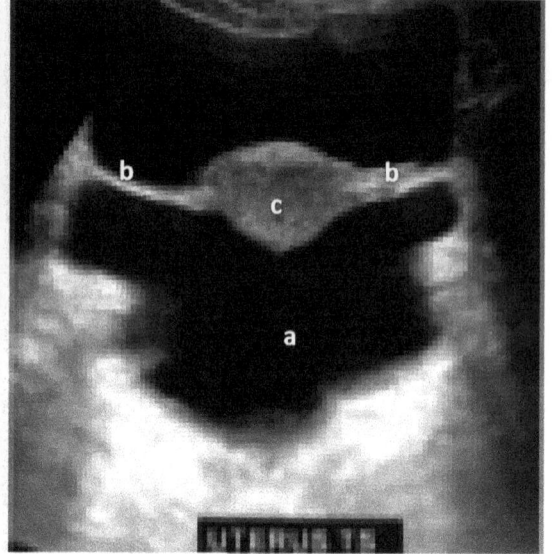

6.25b

a-ascites, b-broad ligament, c- uterus

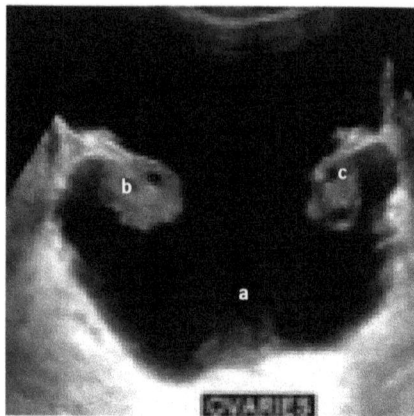

6.25c

a-ascites, b-right ovary, c- follicle in the left ovary

Ultrasound Services in an Early Pregnancy and Acute Gynaecological Unit. Book 2

104

Ultrasound findings: Pelvic ultrasound revealed free fluid in the pelvis but normal uterus and ovaries (6.25a-c).

Impression: Normal anteverted uterus and ovaries. Large quantity of free fluid in the pelvis.

*Abdominal ascites not shown here was noted.

This post menopausal woman was referred with a history of abdominal distension and ascites.

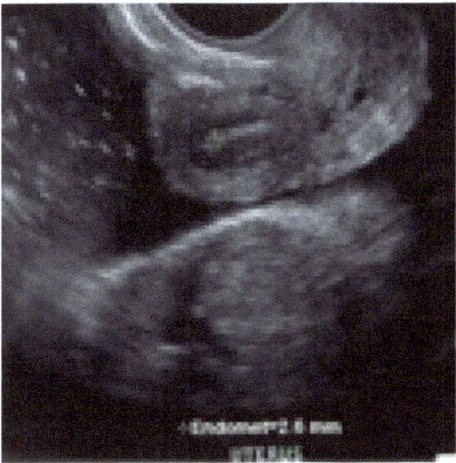

6.26a

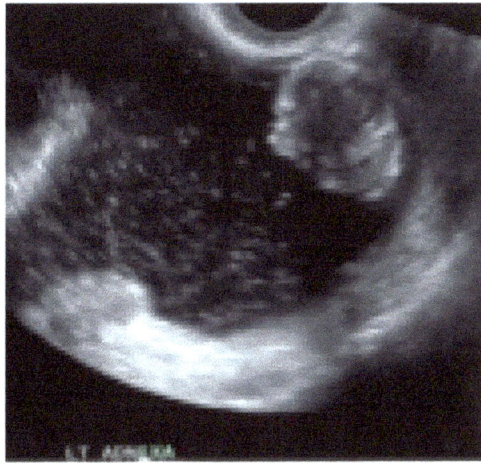

6.26b

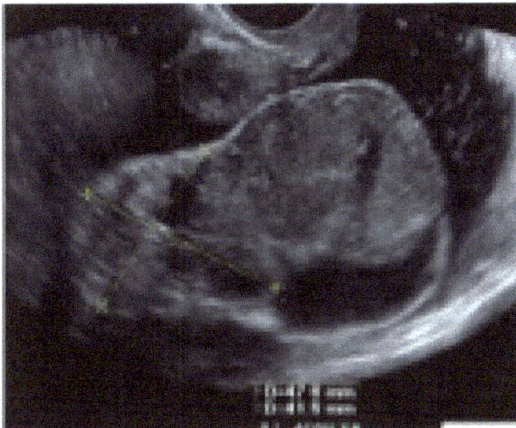

6.26c

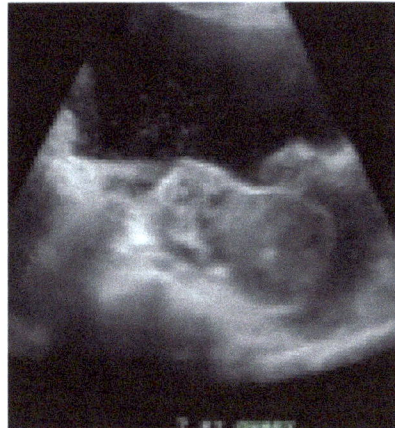

6.26d

Ultrasound Services in an Early Pregnancy and Acute Gynaecological Unit. Book 2

105

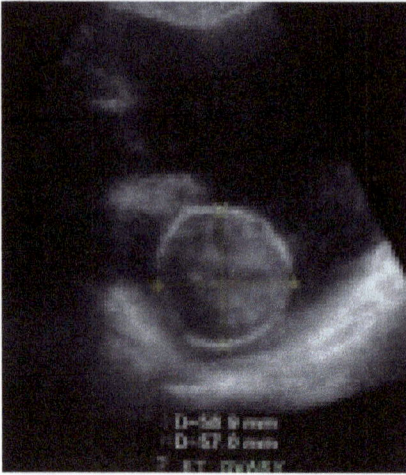

6.26e

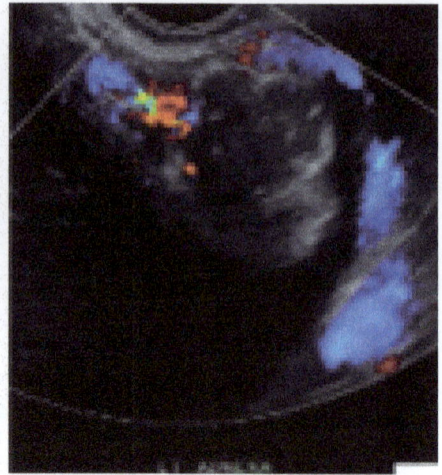

6.26f

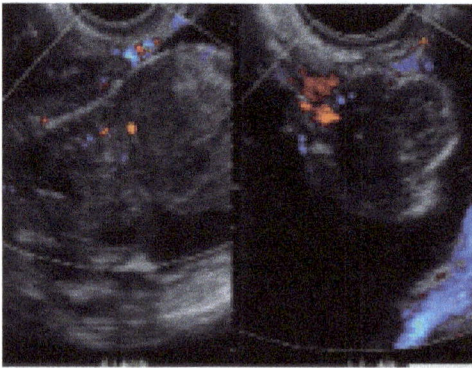

6.26g

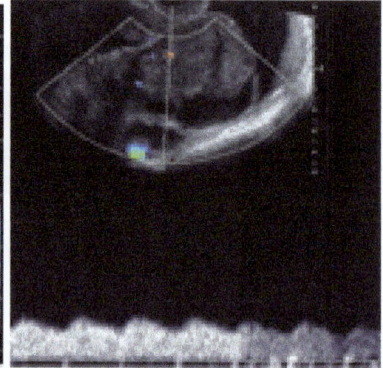

6.26h

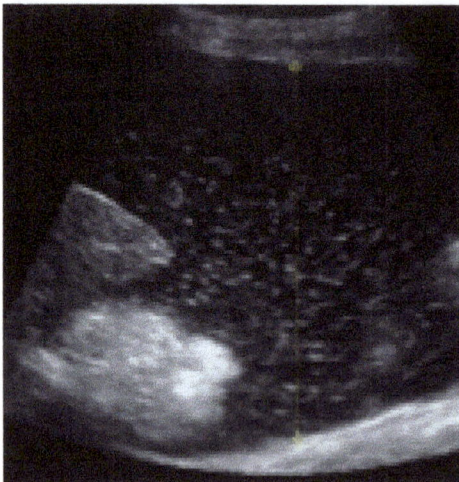

6.26i

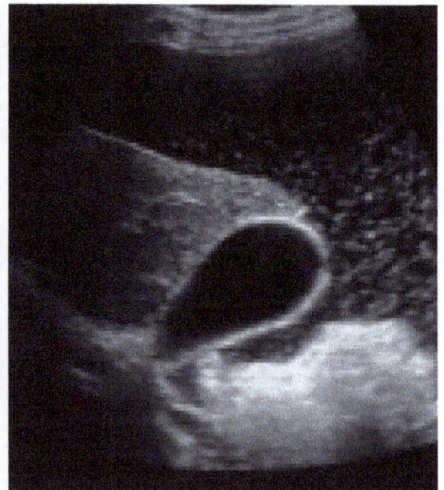

6.26j

Ultrasound Services in an Early Pregnancy and Acute Gynaecological Unit. Book 2

106

Ultrasound findings: Normal atrophic uterus with a 2.6mm endometrium(6.26a). There is a 87 x 53 x 52mm complex mass with vascularity in the right adnexa and a similar structure in the left adnexa measuring 31 x 33 x 26mm (6.26b-h). Both ovaries are not identified. A large quantity of ascites is seen in the pelvis and abdomen (6.26a-j).

Impression: Bilateral complex pelvic masses and pelvic ascites. Further imaging is recommended.

*   Further findings: Patient could not tolerate MRI as she is claustrophobic.
*   CT confirmed pelvic mass. ?of ovarian origin.

Sudden swollen legs

Attempts should be made to exclude any pelvic mass(es) and large fibroids that may cause pressure effect. It is also a good practice to assess the kidneys for hydronephrosis.

Post op complications

The patient could be feeling unwell, with abdominal wound dressings which may make scanning challenging. The patient may be feeling unwell and so making the examination difficult. It is important for the sonographer to scan light-handed and be able to adapt his technique to the need of the patient. With TAS, in most cases there is no need to remove the abdominal dressing but the edges may get wet at the end of the examination with the TAS approach. The soiled dressing can be changed when the patient returns to her ward. Confirm or exclude fluid collections around the area of surgery and ascites in the pelvis or abdomen in addition to providing an answer to the clinical indications. The method of scanning will have to adapt to the type of surgery performed and the clinical questions to be answered.

This woman was referred with a history of abdominal hysterectomy a week earlier.

Ultrasound Services in an Early Pregnancy and Acute Gynaecological Unit. Book 2

107

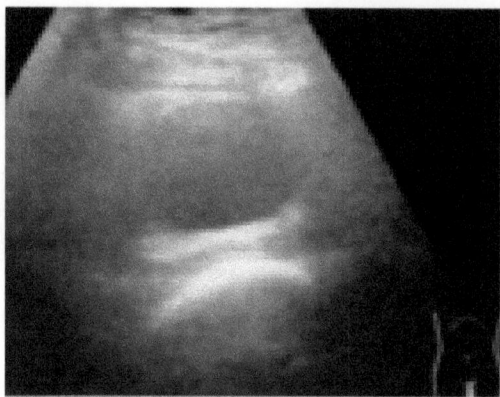

6.27a

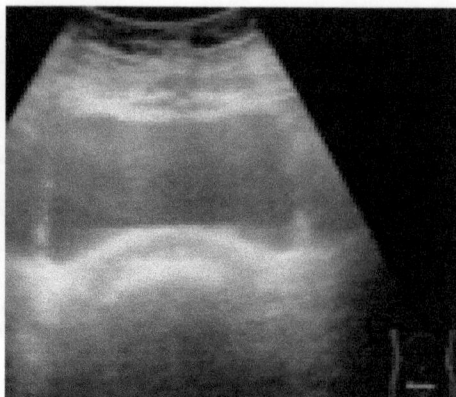

6.27b

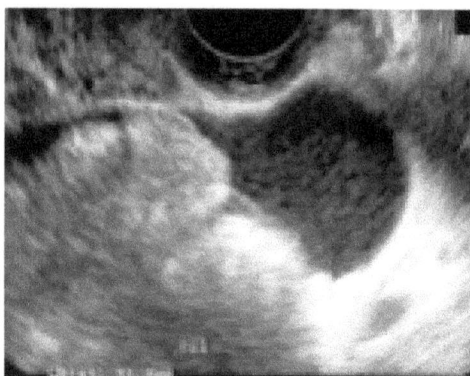

6.27c

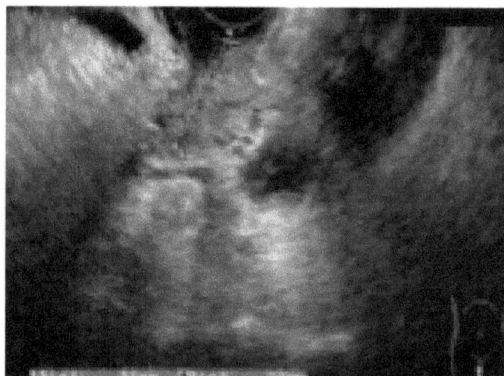

6.27 d

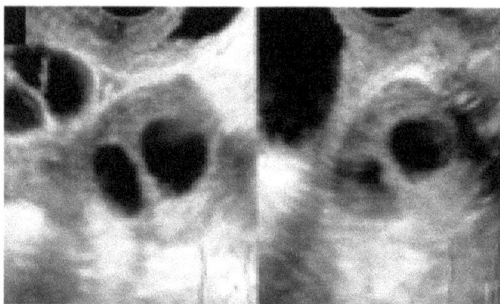

6.27e

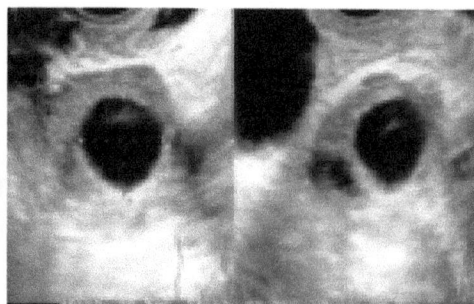

6.27f

Ultrasound Services in an Early Pregnancy and Acute Gynaecological Unit. Book 2

108

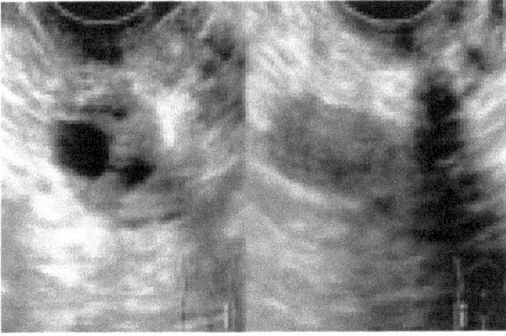

6.27g

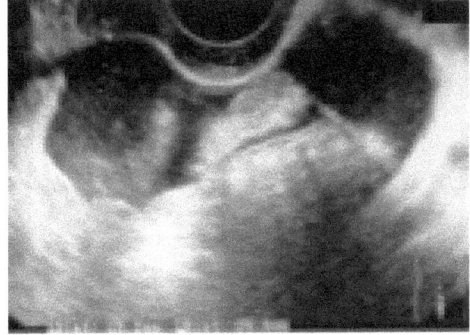

6.27h

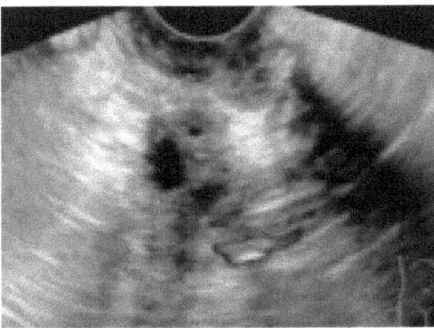

6.27i

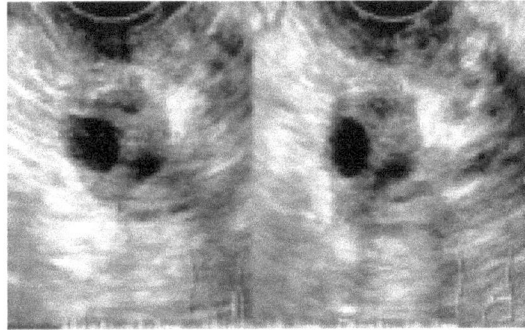

6.27j

Ultrasound findings: Previous total hysterectomy is demonstrated. A vagina stump measuring 32 x 23mm (6.27a-d). The left ovary appears sonographically normal measuring 24 x 19 x 21mm (6.27i& j) and in there are two follicles (6.27e&f). In the right adnexa and in the mid pelvis are some fluid measuring up to 31mm in depth(6.27c &h). The right ovary as best demonstrated (6.27g) appears sonographically normal (measurements not included)

Impression: Previous total hysterectomy noted. Normal appearing ovaries. Low level echo fluid noted bilaterally in the pelvis.

Please refer to chapter five for the following:

Corpus luteum cyst

Follicular cyst

Paraovarian cyst

Haemorrhagic cyst

Dermoid cyst

Ultrasound Services in an Early Pregnancy and Acute Gynaecological Unit. Book 2

109

Mature cystic teratoma

Endometrioma

Multicystic ovary

Polycystic ovary

Complex cyst

Post Menopausal Ovarian cysts or Mass

Ovarian cysts may be found in post menopausal women during routine ovarian screening, secondary to other investigation for other reasons e.g. CT for GIT problems, or because of feeling a mass in the pelvis. Finding such a cyst could be worrying some for the woman and concern for the physician. According the RCOG Guidance 'Ovarian cysts are common in postmenopausal women, although the prevalence is lower than in premenopausal women. Ultrasound is also well established, achieving a sensitivity of 89% and specificity of 73% when using a morphology index'

Which method for Scanning

These patients in most cases are able to eat and drink. It is good to have the patient attend the examination with a full bladder so that a trans-abdominal scan is performed first before embarking on the trans vaginal scan. With the trans abdominal scan, we can obtain a 'helicopter' view of the pelvis which is particularly useful in assessing pathology such as: large fibroid(s), pelvic cyst(s) and other mass(es). There is also a lot of space for the Ultrasonographer to maneuver the trans-abdominal probe. Following this, the patient is asked to empty her urinary bladder for the trans-vaginal scan. Trans-vaginal ultrasound scan (if and where it is not contra-indicated) provides 'close up views' of the pelvic organs. This is helpful where the concern is about fine details with increased sensitivity over transabdominal ultrasound

Technical challenges that the Sonographer may encounter and limit the quality of the ultrasound examination include:
- Very active bowels.
- Overlying bowel gas.
- Intolerance of TV probe.
- High Body mass index (BMI)

Ultrasound Services in an Early Pregnancy and Acute Gynaecological Unit. Book 2

110

- Retroverted and retroflexed uterus.
- Lack of normal landmark e.g. secondary to hysterectomy.
- Limitation or inability of moving the transvaginal probe sufficiently.
- Inability to perform a TVS in patients that is contra-indicated e.g. never been sexually active.

Following the examination, the patient should be offered some dry wipes to use to clean herself and be allowed her privacy in the toilet as she dresses up.

The ultrasound report should be generated after the examination as outlined on Chapter 5.

Whilst the examination is aimed at the finding of a or suspected pelvic mass or cyst, it should cover the uterus, adnexa. If there is ascites, a quick look at the upper abdomen to check for ascites and any other incidental findings is useful. The sonographer should note and document the location of the cyst or mass in relation to the uterus, its size, overall appearance, wall outline – regular or irregular, thin or thick, any septations, any papillary projections, internal echo pattern, evidence of vascularisation around or within the cyst or mass with use of 'Colour flow Doppler'.

Below is the IOTA Group ultrasound 'rules' to classify masses as benign (B-rules) or malignant (M-rules)

B-rules	M-rules
Unilocular cysts	Irregular solid tumour
Presence of solid components where the largest solid component <7 mm	Ascites
Presence of acoustic shadowing	At least four papillary structures

Ultrasound Services in an Early Pregnancy and Acute Gynaecological Unit. Book 2

111

Smooth multilocular tumour with a largest diameter <100 mm	Irregular multilocular solid tumour with largest diameter ≥100 mm
No blood flow	Very strong blood flow

Management of Suspected Ovarian Masses in Premenopausal Women

Ó RCOG Green-top Guideline No. 62 .Available @https://www.rcog.org.uk/globalassets/documents/guidelines/gtg_62.pdf

This postmenopausal woman was referred with a clinical history of right adnexal mass. The right ovary was seen and appeared normal. The left ovary was not seen. Below are some other ultrasound findings.

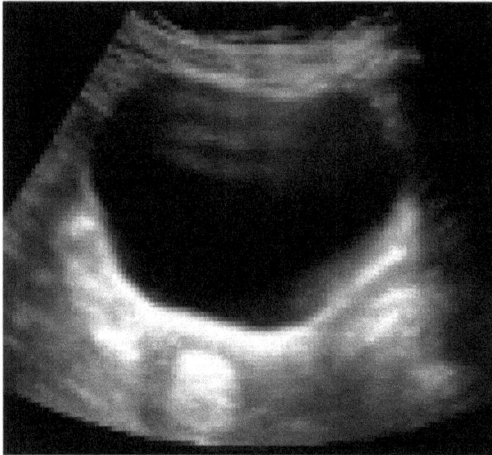

6.28a

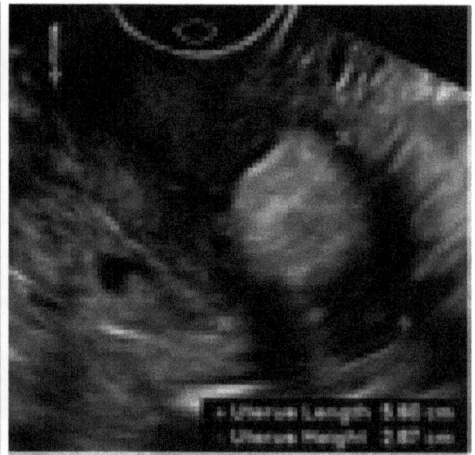

6.28b

Ultrasound Services in an Early Pregnancy and Acute Gynaecological Unit. Book 2

112

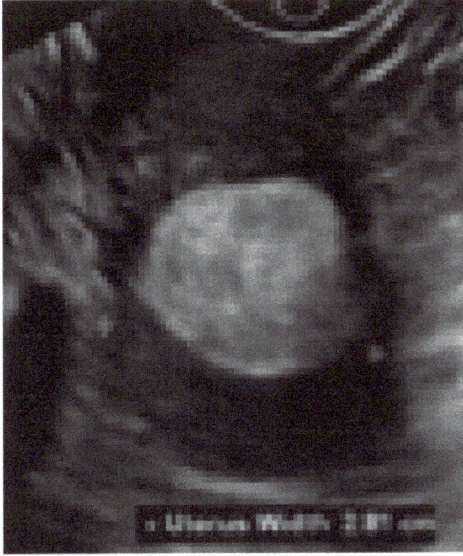

6.28c

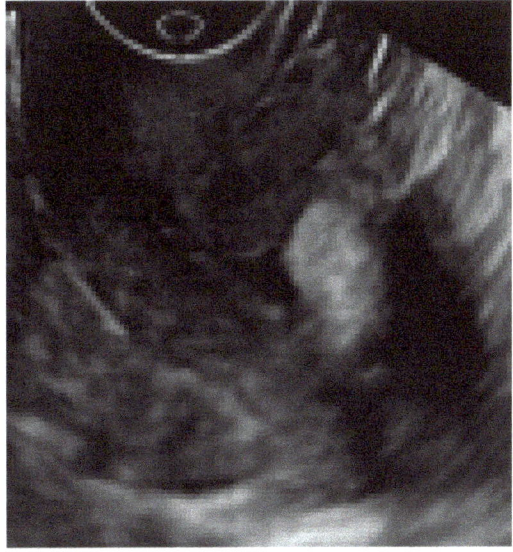

6.28d

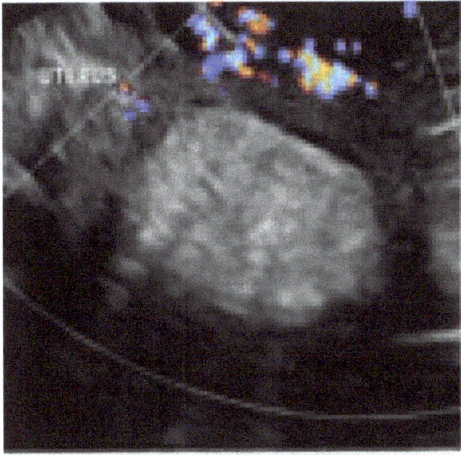

6.28e

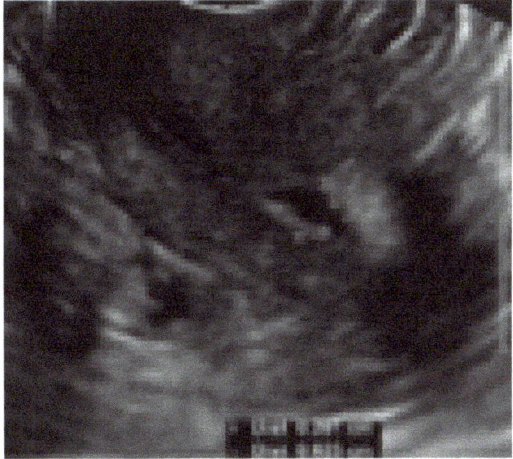

6.28f

Ultrasound findings: Retroverted uterus measuring approx. 56 x 29 x 26mm. (6.28a-c) Adjacent to the endometrial cavity in the fundus but in the myometrium is an approx. well defined avascular echogenic structure measuring 29 x 22 x 19mm (6.28a-e). There is some free fluid in the endometrial cavity and the corrected endometrial thickness is 4mm which is still within normal limits for a post meonopausal woman (6.28f).

Ultrasound Services in an Early Pregnancy and Acute Gynaecological Unit. Book 2

113

Impression: Lipoleiomyoma within the fundal myometrium.

Small free fluid is noted in the endometrial cavity. .

- Differentials – uterine myomas.

Lipoleiomyoma - Experts claim that:

- Lipoleimyomas are uncommon with incidence that varies from 0.03 – 0.2%.
- Are uncommon benign tumours or neoplasms of the uterus.
- May be seen in overweight and menopausal patient who are also prone to gall bladder disease.

Post cornual pregnancy treatment:

Following cornual pregnancy treatment, a patient may be referred for a scan especially following puncture and injection (usually by methotrexate). Primarily the scan aims at confirming the abscence of FHB and check that the size is reduced when compared with the pre treatment scan measurements.

This woman was referred for a scan some days post cornual pregnancy treatment. Both ovaries were not identified. Below are the ultrasound findings,

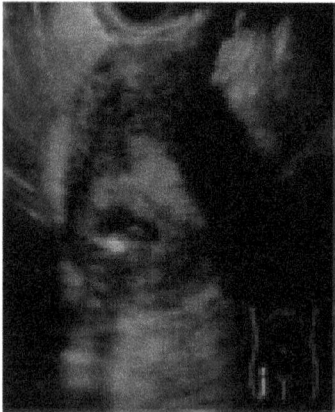 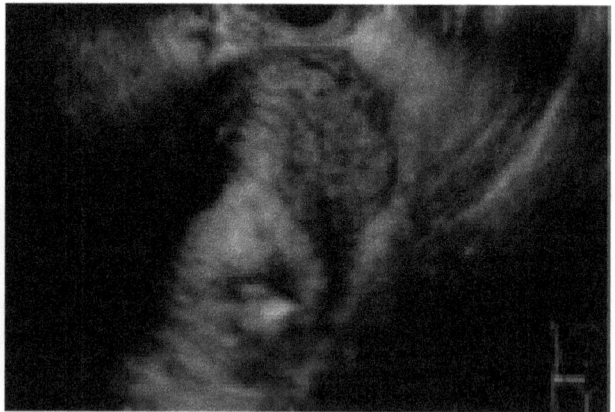

6.29a   6.29b

Ultrasound Services in an Early Pregnancy and Acute Gynaecological Unit. Book 2

114

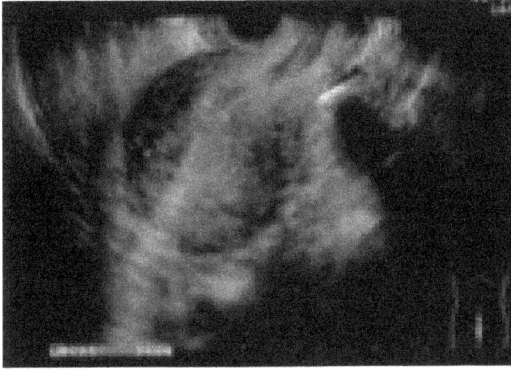

6.29c

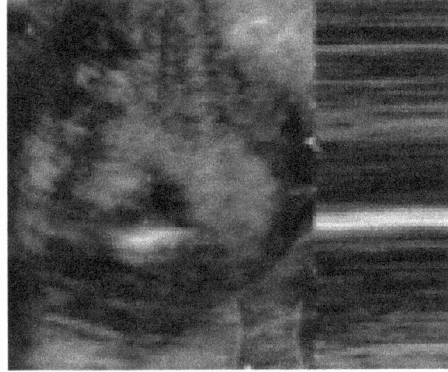

6.29d

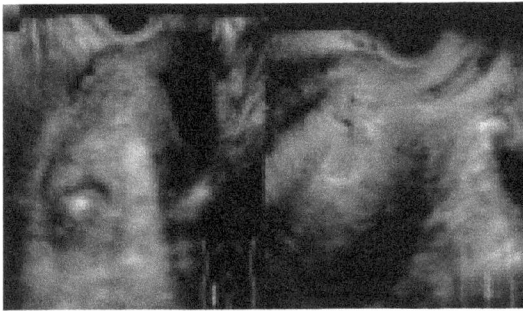

6.29e

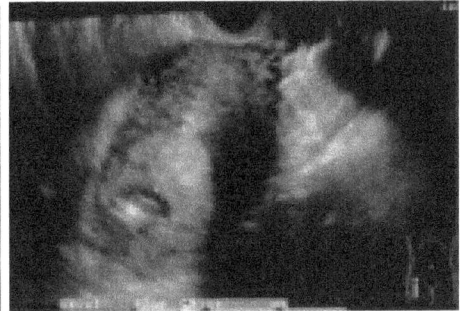

6.29f

Ultrasound findings: An anteveted uterus with a 34mm thick endometrium (6.29c). Previously noted cornual pregnancy in the right horn is seen but a collapsed sac and no EHB or FHB is noted. (6.29a-b & c-f)

Post delivery complications

Referral may be made within a few days to few weeks post delivery. In most cases, the clinicians want to know if there is any RPOC that might be causing prolonged bleeding or clots or infection. The endometrium and cervical canal needs to be assessed for RPOC and free fluid. Identified RPOC should be measured and its location in relation to the uterus be mentioned in the report. Any free pelvic fluid or ascites needs to be documented and measured. It is not unusual not to be able to locate the ovaries during such ultrasound examination. The scan could also be used to check for hematoma around the c/s area if the delivery was by caesarian section. The technique may have to be modified in order to give an explanation for the reason for the scan. It may also be done because of No pv bleed post delivery.

Ultrasound Services in an Early Pregnancy and Acute Gynaecological Unit. Book 2

115

This woman was referred with a history of swollen c/s site six weeks post delivery. Both ovaries were not identified. TVS was not indicated in this woman due to the position or location of her problem.

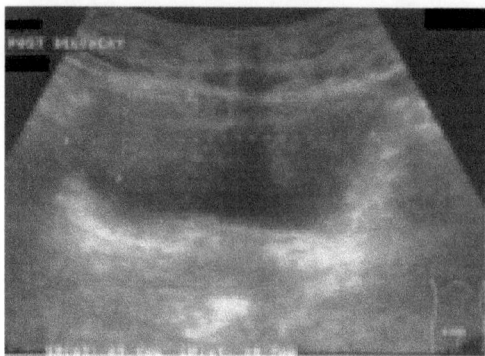

6.30a

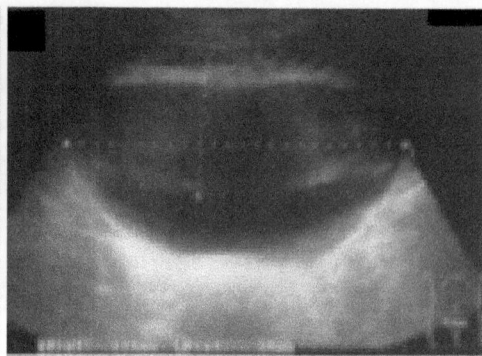

6.30b

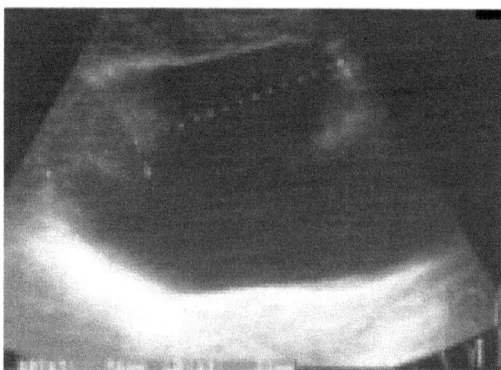

6.30c

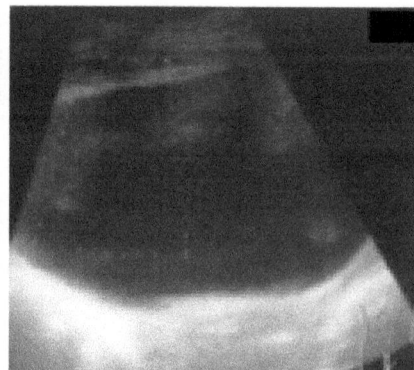

6.30d

The woman was tender in the area of the ultrasound findings. In the area of caesarean section was a 96 x 114 x 32mm collection (6.30a-c). There is no blood flow in this collection. ?blood, ?abcess. (6.30d)

This woman was referred with a history of 10/52 Post c/s continuing pain in the RIF and tenderness. No temperature, not systematically unwell, no mass felt in the RIF and on antibiotics. ?adnexal cause, ?retained products.

Ultrasound Services in an Early Pregnancy and Acute Gynaecological Unit. Book 2

116

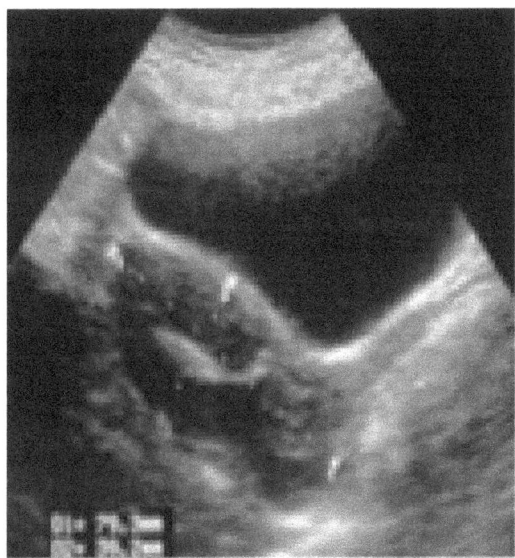

6.31a

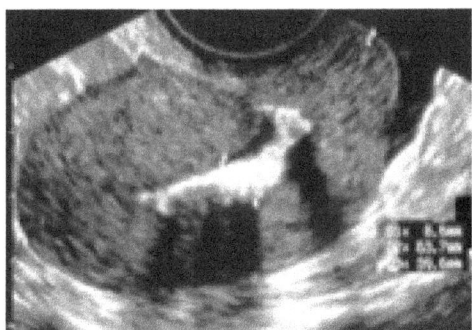

6.31b

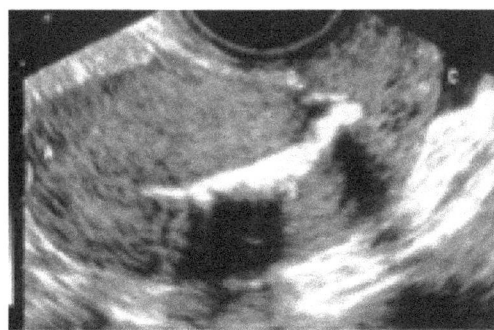

6.31c

a - Fundal myometrium, b- Previous C/S scar, c - Fluid in the POD

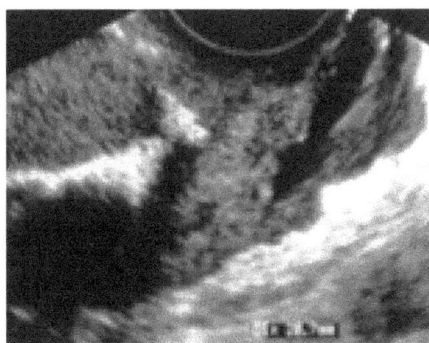

6.31d

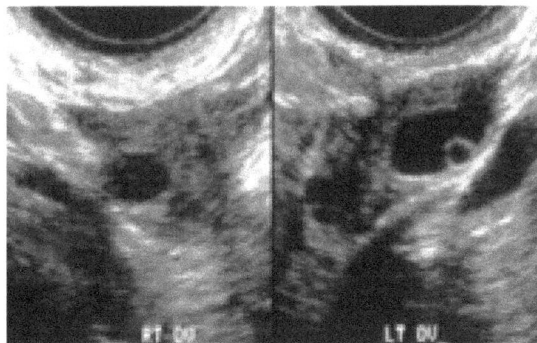

6.31e

Ultrasound Services in an Early Pregnancy and Acute Gynaecological Unit. Book 2

117

Ultrasound findings: An a/v uterus measuring approx. 79 x 39 x 60mm with a 9.6mm endometrium (6.31 a-b). The endometrium is filled with echogenic materials that has posterior acoustic shadowing (6.31a-d). Both ovaries appear sonographically normal (6.31e). Previous c/s scar is noted- arrow (6.31a-d). Some fluid is seen in the POD (6.31a-d).

Impression: RPOC. GIT problems including appendicitis can not been excluded.

This woman was referred with a history of 9/7 post natal bleeding. Forceps delivery. Passed 2 large clots. Both ovaries were not identified on ultrasound.

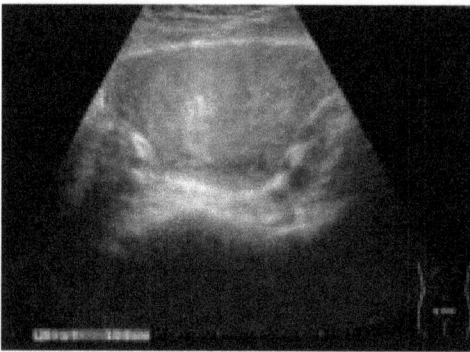

6.32a

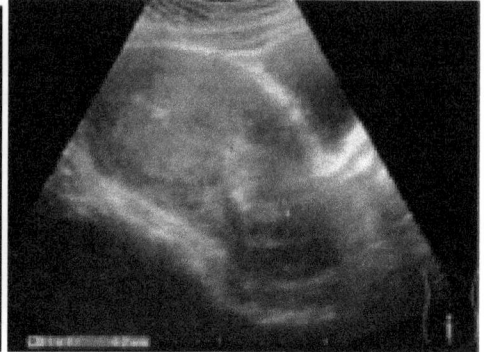

6.32b

Uterus measurement – 150 x 80 x 195mm

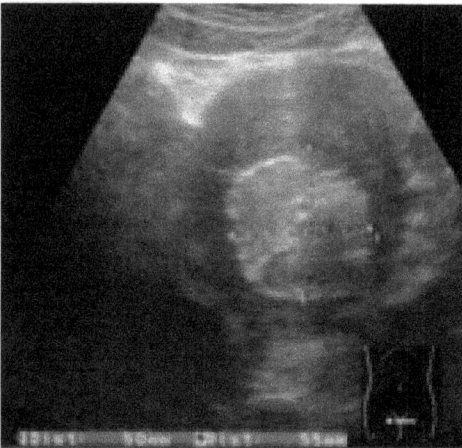

6.32c

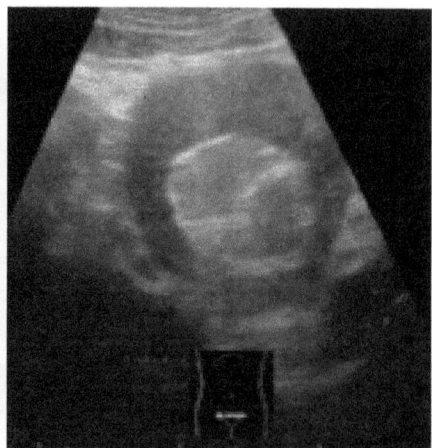

6.32d

Ultrasound Services in an Early Pregnancy and Acute Gynaecological Unit. Book 2

118

Ultrasound findings: An A/V uterus with a thickened endometrium (6.32b) (measurement is not included). There is an approx.. 42 x 50 x 55mm echogenic structure in the cervical canal (6.32b-c). It is an avascular entity (6.32d).

Impression: Ultrasound appearances is suggestive of RPOC.

This woman was referred with a history of acute abdomen 12days post C/S.

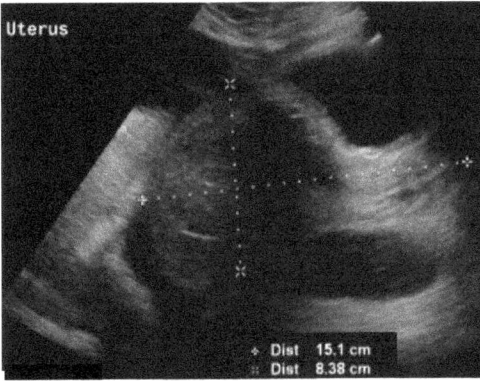

6.33a

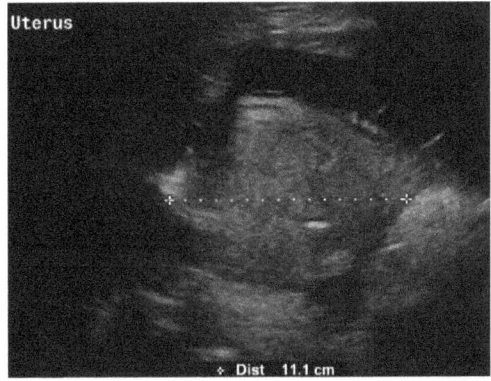

6.33b

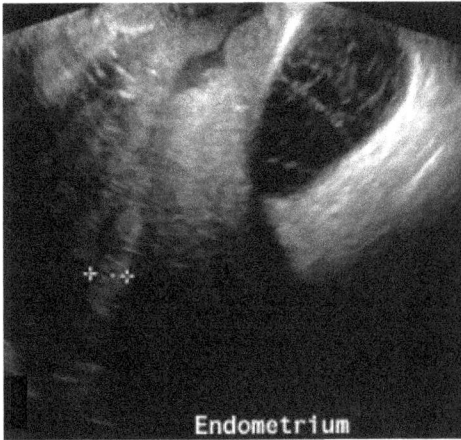

6.33c

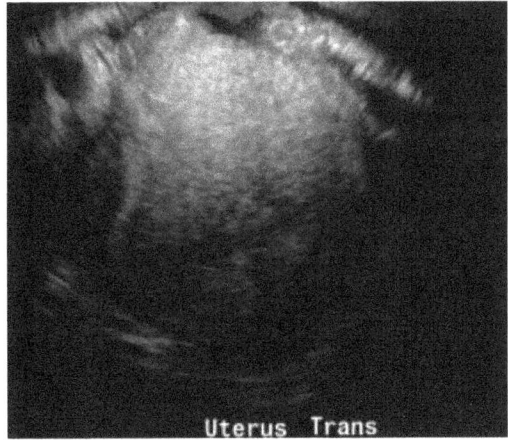

6.33d

Ultrasound Services in an Early Pregnancy and Acute Gynaecological Unit. Book 2

119

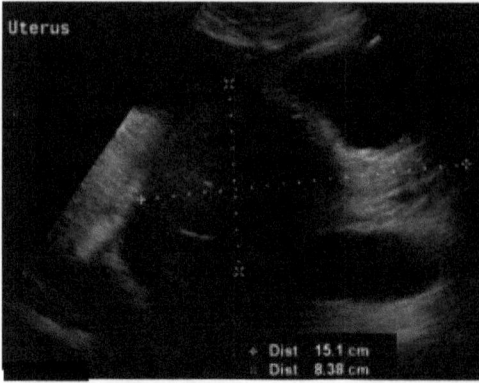

6.33e

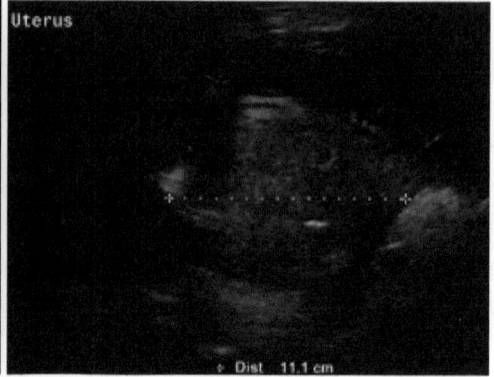

6.33f

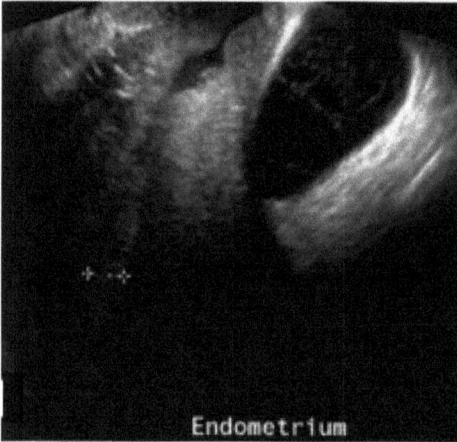

6.33g

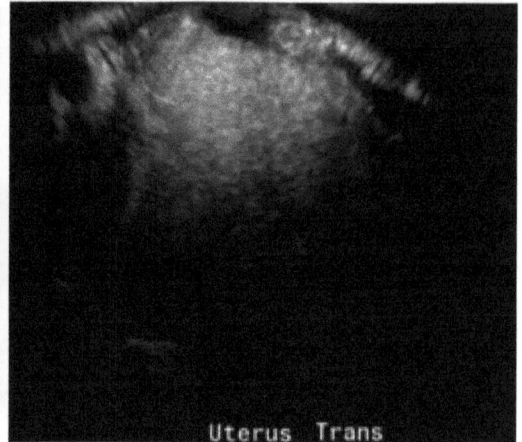

6.33h

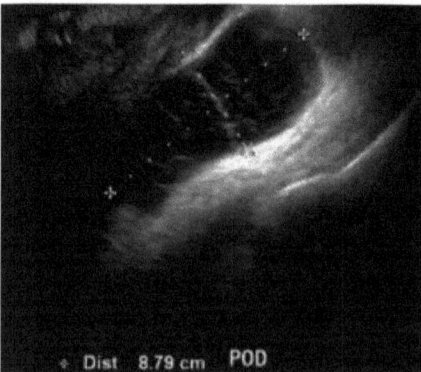

6.33i

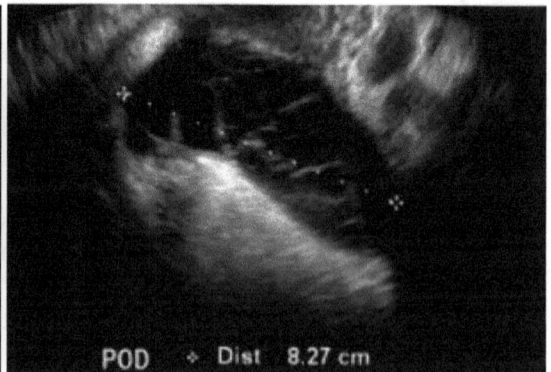

6.33j

Ultrasound Services in an Early Pregnancy and Acute Gynaecological Unit. Book 2

120

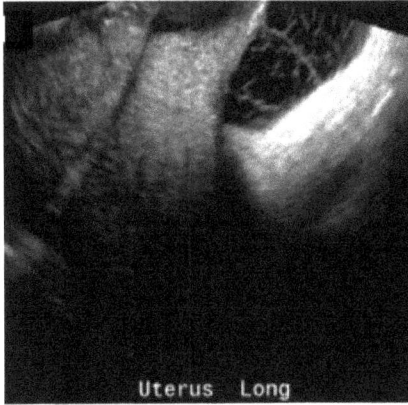
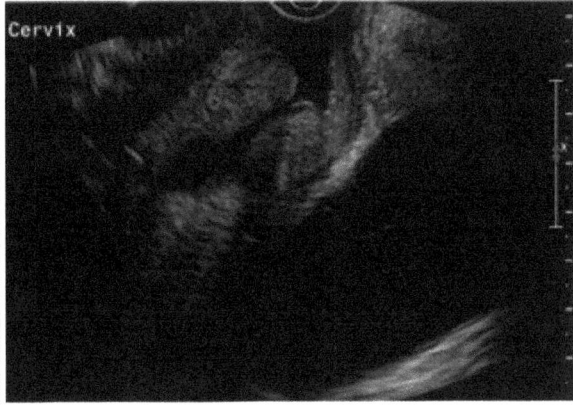

6.33k   **6.33l**

Ultrasound findings: A post partum uterus measuring approx. 15 x 11 x 8.4cm. The endometrium is 12mm with no evidence of RPOC. There is some free fluid at the level of the lower endometrial cavity, in the cervical canal and vagina. There is a 8.8 x 3.8 x 8.2cm low level echoed haemorrhagic fluid in the POD. Both ovaries have not been demonstrated.

Impression: A defect in the caesarean section site has not been demonstrated on ultrasound. There is haemorrhagic collection in the POD

Suspected ovarian cysts

An ovarian cyst is a fluid filled sac in the ovary. The cyst could be a functional cyst which is related to the woman's cycle or pathological cyst which is not menstrual cycle dependent. It may have a thin or thick wall, it will be well defined, with posterior enhancement or may not. To interpret a cystic appearance, the woman's age, LMP or approximately where she is in her menstrual cycle is essential. Is the cyst within or outside the ovary? Attempts should be made to identify both ovaries in the woman who has not had any pelvic operation or oophorectomy. The ovaries should be assessed for size, echo pattern and location. No ovary should be more that twice the size of the other one. As any cyst may need further assessment and monitoring, it is always good practice to document ovarian volumes and the echo pattern at the initial and every follow up scan. Attempts should be made to exclude or confirm ovarian torsion. Any found cysts, masses should be assessed with Dopplers to confirm or refute whether the cyst or mass is vascular or not.

Please refer to chapter 5 on the information required once a cyst has been found.

Ultrasound Services in an Early Pregnancy and Acute Gynaecological Unit. Book 2

121

This woman was referred with a history of Ca breast, ? ovarian pathology. Both ovaries were not identified during this examination.

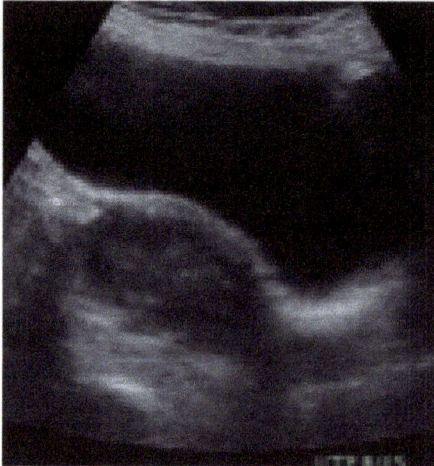

6.34a

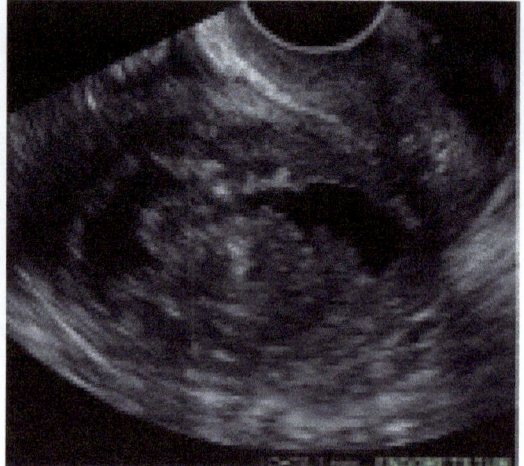

6.34b

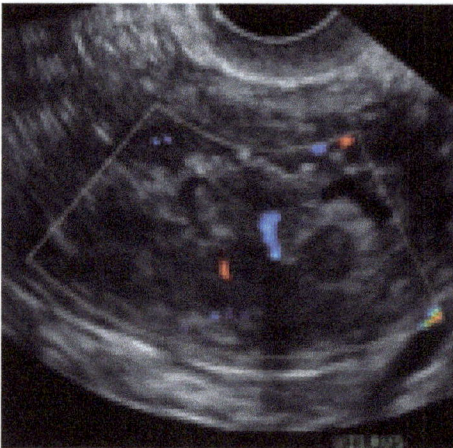

6.34c

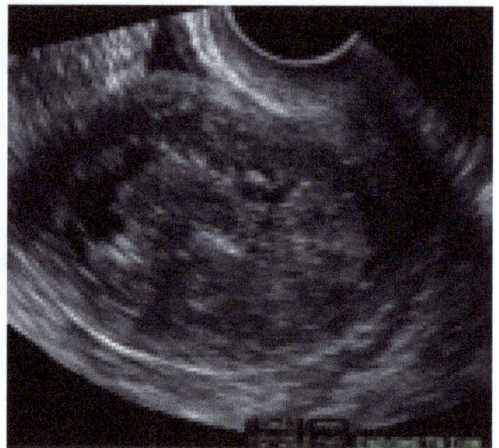

6.34d

Ultrasound Services in an Early Pregnancy and Acute Gynaecological Unit. Book 2

122

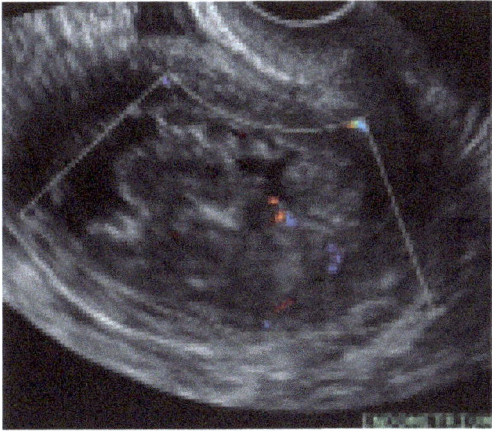

6.34e

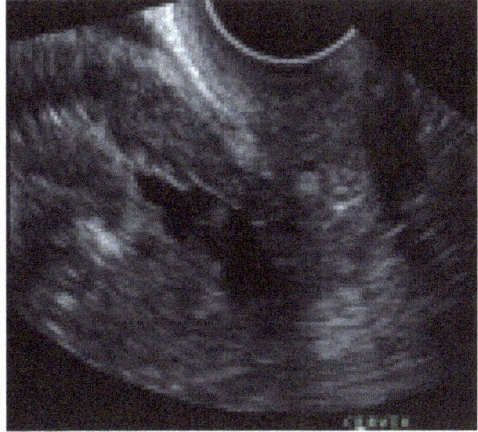

6.34f

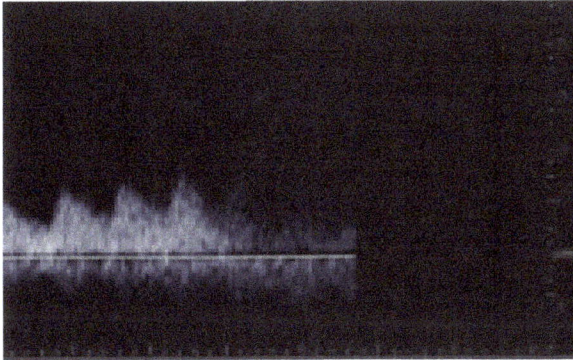

6.34g

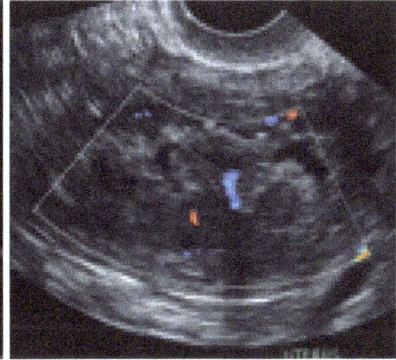

6.34h

Ultrasound findings: The endometrial cavity is grossly distended measuring 29mm.(6.34b) There appears to be loss of contour between the endometrial/ posterior myometrial border (6.34a-h). Within the cavity there is a ill-defined isoechoic mass which is irregular in outline and is surrounded by an area of fluid. Vascularity is seen in this mass with colour Doppler with low resistance arterial flow is also noted (6.34 b -h)

Impression: The endometrial cavity is grossly distended with an ill-defined isoechoic mass with low resistance arterial flow. There appears to be a loss of contour between the endometrial and posterior myometrial border. Further imaging is recommended.

Ultrasound Services in an Early Pregnancy and Acute Gynaecological Unit. Book 2

123

Sudden generalized or local pelvic pain

Before embarking on performing the examination it is good to ask the woman to describe the type of pain, what sparked the pain off, the duration of the pain, find out if it has any bearing with her menstrual cycle or meals. Ask the woman to pin point the area of her worst pain. Generalised pain will mean searching the whole pelvis thoroughly for the evidence and cause for pain. Confirm or exclude dilated pelvic blood vessels which can be an indication of pelvic congestion syndrome that can cause pelvic pain. A normal gynecology scan cannot exclude GIT problems. Confirm or exclude PID which can cause pain, ovarian cysts, ovarian torsion. PID, pedunculated fibroid torsion, KUB or urinary bladder problems, overlying bowel gas. The possibility of an ectopic pregnancy should not be ignored in a sexually active patient. As in other scans, the LMP needs to be established before commencing the scan so that the ultrasound findings can be better interpreted. If the pain is localised, the woman should be encouraged to pinpoint the area of her pain with her finger so that the sonographer can assess the area. Seeing a normal right ovary in a woman with RIF pain should make the sonographer think of the possibility of appendicitis.

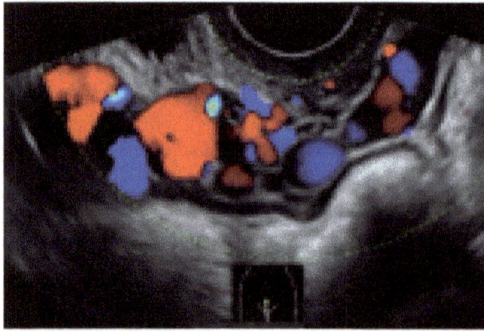 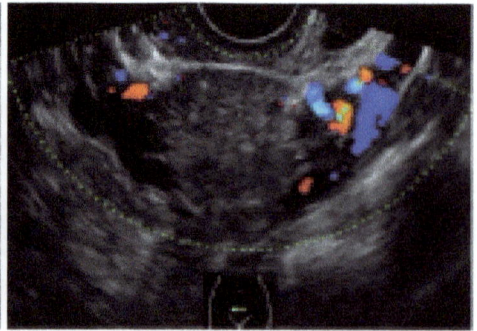

| 6.35a | 6.35b |

The above shows dilated pelvic vessels in a non pregnant pelvis (pelvic varices).

This woman was referred for a pelvic scan by the medical clinicians with a history of sudden onset of lower abdominal pain, stabbing, radiating to the back, nausea, tender RIF. Normally has irregular periods. ?appendicitis, ?urology cause, ?gynaecology cause. LMP – 1 week ago.

Ultrasound Services in an Early Pregnancy and Acute Gynaecological Unit. Book 2

124

Below are the ultrasound findings of her pelvis and in the area of her pain.

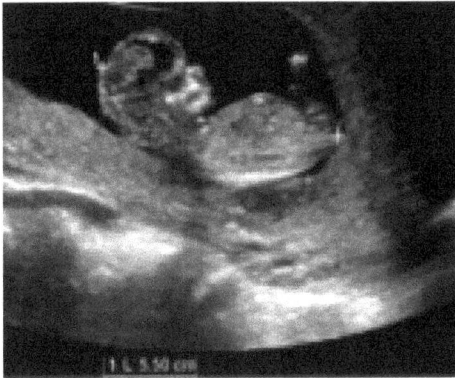

6.36a

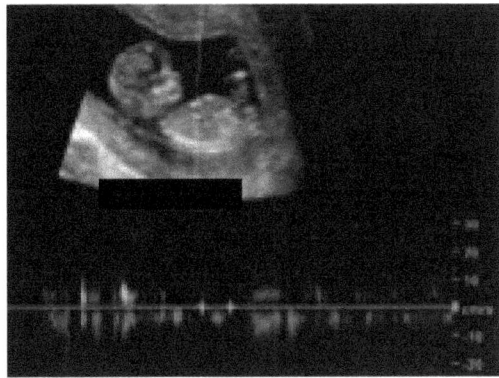

6.36b

Ultrasound findings- there is a single intrauterine pregnancy. FHB and movement were seen. CRL = 55mm = 12/40. The fetal head is seen in the RIF in the area of the patient's pain. Both ovaries were not seen. TVS declined. GIT problems especially appendicitis could not be excluded.

Impression: Intrauterine singleton pregnancy.
The above is a case of 'social bad news' as the patient was oblivious of her pregnancy before the pelvic scan.

This woman was referred with a history of LIF pain for 3/7. Below are the images on Day 40.

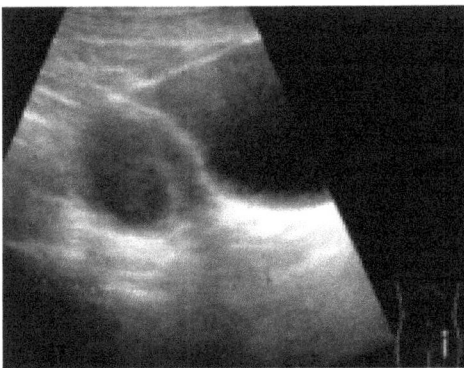

6.37a

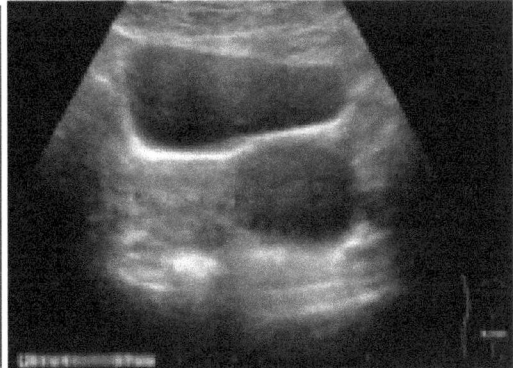

6.37b

Ultrasound Services in an Early Pregnancy and Acute Gynaecological Unit. Book 2

125

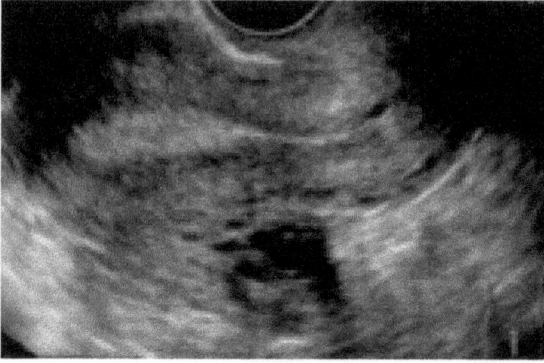

6.37c

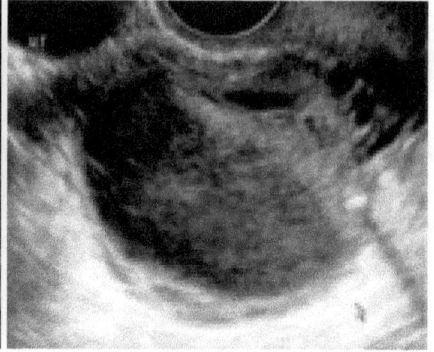

6.37d

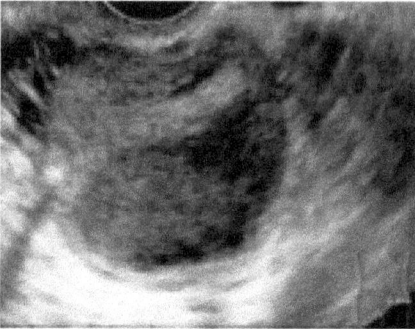

6.37e

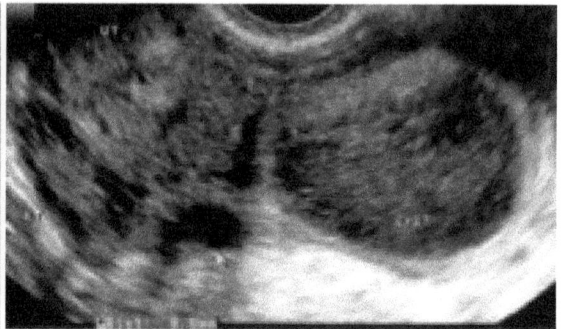

6.37f

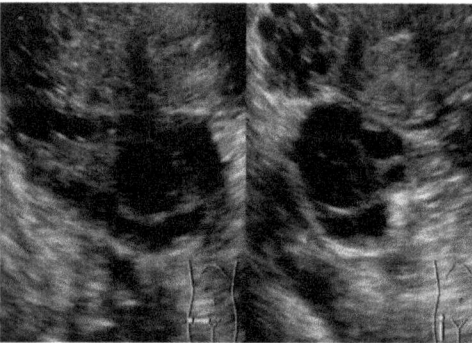

6.37g

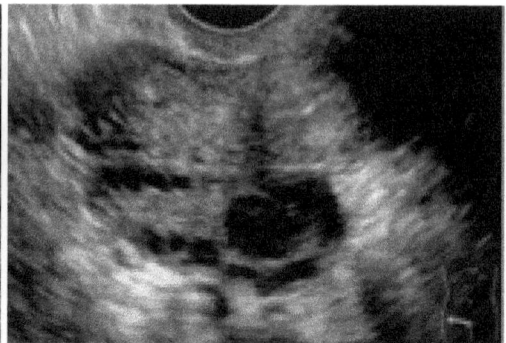

6.37h

Ultrasound findings – The anteverted uterus appears sonographically normal with a luteal phase endometrium – measurement not included (6.37c). The right ovary appears polycystic (6.37g –h). In the LIF is an approx.49 x 46 x48mm complex but predominantly low level echo cystic lesion that also had a 8mm hyperechoic band and two echogenic foci (6.37a-b,& d-f).

Ultrasound Services in an Early Pregnancy and Acute Gynaecological Unit. Book 2

126

Impression: Normal a/v uterus and endometrium. Right PCO. Left complex cyst, ?haemorrhagic cyst, ?endometrioma, ?dermoid. Suggest a follow up scan in six weeks time or in other menstrual phase to re-assess the left ovary.

* re-assessing the ovary in another menstrual phase or in six weeks from then is to be able to confirm or refute the type of LIF mass. Dermoids and endometriomas don't change appearance whereas a haemorhagic cyst will likely change its size and its appearance during the next menstrual phase.

This woman was referred with a history of LIF pain. She is known to have a 28days cycle. She is on metformin. Below are some of the images done on day 22 of her cycle. Not shown here was a normal anteverted uterus with a 4.5mm endometrium thickness.

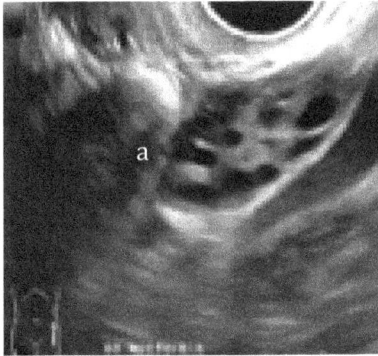

6.38a

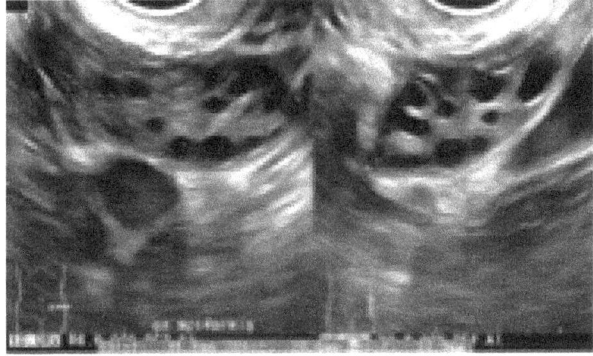

6.38b.   35 x 19 x 34mm

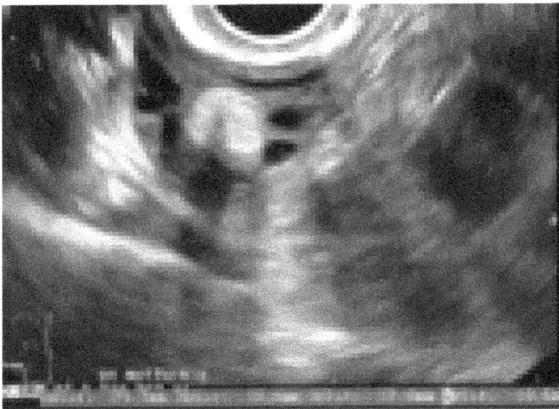

6.38c 25 x 31 x 37mm

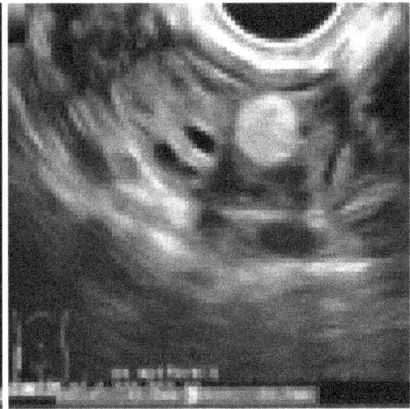

6.38d 11 x 12 x 11mm

Ultrasound Services in an Early Pregnancy and Acute Gynaecological Unit. Book 2

127

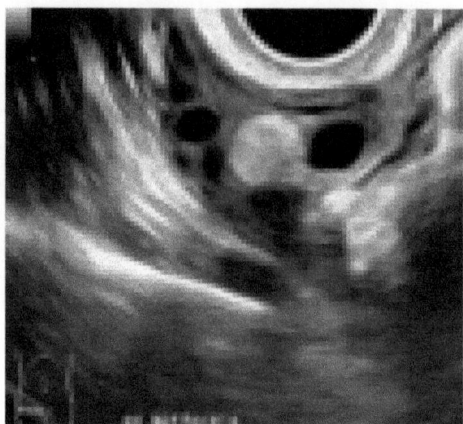

6.38e

Ultrasound findings: Uterus findings as stated above.

The left ovary (6.38b) had an ovarian volume of 3.5 x 1.9 x 3.4cm x 0.5233 = 11.2mls and the right ovary a 2.5 x 3.1 x 3.7cm x 0.5233 = 15mls ovarian volume. On the right (6.38 c-e) is a hyperechoic slightly irregular structure with some shadowing within the right ovary measuring approx. 11 x 11 x 12mm.

Impression: Bilateral multicystic ovaries and dermoid cyst in the right ovary.

Note the overlying bowel gas on the left – a- in 6.38a. This was in the area of patient's pain.

Ultrasound sometimes cannot find the cause of pelvic pain. It is important that the status of the normal ovaries, uterus etc. be documented as it would help to re think of other possible causes of the pain.

Metformin is a diabetes medicine sometimes used for lowering insulin and blood sugar levels in women with polycystic ovary syndrome (PCOS). This helps regulate menstrual cycles, start ovulation, and lower the risk of miscarriage in women with PCOS. Like any other drug, it has side effects including increased abdominal distension.

'KISSING OVARIES'

This woman was referred for a scan with a history of sharp LIF pain radiating to the back and thighs. LMP 37months before. A normal uterus with a 9.5mm endometrium was seen not shown here. Partially joined together are the ovaries as best seen.

Ultrasound Services in an Early Pregnancy and Acute Gynaecological Unit. Book 2

128

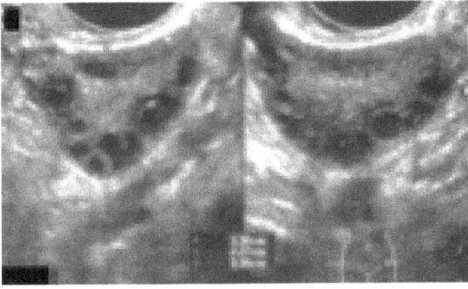

6.39a

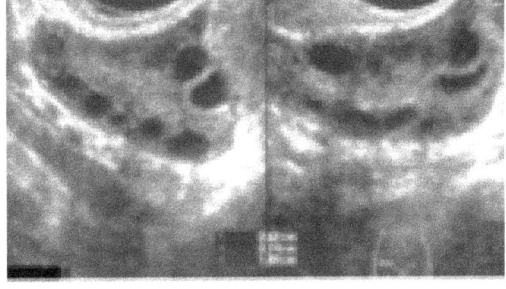

6.39b

Ultrasound findings: Both ovaries appear sonographically polycystic. The right ovarian volume is 13.2mls (6.39b) and the left ovarian volume is 13.9mls.(6.39a)

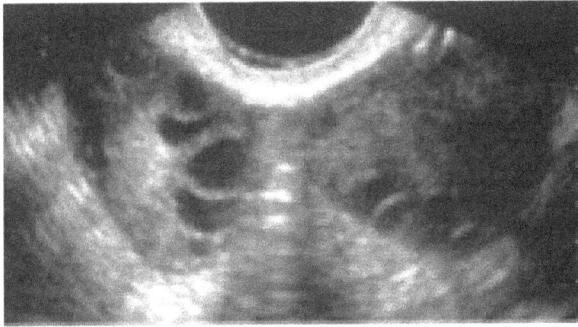

6. 39c

The above could be described as 'Kissing ovaries'.

'Kissing ovaries' is a condition where both ovaries are partly or completely joined together and are stabilized behind the pouch of Douglas. Experts believe that finding 'kissing ovaries' on ultrasound is strongly associated with the presence of endometriosis and is a marker of the most severe form of this disease.

*Occassionally with patients having fertility treatment, both ovaries with multiple big follicles may be seen in the POD, due to the weight of the multiple follicles in the ovaries, but the ovaries are not joined together. In such an instance that is not 'kissing ovaries'.

Ultrasound Services in an Early Pregnancy and Acute Gynaecological Unit. Book 2

129

No menstrual period and –ve pregnancy test result

Particular attempt should be made to assess and measure the endometrium, exclude very thin endometrium in relation to the woman's menstrual cycle. The ovaries should be assessed for size and echo texture or pattern. PCO or un ruptured cyst or other cysts that can sometimes be the cause for no menstrual period. At other times it could be very thin endometrium which is too thin to be shed.

This woman in her thirties was referred for a scan with a history of -ve pregnancy test result. No periods for over 15years.

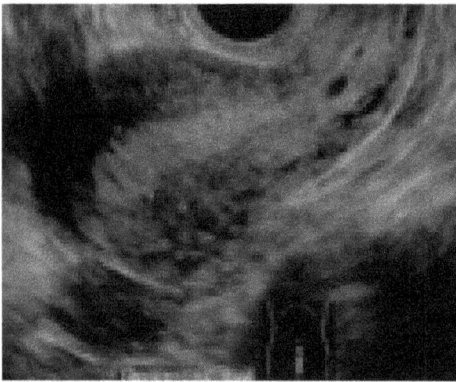

6.40a

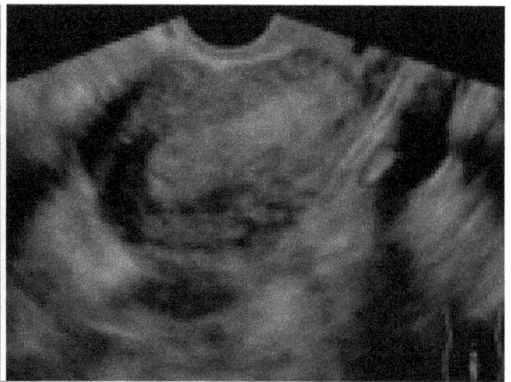

6.40b

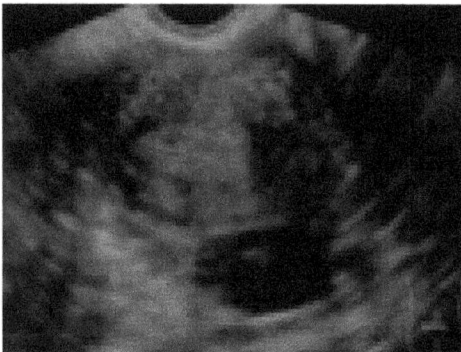

6.40c

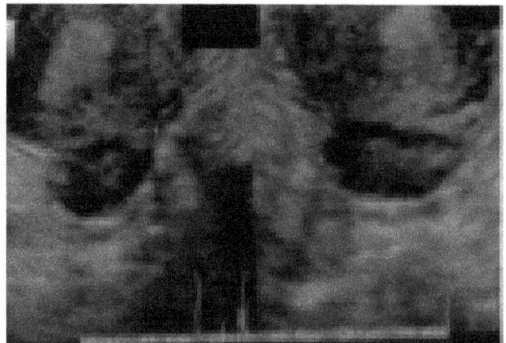

6.40d

Ultrasound Services in an Early Pregnancy and Acute Gynaecological Unit. Book 2

130

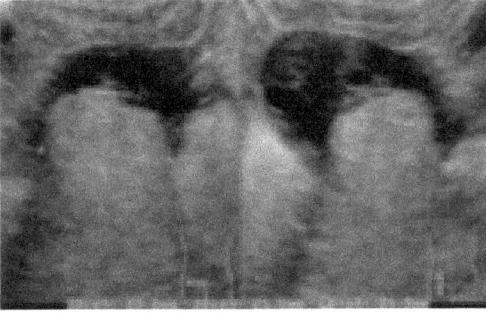 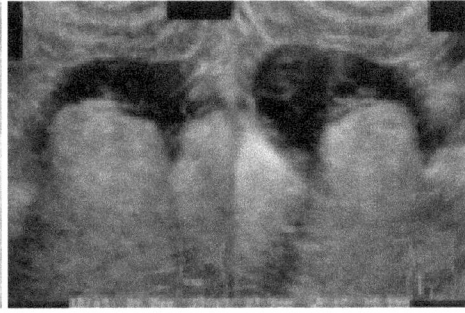

6.40e   **6.40f**

Ultrasound findings: A normal size anteverted uterus with a 15mm endometrium and possible tiny cystic entities in it. (6.40a-b) The right ovarian volume = 17.5mls and a solid echogenic structure in it measuring 24 x 21 x 21mm (6.40e-f). The left ovary appears polycystic with a volume of 10.4mls (6.40c-d).

Impression Thickened endometrium, Bilateral PCO. In the right ovary is a dermoid cyst.

Calcified mass in the ovary

Sometimes a calcified mass may be seen in the ovary. There is a calcified rim surrounding a hypoechoic lesion in the ovary with no acoustic shadows posterior to the mass. These ultrasound findings is suggestive of a calcified dermoid cyst. The differentials being ovarian fibroma with rim calcification.

This woman was referred for a scan with a history of pelvic pain.

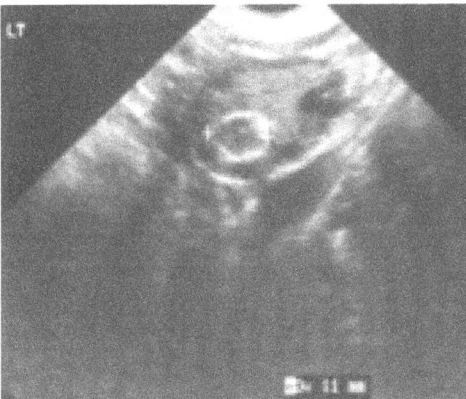 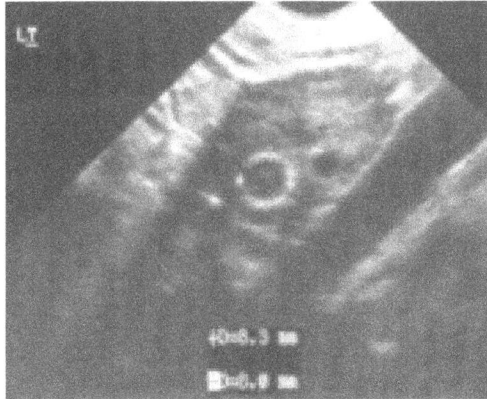

6.41a   **6.41b**

Ultrasound Services in an Early Pregnancy and Acute Gynaecological Unit. Book 2

131

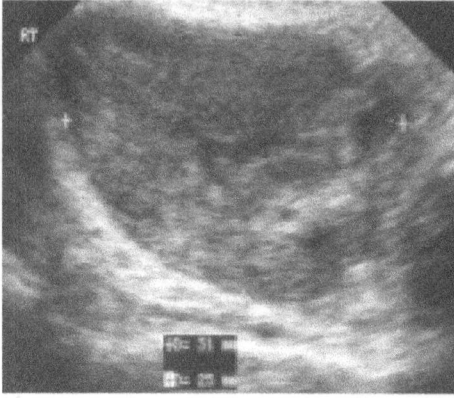

6.41c

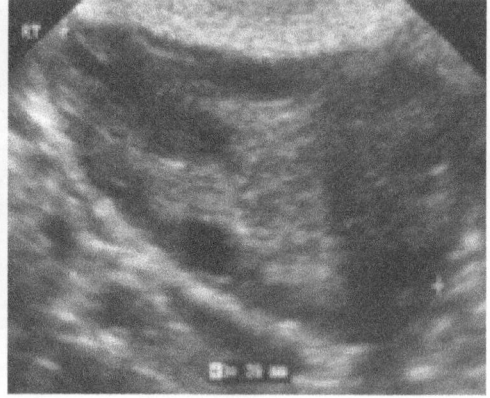

6.41d

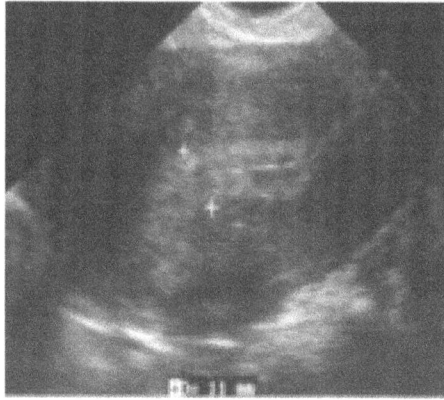

6.41e

Ultrasound findings: An anteverted uterus with a 11mm luteal phase endometrium. (6.41e). There is a 11 x 8 x 8mm hypoechoic lesion with rim calcifications in the left ovary (6.41 a-b). Left ovarian measurements have not been included. The right ovarian volume is 3.9 x 3.1 x 2.5 x 0.5233 =15.8mls (6.41 c-d).

Impression: Calcified dermoid of the left ovary or left ovarian fibroma with rim

Ultrasound Services in an Early Pregnancy and Acute Gynaecological Unit. Book 2

132

Here are some tips:

	Clinical Indication	Added Tips or what to assess carefully
1	Abnormal pv. Bleeding	Assess the endometrium and cervix for space occupying lesion, Exclude urinary bladder abnormality.
2	Abdominal bloating	Assess the uterus and ovaries. Confirm or exclude any pelvic mass or cysts. Confirm or exclude pelvic or abdominal ascites. Confirm or exclude excessive bowel gas.
3	Following fertility treatment	Confirm or rule out OHSS, Ectopic and heterotopic pregnancy. Check the upper abdomen to confirm or exclude ascites.*
4	Generalized or localised sudden pelvic pain	Ask the patient to put a finger over the most painful part of the pelvis. Scan carefully and thoroughly the structure below the patient's identified area of pain.
5	Heavy bleeding	Confirm or exclude fibroids, size and position, adenomyosis. Exclude incorrectly positioned IUCD using 3D if and where possible, polyps, and any other endometrial pathology.
6	IMB	Exclude polyps, assess and measure ovaries
7	Irregular bleeding	Exclude polyps and space occupying lesions and assess the ovaries.

Ultrasound Services in an Early Pregnancy and Acute Gynaecological Unit. Book 2

133

8	Missing IUCD	Confirm from the patient the type of the missing IUCD if she knows. Confirm or exclude the presence of an IUCD in the uterus, if the IUCD is correctly or incorrectly positioned in the positioned in the uterus using 3D if and where possible,. *Be aware of uterine perforation. * Where the IUCD is not identified and a pregnancy test result is negative, suggest further pelvic imaging e.g. plain X-Ray of the abdomen.
9	Pain in a patient with known cyst	Assess and measure cyst. Exclude or confirm ovarian torsion. Compare the measurements and echo pattern obtained with the previous ones.
10	Pains in patient with known pedunculated fibroid	Assess and measure the fibroid. Exclude or confirm torsion or red degeneration. Red degeneration should not normally cause pain in a non pregnant woman. Include the location(s) of the fibroid(s)
11	Post Cornual pregnancy	Confirm no EHB or FHB. Assess gestational sac size.
12	Post delivery	Confirm or exclude RPOC, fluid collections if it is post C/S
13	PMB	Assess the endometrium, measure and confirm or exclude polyps, ca. of the endometrium, hyperplasia. Depth of the fluid in the endometrium if any should not be included in the endometrial thickness. Assess the woman's urinary bladder and ovaries.

Ultrasound Services in an Early Pregnancy and Acute Gynaecological Unit. Book 2

134

14	Post menopausal ovarian cyst or mass	Identify ovaries in relation to the cyst/mass. Assess the size, margins and content of the cyst or mass. Confirm vascularity around and within the ?mass or cyst. Assess the kidneys to exclude hydronephrosis. Confirm or exclude any pelvic or abdominal ascites. Suggest further imaging modalities e.g. MRI where necessary.
15	Post miscarriage	Confirm or exclude RPOC. Assess the ovaries. Is there any uterine abnormality? If there is a uterine abnormality, check the kidneys for any abnormality.
16	Post surgical (op) complications	Confirm or exclude fluid collections and abscess around the wound bed. Check the upper abdomen to confirm or exclude ascites.
17	Post TOP	Confirm or exclude, embryo or fetus or RPOC.
18	Suspected ovarian cysts	Be aware of ovarian torsion. Measure ovaries and document measurements. Describe the nature or pattern of the cyst and confirm or refute vascularity with Doppler's.

Ultrasound Services in an Early Pregnancy and Acute Gynaecological Unit. Book 2

135

Chapter conclusion

A good and sound knowledge of the female normal anatomy or variant is essential for the gynaecology ultrasound. As the ultrasound appearances changes with the phase of the menstrual cycle, an understanding and appreciation of these changes will enhance the ultrasound interpretation of the examination.

Where and when possible, an ultrasound diagnosis and differentials should be made. However a detailed description may be useful especially, where the ultrasound images obtained or findings are complex and does not fit into any particular condition.

Feedback from colleagues (Gynaecologists, Nurses, Histology or MDT meetings) should be positively embraced. It helps with learning and confidence.

As it is not usual for the same patient to be seen by the same Sonographer on each visit, documentation in terms of the images stored and ultrasound report should always be available for the next Sonographer to access for comparison if need be.

Ultrasound Services in an Early Pregnancy and Acute Gynaecological Unit. Book 2

136

CHAPTERS 5 & 6
FURTHER READING:

BOOKS:

Bates J (ed) 1997 Practical Gynaecological Ultrasound. Greenwich Medical Media, London

Ola-Ojo O.O 2017 NT Scanning for the Beginner. Protokos Publishers. London

Ola-Ojo O.O 2005 Obstetrics and Gynaecological Ultrasound: A Self Assessment Guide. Elsevier Churchill Livingstone. Edinburgh

Ola-Ojo O.O 2017 Ultrasound Services in an Early Pregnancy and Acute Gynaecological Unit, Book 1. Protokos Publishers. London

Articles:

Baby Centre. 2013. Abnormalities of the uterus and fertility. http://www.babycentre.co.uk/a1038163/abnormalities-of-the-uterus-and-fertility#ixzz2XMnrwoWT

Barloon TJ, Brown BP, Abu-Yousef MM et.al. Paraovarian and paratubal cysts: preoperative diagnosis using transabdominal and transvaginal sonography. J Clin Ultrasound, 24 (1996), pp. 22–117

Bell D.J and Radswiki et al. Peritoneal inclusion cyst https://radiopaedia.org/articles/peritoneal

Ganzone G, Parlato M, Triolo L. 2007. 2D-3D Ultrasound in the diagnosis of uterine malformations. Donald School Journal of Ultrasound in Obstetrics and

Ultrasound Services in an Early Pregnancy and Acute Gynaecological Unit. Book 2

137

Gynaecology, July - Sept 2007: 1 (3); 77-79

George T. M, Lieberman G. November 2008 Imaging Ovarian endometriomas Gynecol Obstet Invest, 12 (1981), pp. 1–10

George T.M Imaging Ovarian Endometriomas - Lieberman's eRadiology http://eradiology.bidmc.harvard.edu/LearningLab/genito/George.pdf

Hacking C, Yang N. et al. 2014. Septate uterus, https://radiopaedia.org/articles/septate-uterus

Kim J.S, Woo S.K, Suh S.J, et.al. 1995 Sonographic diagnosis of paraovarian cysts: value of detecting a separate ipsilateral ovary. Am J Roentgenol, 164 (1995), pp. 4–1441 -1444

Kyland G, 2016 Accurate detection of IUD placement using 3D ultrasound. https://sononotes.com/category/obgyn-ultrasound

Lin, PC.. Reproductive outcomes in women with uterine anomalies. Journal of Women's Health. 2004 Jan-Feb;13(1):33-39.

Morgan M. A, Yang N. et al. Septate uterus. Available at: http://radiopaedia.org/articles/septate-uterus

Moyle P. L, Kataoka M.Y , Nakai A, et.al. Non ovarian Cystic Lesions of the Pelvis. http://pubs.rsna.org/doi/full/10.1148/rg.304095706

Payne J. Menopause including HRT http://www.patient.co.uk/health/menopause-and-hrt.htm

RCOG. Management of Suspected Ovarian Masses in Premenopausal Women RCOG Green-top Guideline No. 62. https://www.rcog.org.uk/globalassets/documents/guidelines/gtg_62.pdf

Rezaee A, Weerakkody Y et al. Paraovarian cyst. https://radiopaedia.org/

Ultrasound Services in an Early Pregnancy and Acute Gynaecological Unit. Book 2

138

articles/paraovarian-cyst-1

Steinback F, Kauppila A. Development and classification of paraovarian cysts: an ultrastructural study.

The American College of Obstetricians and Gynecologists. Committee opinion no 274. Nonsurgical diagnosis and management of vaginal agenesis. Obstet Gynecol100(1):213-6 . ACOG 2002.

Ultrasound Image Gallery. Ultrasound images of ovarian tumours. http://www. ultrasound-images.com/ovarian-masses/#Calcific%20masses%20of%20 the%20ovary

Veldhuis W, Smithuis R, Oguz Akin O et.al Ovarian Cysts - Common lesions in Radiology. http://www.radiologyassistant.nl/en/p4cdf9b5de7d3b/ovarian-cysts-common-lesions.html

Wikipedia. Uterine fibroid. https://en.wikipedia.org/wiki/Uterine_fibroid

Williams P.L, Dubbins, P.A, Defriend D.E. Ultrasound in the diagnosis of ovarian dermoid cysts: a pictorial review of the characteristic sonographic signs http://ult.sagepub.com/content/19/2/85.full

Ultrasound Services in an Early Pregnancy and Acute Gynaecological Unit. Book 2

139

CHAPTER 7

101 Case presentations and Quiz

The aim of this chapter is to present some cases for you to test your knowledge in some of the areas covered in the previous chapters of Books 1 and 2. The answers are provided in the next chapter. The cases have not been grouped under gynaecology or obstetrics. They have been deliberately mixed to reflect what mostly happens in a typical EPAGU ultrasound setting. The best obtainable images have been presented. As protocols and the charts may vary from hospital to hospital, please reflect your answers in line with your own departmental protocols and charts in mind.

1

   a.   Identify A – J below.
   b.   Approximately how old is this embryo?
   c.   Which structures are shown in 7.1b
   d.   What is the difference in the Doppler box in 7.1d and 7.1e?

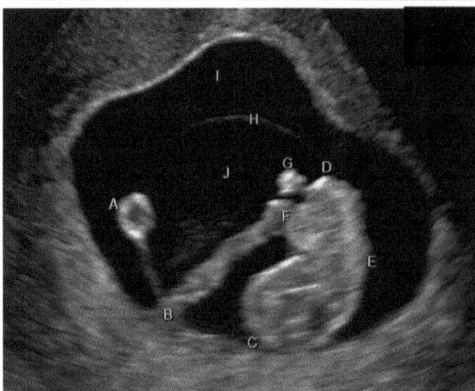 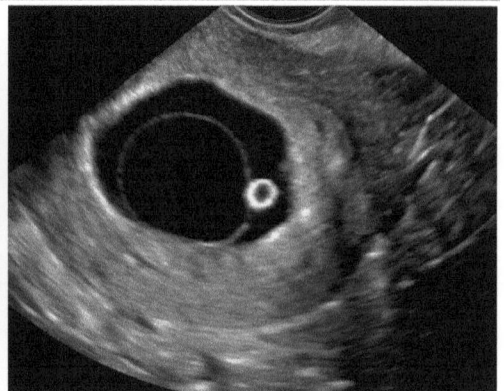

      7.1a   **7.1b**

Ultrasound Services in an Early Pregnancy and Acute Gynaecological Unit. Book 2

140

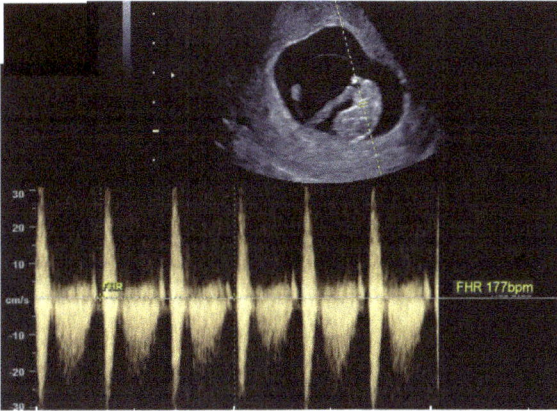
7.1c

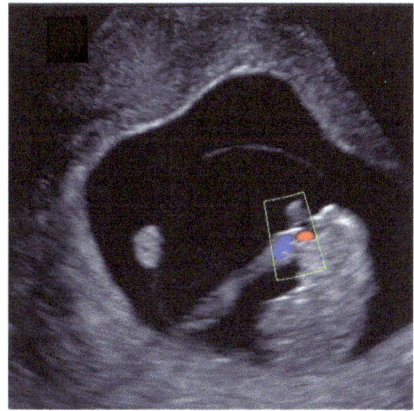
7.1d

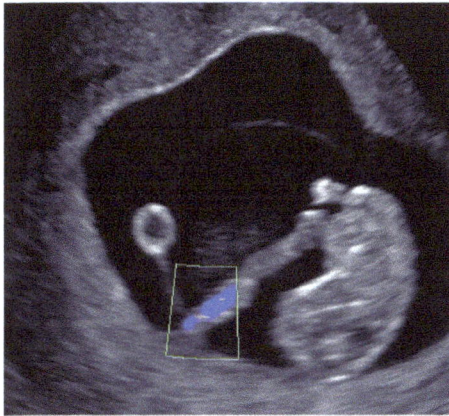
7.1e

2

7.2a TS showing lower limbs at 12+4/40. Can you identify a-d ?

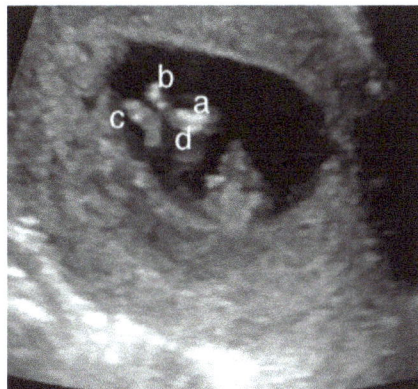
7.2a

Ultrasound Services in an Early Pregnancy and Acute Gynaecological Unit. Book 2

141

7.2b

TS at the level of the fetal thorax showing both hands and face at 12+4/40.
Identify a-d.

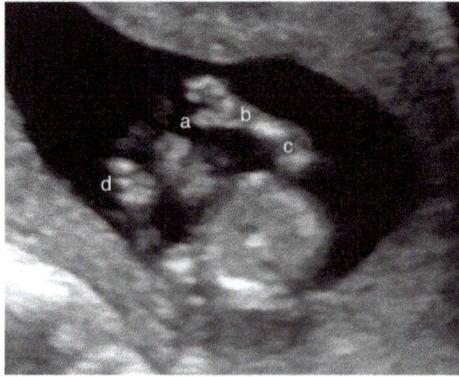

7.2b

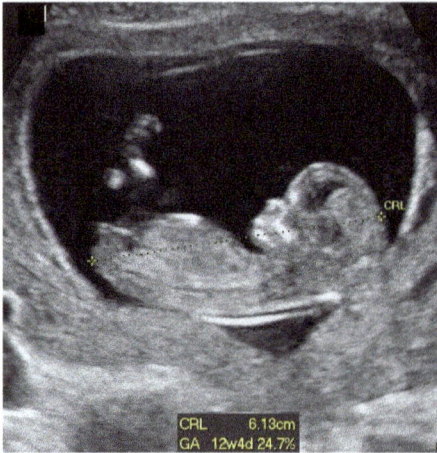

7.2c

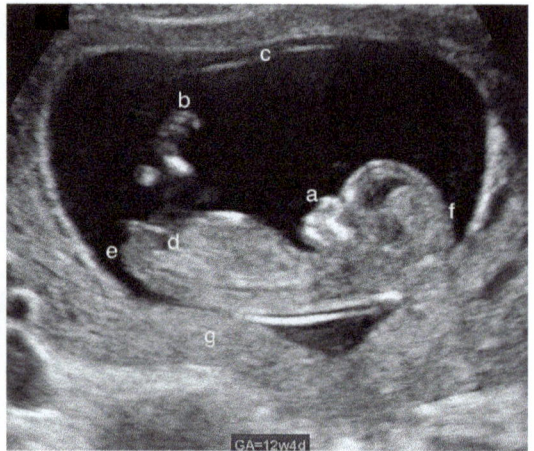

7.2d

Identify a-g.

Ultrasound Services in an Early Pregnancy and Acute Gynaecological Unit. Book 2

142

In the following images, identify the fetal parts and the views/ sections.

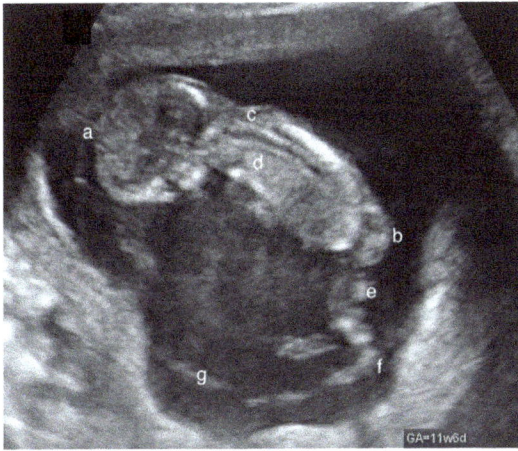

7.2e

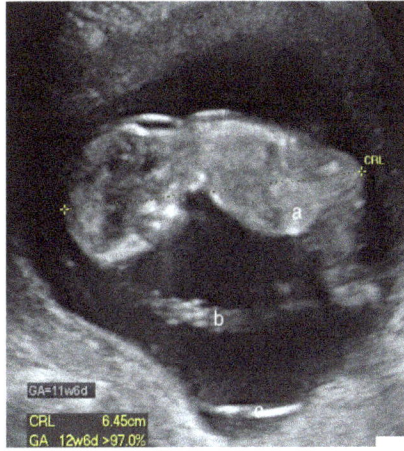

7.2f

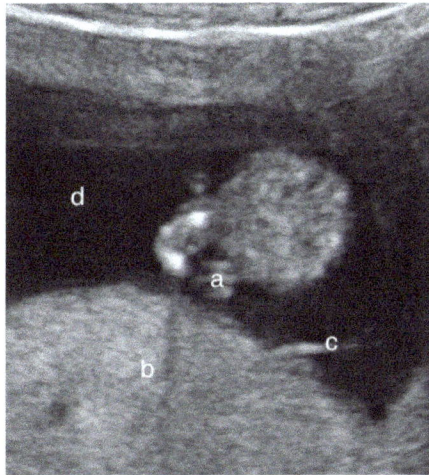

7.2g

Ultrasound Services in an Early Pregnancy and Acute Gynaecological Unit. Book 2

143

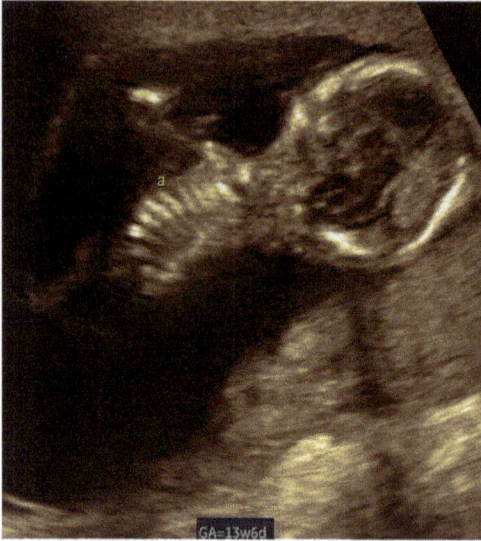

7.2g

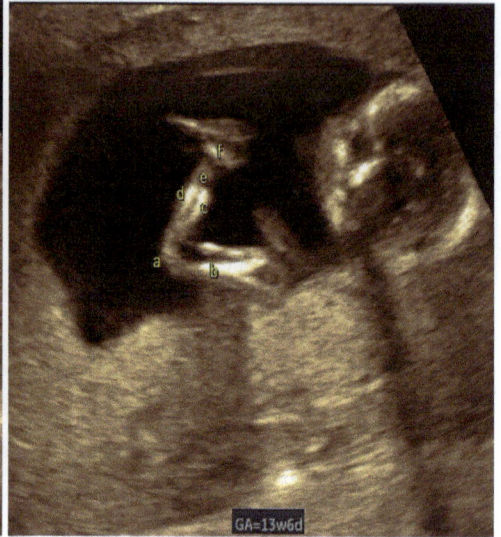

7.2h

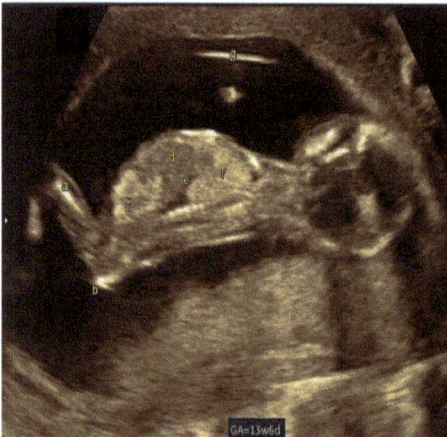

7.2i

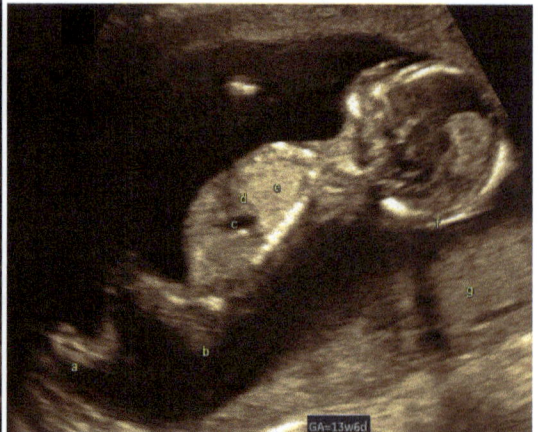

7.2j

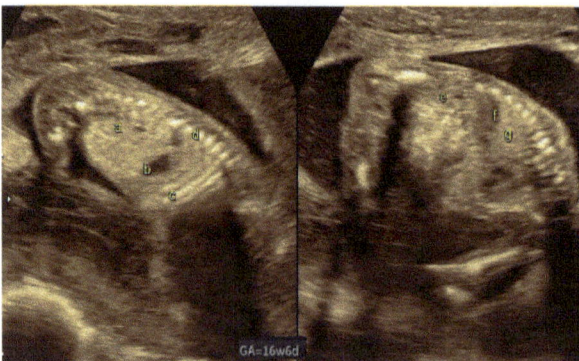

7.2k

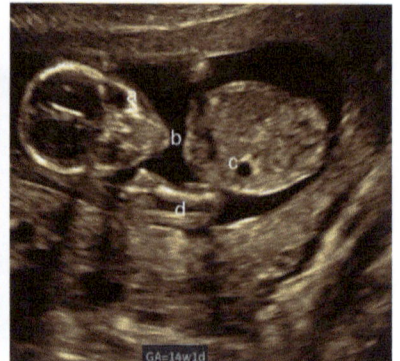

7.2l

Ultrasound Services in an Early Pregnancy and Acute Gynaecological Unit. Book 2

144

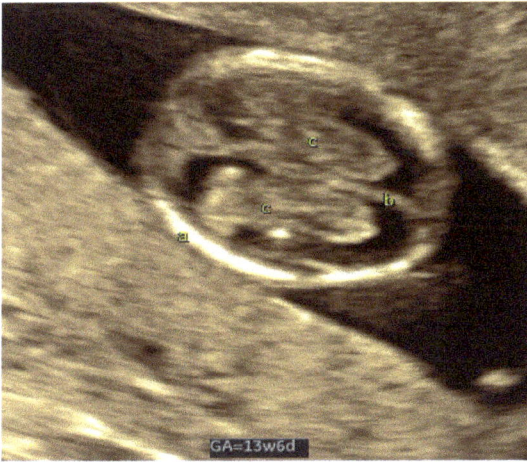
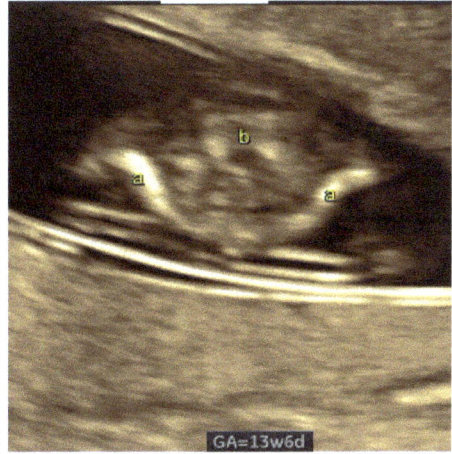

7.2m 7.2n

7.3a

Patient referred with a history of light pv bleed for 1/7 and LIF pain.

Can you identify any unusual ultrasound appearances in this ultrasound appearance? GA by CRL = 21mm = 9/40. EHB not shown here was seen in the embryo.

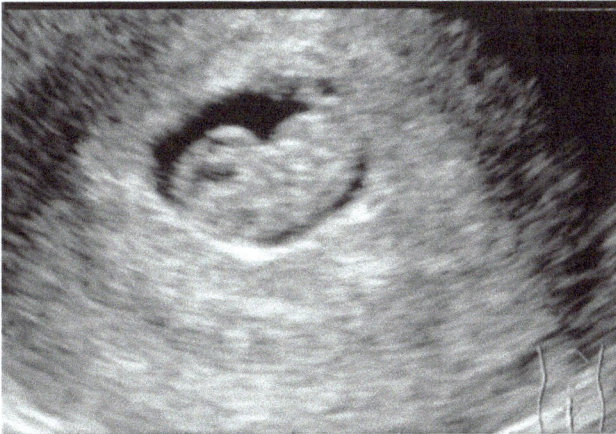

7.3b

GA by CRL = 9/40. EHB not shown here was seen in the embryo.

Ultrasound Services in an Early Pregnancy and Acute Gynaecological Unit. Book 2

145

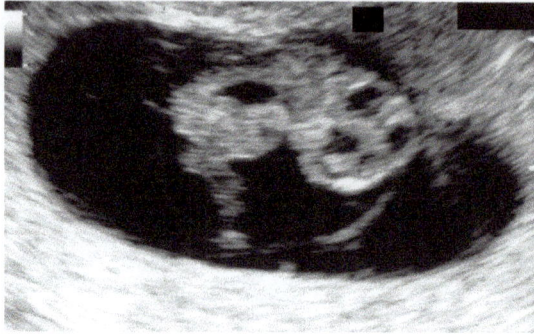

7.3c

Can you identify any unusual ultrasound appearance in this ultrasound appearance?

7.4
In the following images, identify the fetal parts and the views or sections.

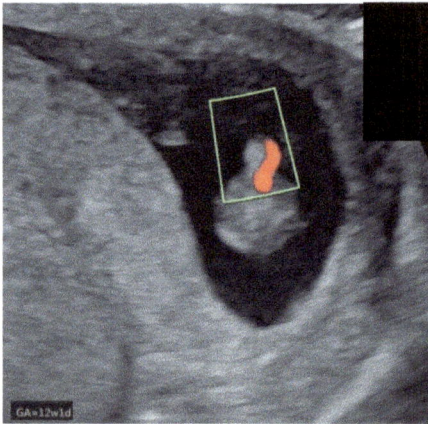

7.4a

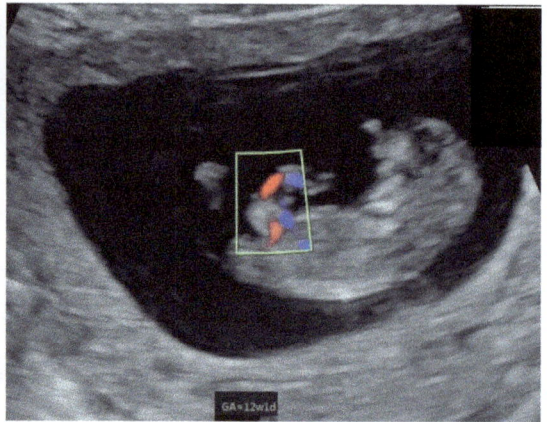

7.4b

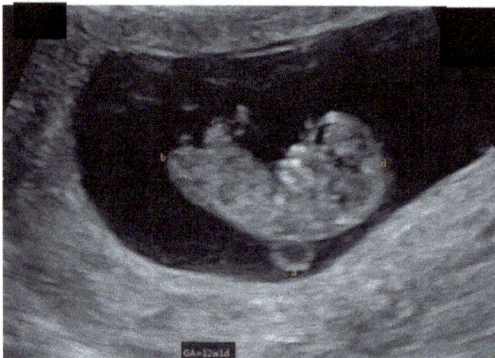

7.4c

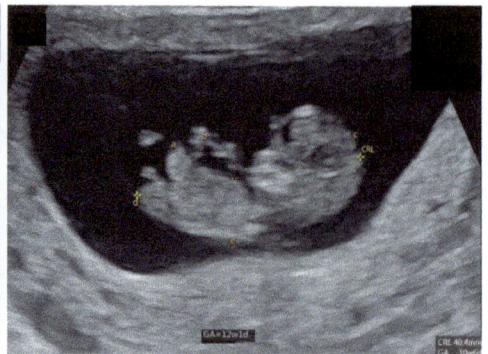

7.4d

Ultrasound Services in an Early Pregnancy and Acute Gynaecological Unit. Book 2

146

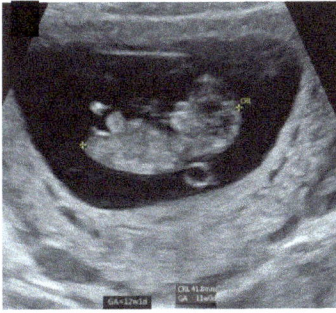
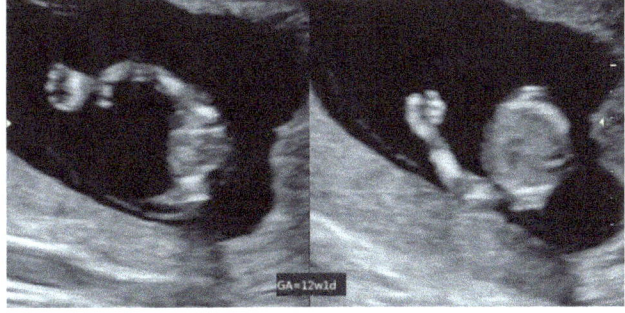

7.4e **7.4f**

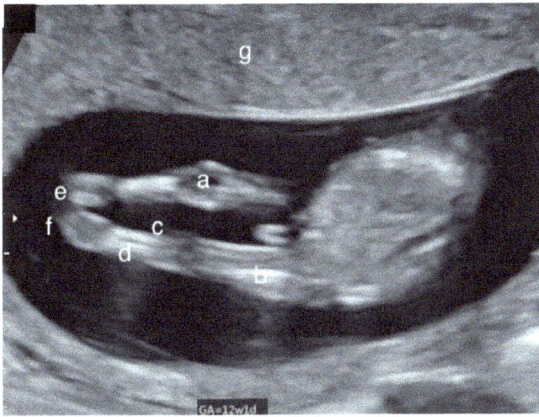
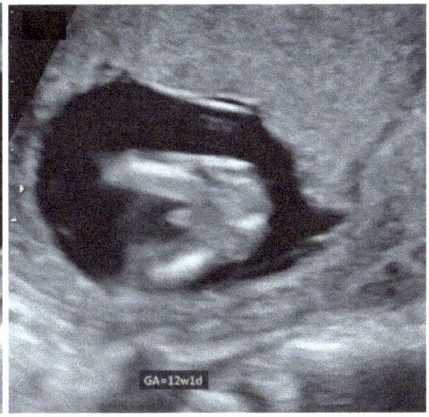

7.4g **7.4h**

7. i How old is this fetus?
   j. What does the Sonographer need to do and why?

7.5
This patient was referred for a dating scan.

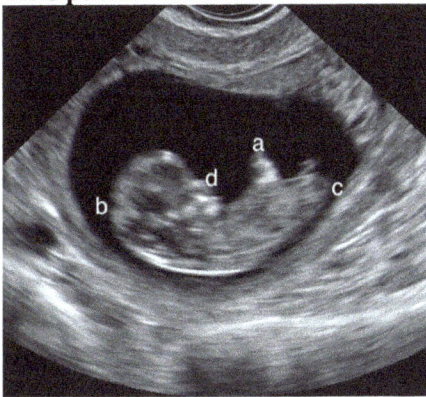
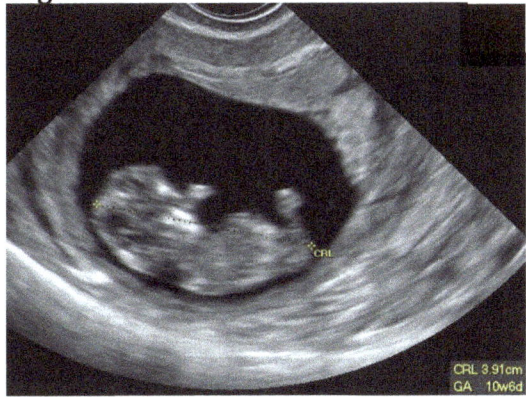

7.5a **7.5b**

Ultrasound Services in an Early Pregnancy and Acute Gynaecological Unit. Book 2

147

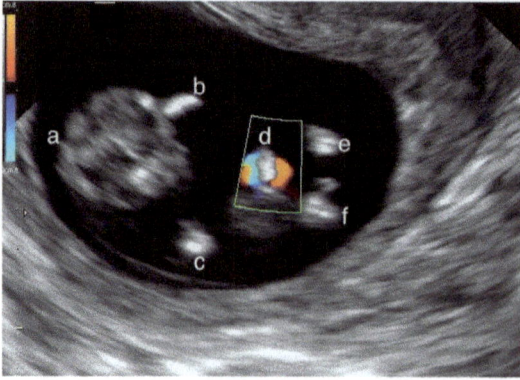

7.5c

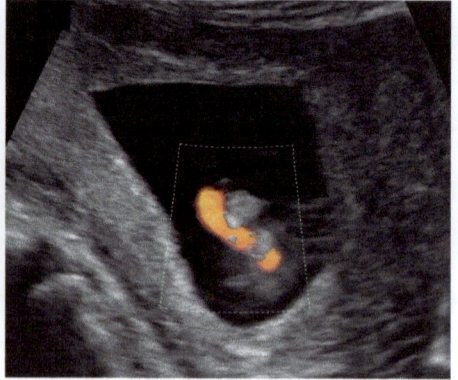

7.5d

a. Identify a-d in 7.5a and a-f in 7.5c

b. Is there anything wrong with this fetus?

7.6

This woman was referred at 11/40 with a history of pv bleed for 1/7. FHB and movements not shown were seen.

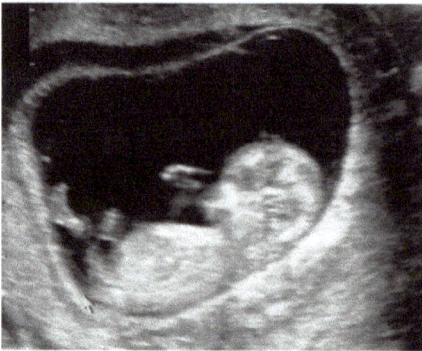

7.6a

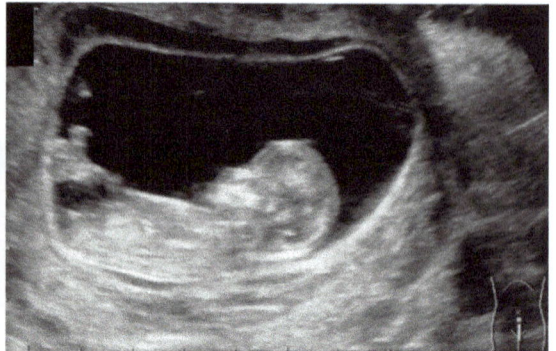

7.6b

Ultrasound Services in an Early Pregnancy and Acute Gynaecological Unit. Book 2

148

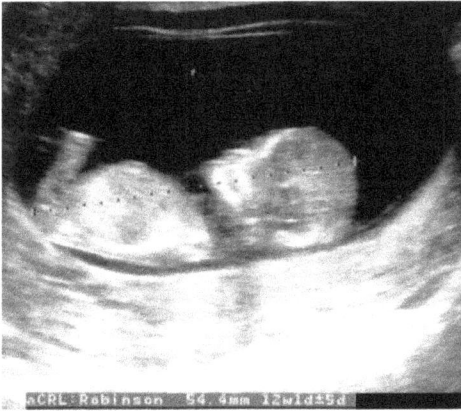
7.6 c

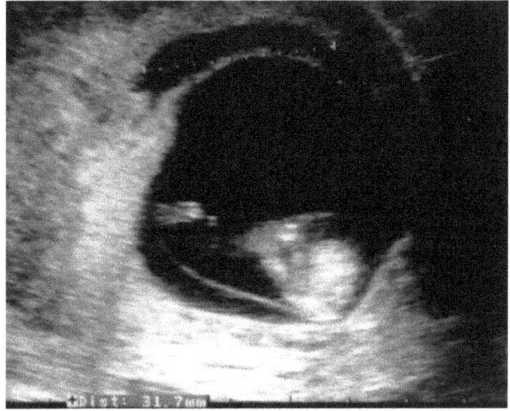
7.6d

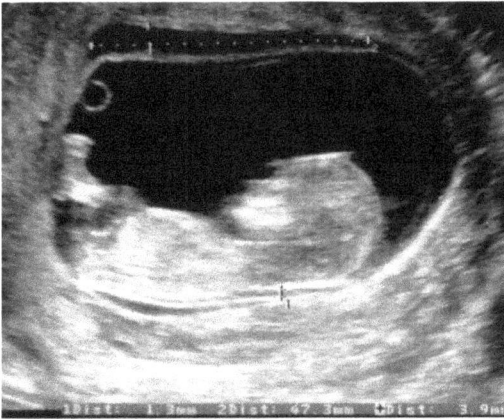
7. 6e

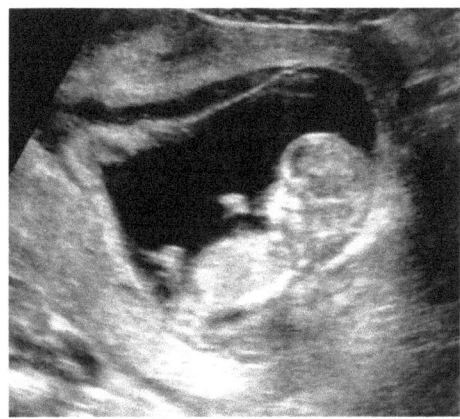
7.6 f

a. Is there any ultrasound identifiable cause or reason for this woman's pv bleeding?
b. What else will the sonographer have to do?
c. Write an ultrasound report.
d. In what way may the ultrasound findings affect this pregnancy?

7.7
This woman was referred with a history of known IUCD in situ plus positive pregnancy test result. GA by LMP = 4 +3/40

Ultrasound Services in an Early Pregnancy and Acute Gynaecological Unit. Book 2

149

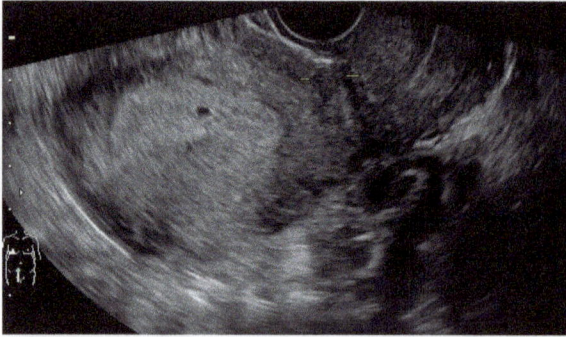

7.7a

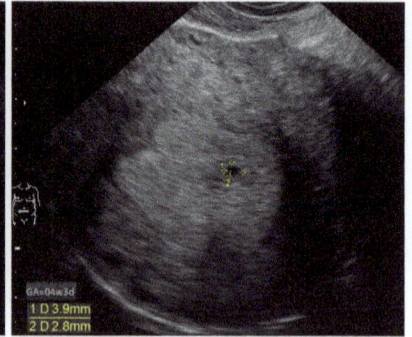

7.7b

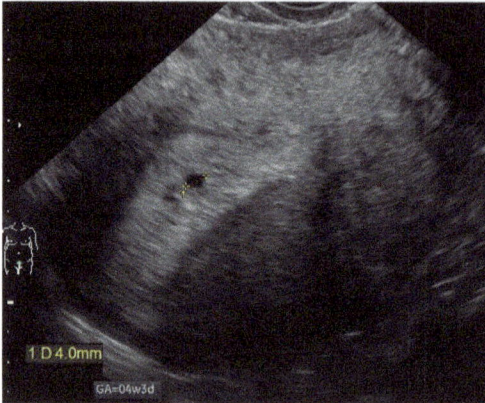

7.7c

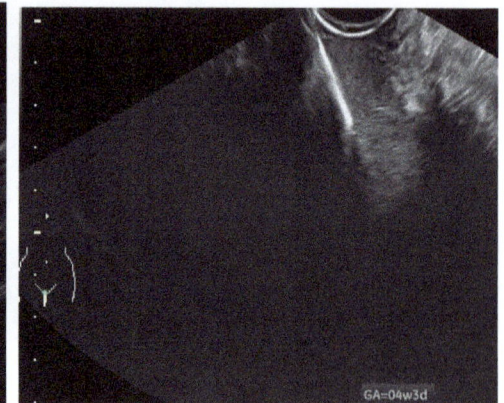

7.7d

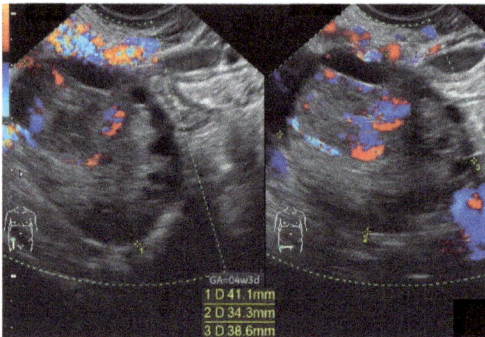

7.7e

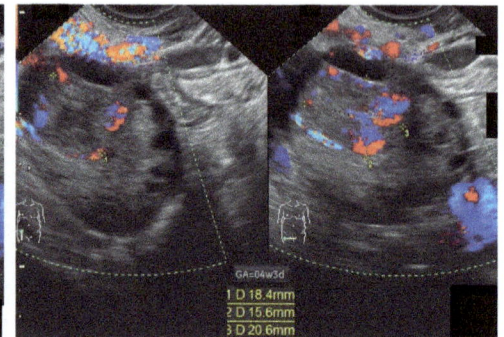

7.7f

Ultrasound Services in an Early Pregnancy and Acute Gynaecological Unit. Book 2

150

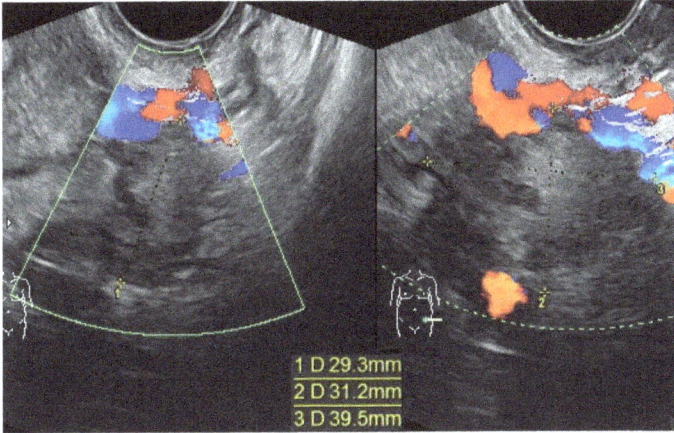

7.7g

| 1 D 29.3mm |
| 2 D 31.2mm |
| 3 D 39.5mm |

a. What pregnancy number is this at least?

b. Which type of IUCD was inserted?

c. Where is the IUCD?

d. Why and how could a woman having an IUCD in situ get pregnant?

e. Write the ultrasound report

7.8

This woman was referred with a history of maternal anxiety. Natural conception. Previous left salpingectomy secondary to left ectopic pregnancy. Below are images of her uterus and ovaries.

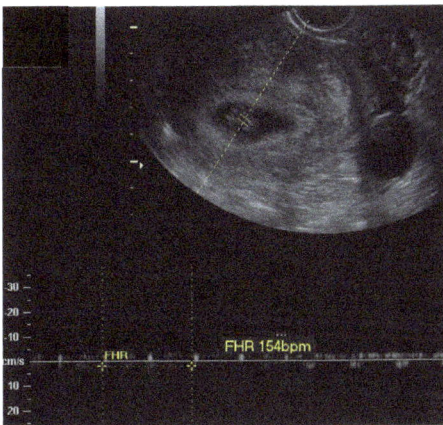

7.8a

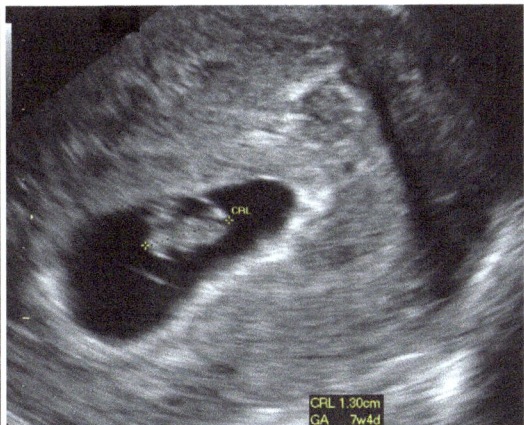

7.8b

Ultrasound Services in an Early Pregnancy and Acute Gynaecological Unit. Book 2

151

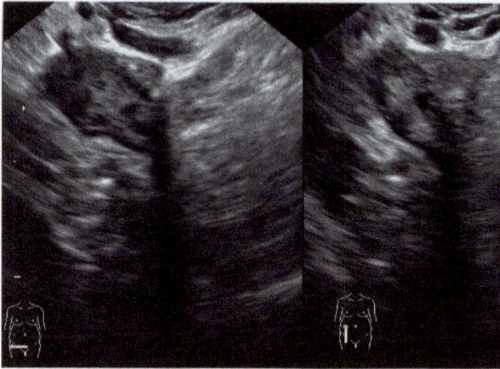
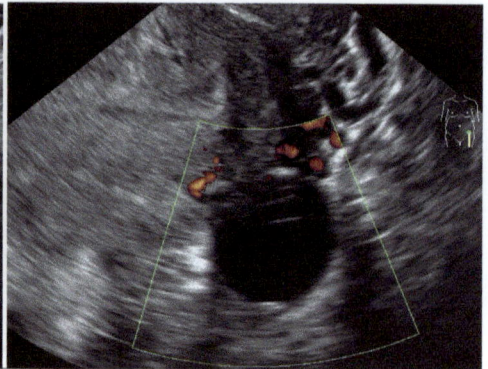

7.8c　　　　　　　　　　**7.8d**

a. Which ovary produced the egg for this conception?

b. By which mechanism did the woman get pregnant?

c. Write the ultrasound report

7. 9

7.9a is from a patient and 7.9b-c is from another patient. Heart beats were seen in all the embryos.

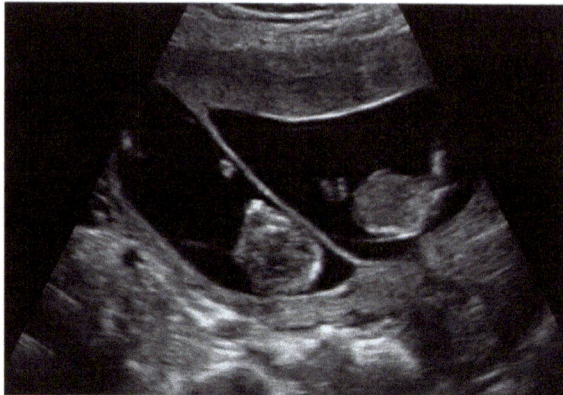

7.9a

Ultrasound Services in an Early Pregnancy and Acute Gynaecological Unit. Book 2

152

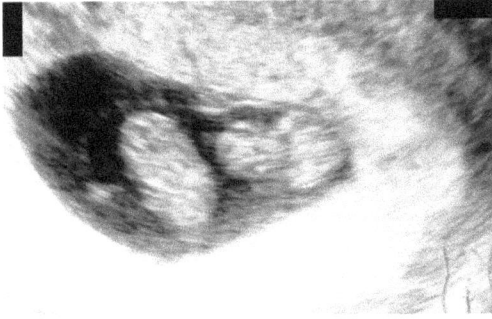

7.9b

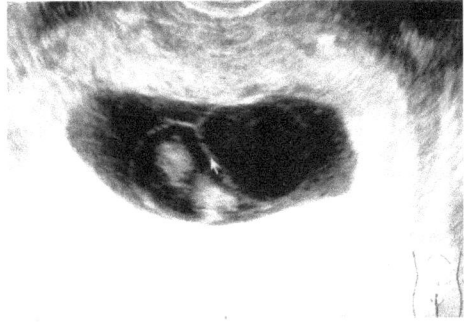

7.9c

a. Is there any similarities between these pregnancies?

b. Are there any differences between the pregnancies and why or what?

7.10
This is a follow up scan for viability. GA by LMP = 8+4/40.

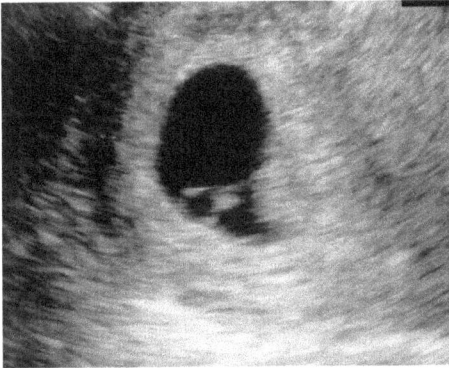

7.10a

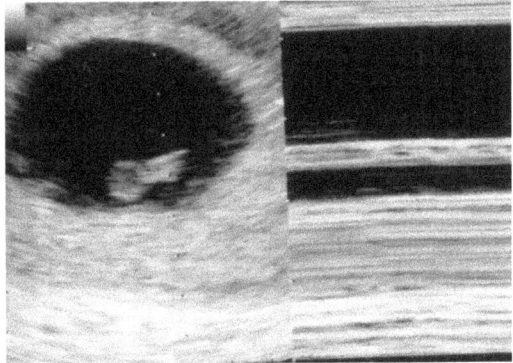

7.10b

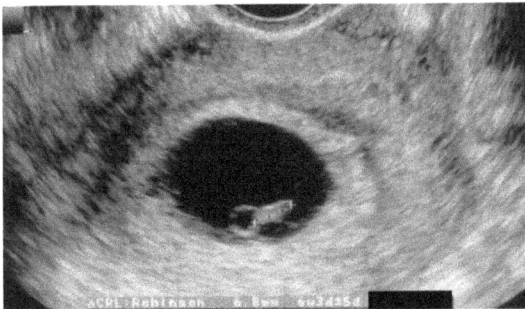

7.10c

Ultrasound Services in an Early Pregnancy and Acute Gynaecological Unit. Book 2

153

a. Write the ultrasound report.
b. Why is the CRL not matching the GA by LMP?
c. What will the role of ultrasound be in the management of this pregnancy?

11

This woman was referred with a history of RIF pain. ?Ectopic pregnancy at 6/40. This was a natural conception.

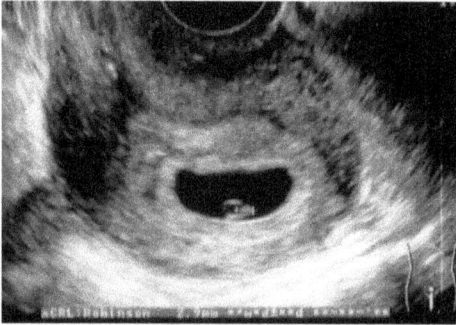

7.11a

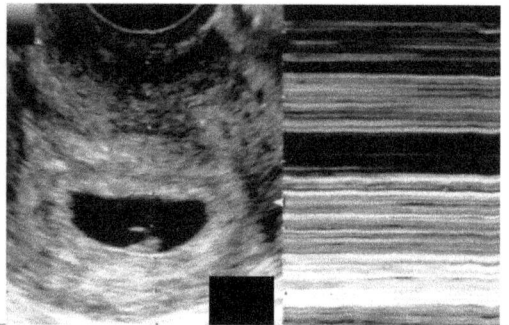

7.11b

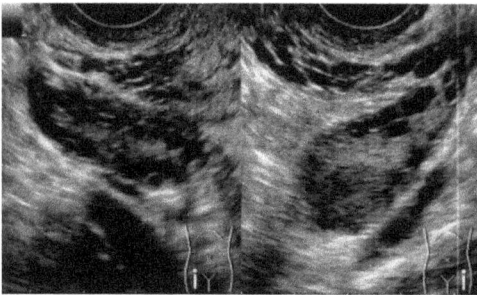

7.11c

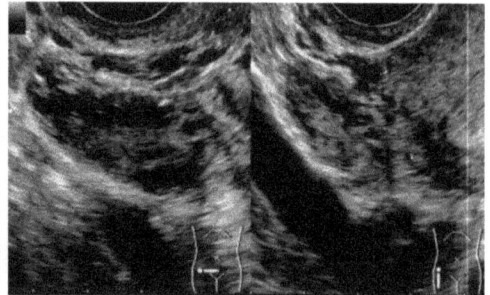

7.11d

a. Do you think this is an ectopic pregnancy?
b. Describe the ultrasound appearances of the ovaries.
c. Is there any ultrasound cause for RIF pain found on this scan?
d. What else needs to be excluded?

12

This woman was referred for a scan with a history of pain.

Ultrasound Services in an Early Pregnancy and Acute Gynaecological Unit. Book 2

154

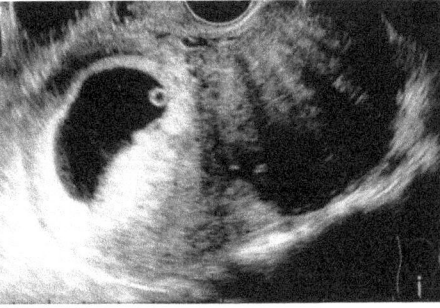

7.12a

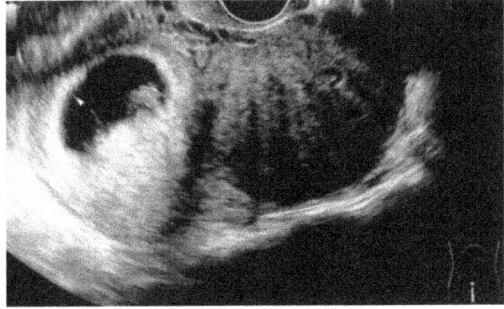

7.12b

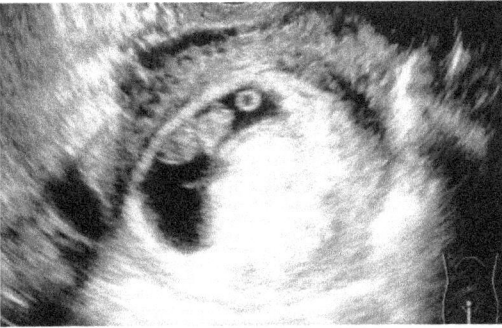

7.12c

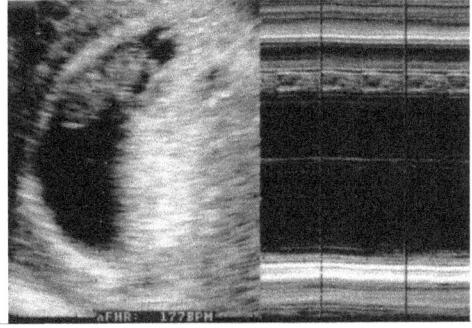

7.12d

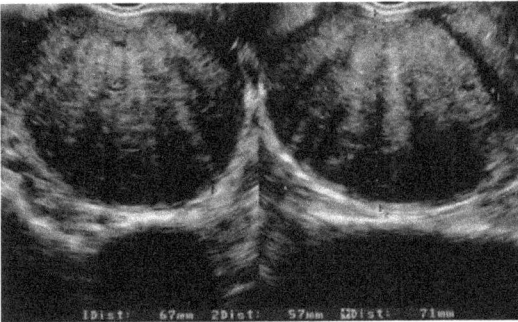

7.12e

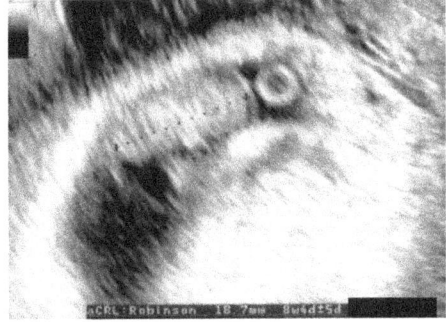

7.12f

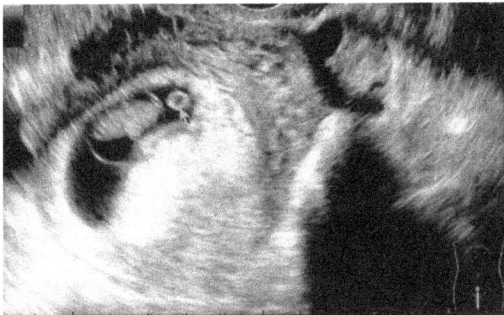

7.12g

Ultrasound Services in an Early Pregnancy and Acute Gynaecological Unit. Book 2

155

a. Write the ultrasound report.
b. Is there any significant finding that may affect this pregnancy later?
c. What is the role of ultrasound in the future management of this pregnancy?

13
This woman was referred with a history of pv bleed.

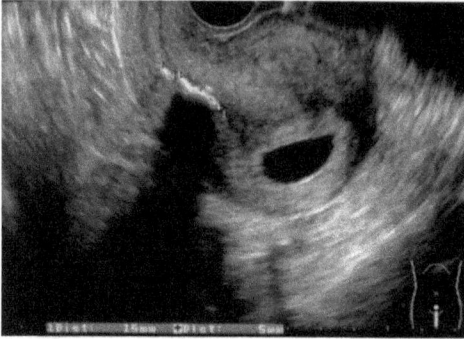
7.13a

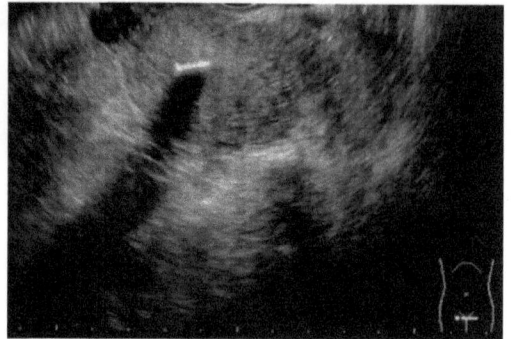
7.13b

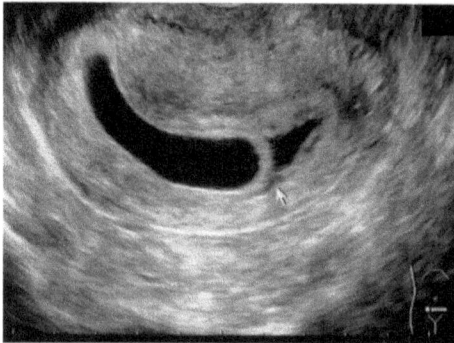
7.13c

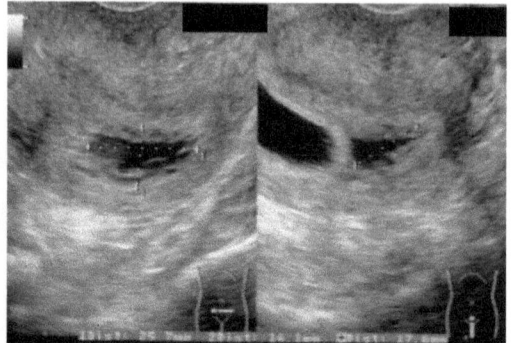
7.13d

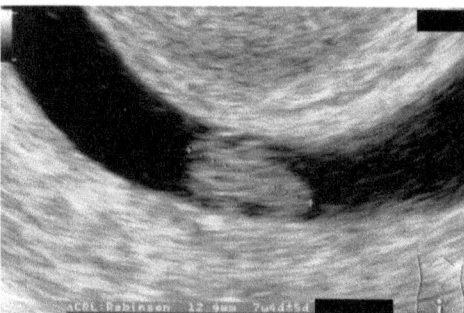
7.13e

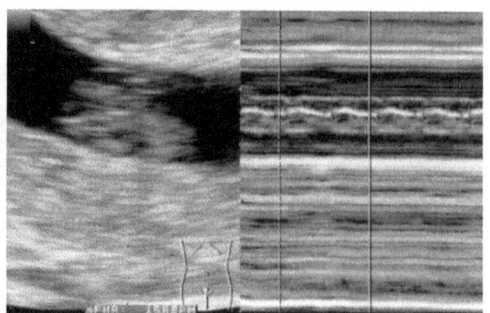
7.13f

Ultrasound Services in an Early Pregnancy and Acute Gynaecological Unit. Book 2

156

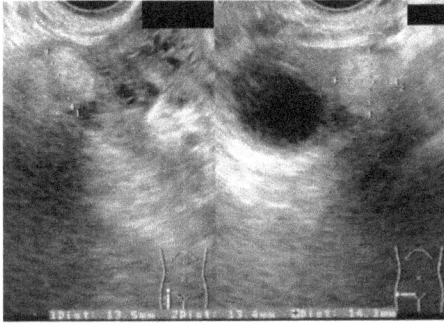
7.13g

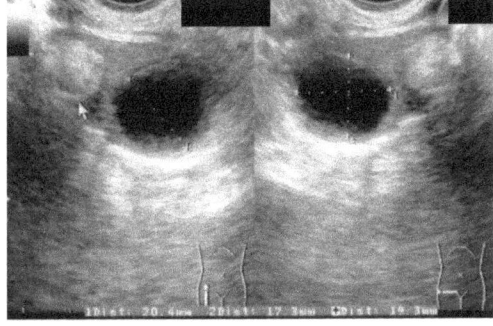
7.13h

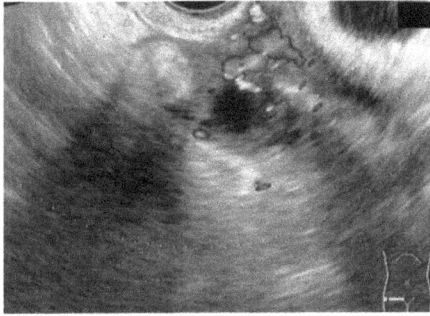
7.13i

a. Write the ultrasound report.

14

This woman was referred with a history of 5 weeks post c/s bleeding. Both ovaries not shown here were seen and appeared sonographically normal.

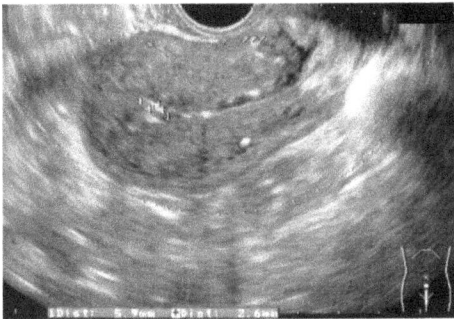
7.14a

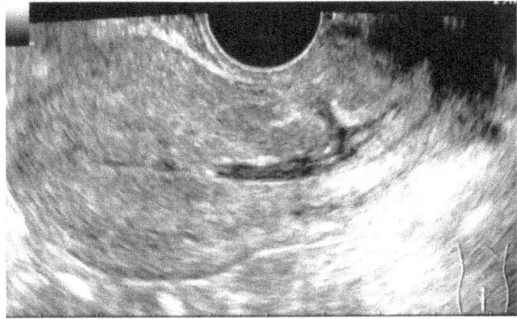
7.14b

Ultrasound Services in an Early Pregnancy and Acute Gynaecological Unit. Book 2

157

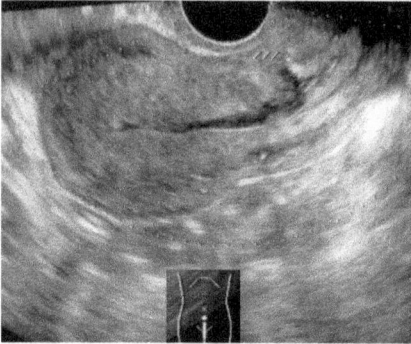

7.14 c

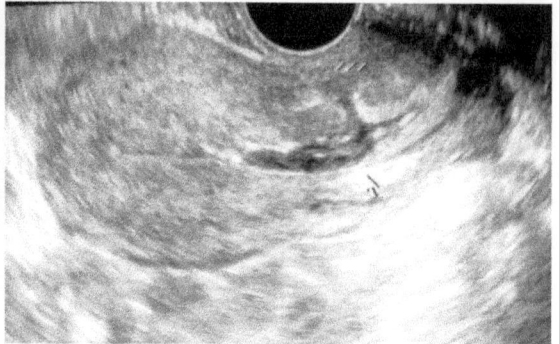

7.14d

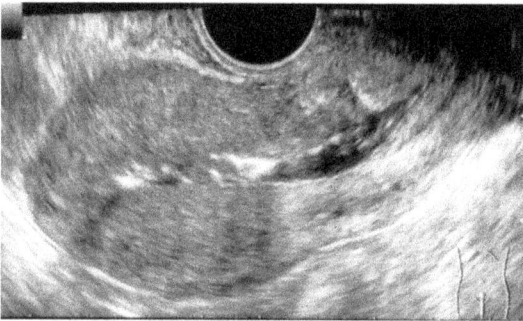

7.14 e

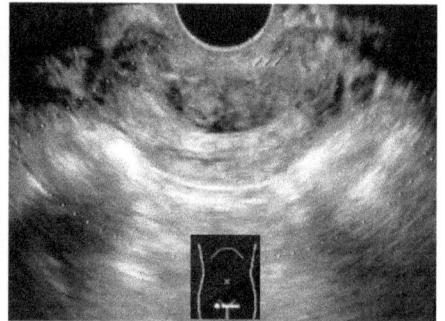

7.14f

Write the ultrasound report.

15
This woman was referred with a history of RIF pain.

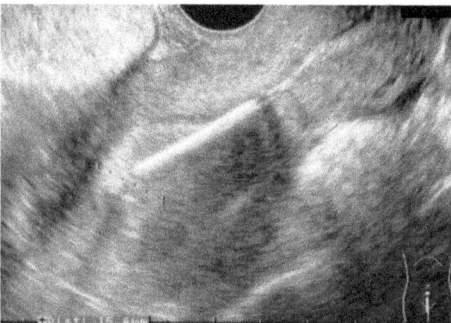

7.15a

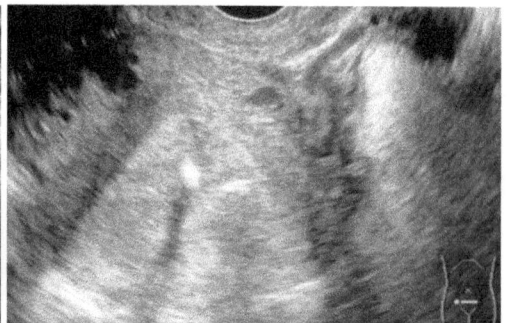

7.15b

Ultrasound Services in an Early Pregnancy and Acute Gynaecological Unit. Book 2

158

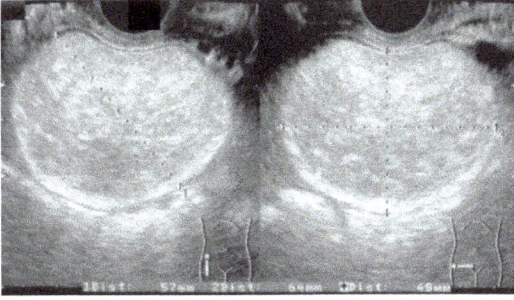

7.15c

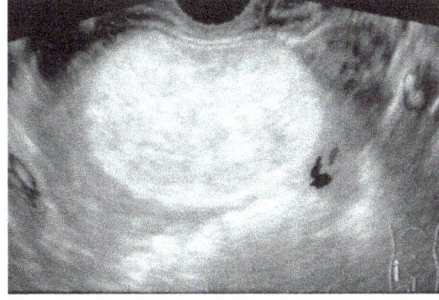

7.15d

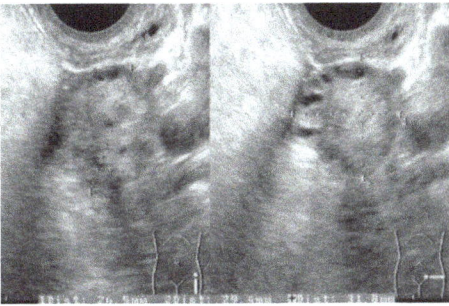

7.15e

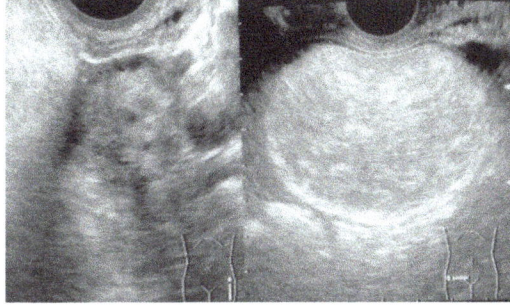

7.15f

a. Write the ultrasound report

b. Can this scan exclude all the possible causes of her pain?

16

This woamn had a scan because of pv spotting , FHB were seen but not shown here. CRL = GA by LMP.

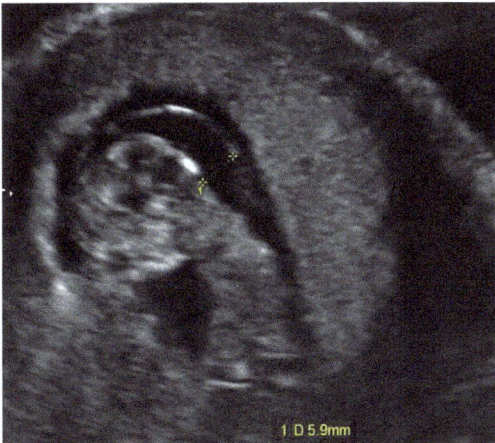

1 D 5.9mm

7.16a

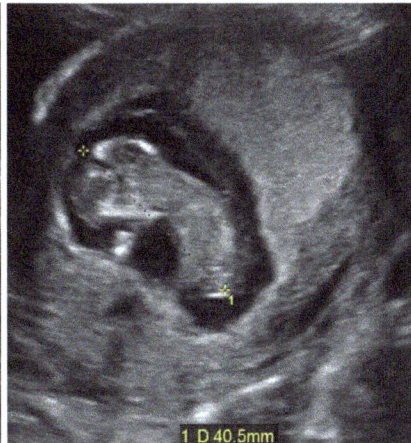

1 D 40.5mm

7.16b

Ultrasound Services in an Early Pregnancy and Acute Gynaecological Unit. Book 2

159

a. Describe the ultrasound appearances
b. Will this woman be requiring another scan before the anomaly
   scan? Why or why not?
c. What challenges or disadvantages or advantages may be
   experienced during such ultrasound examination?

**17.   This patient was referred because of pv bleed. GA by LMP =
16+1/40. A singleton pregnancy was seen. Fetal measurements not shown
= date. Below are the other findings.**

a. Identify a-c in 7.17a
b. Identify a-b in 7.17i
c. Identify a-e in 7.17j
d. How was the patient scanned?
e. Describe the ultrasound findings

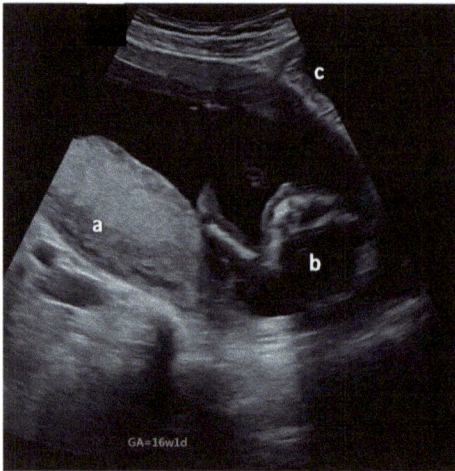

7.17a

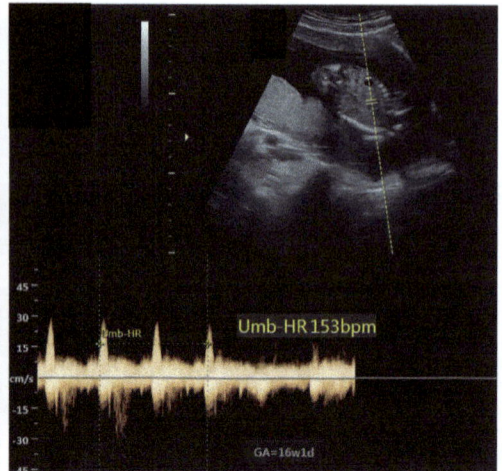

7.17b

Ultrasound Services in an Early Pregnancy and Acute Gynaecological Unit. Book 2

160

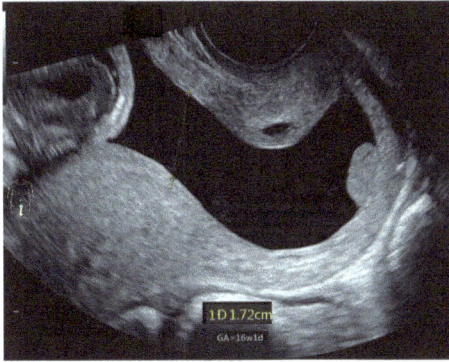

7.17c

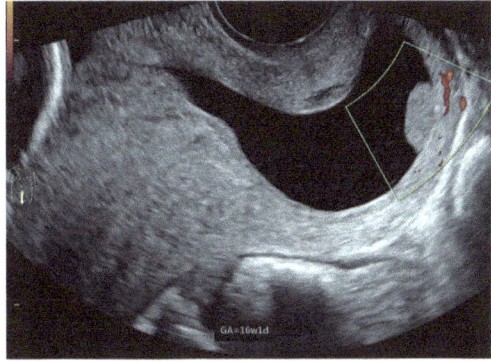

7.17d

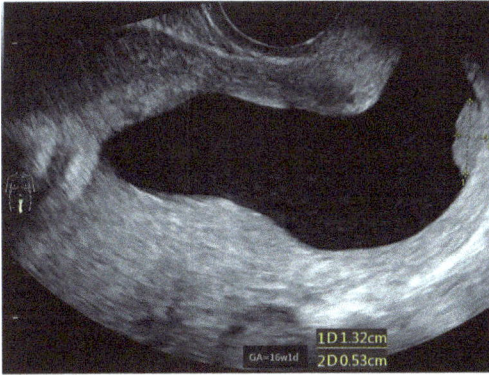

7.17e

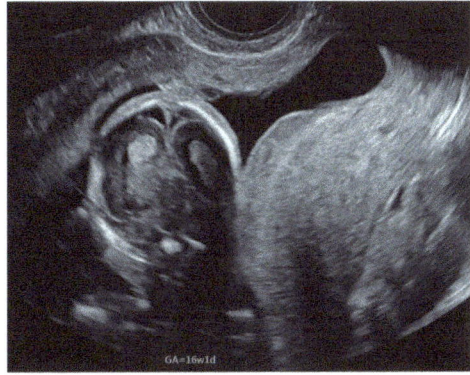

7.17f

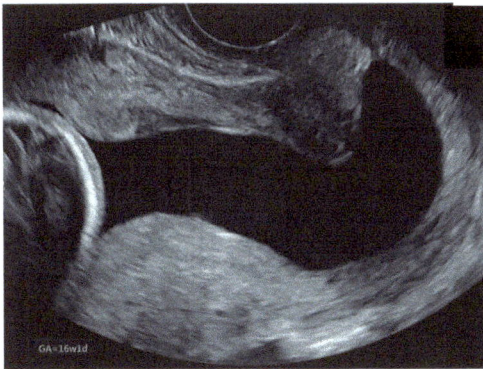

7.17g

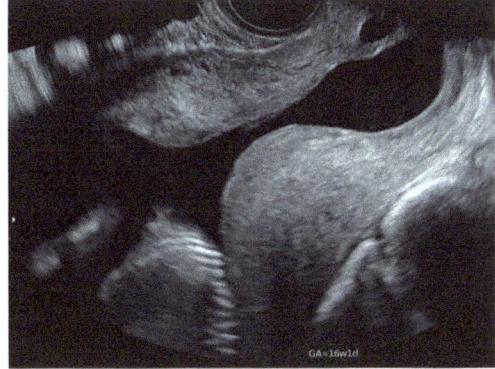

7.17h

Ultrasound Services in an Early Pregnancy and Acute Gynaecological Unit. Book 2

161

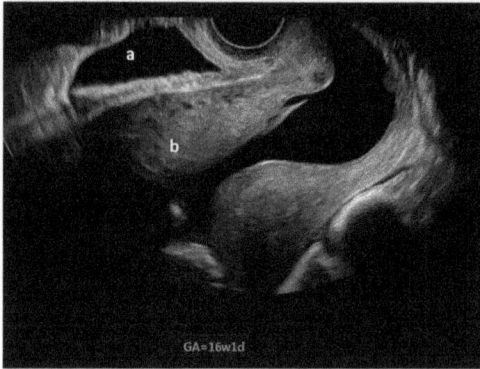

7.17i

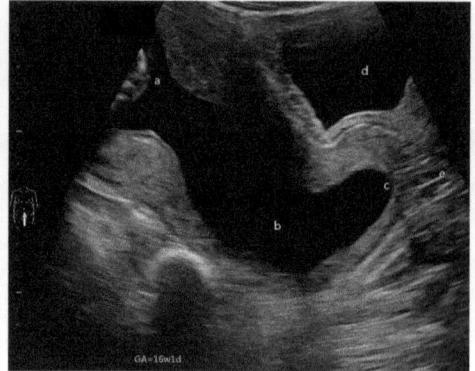

7.17j

18

a. What is HCG?

b. What is the beta hCG test?

c. How is qualitative beta hCG expressed?

d. When and how is beta hCG used in pregnancy?

19

A dating scan at 14/40 revealed this. No history of pvb in this pregnancy. Both ovaries appear sonographically normal. The couple are not keen on the NT screening test.

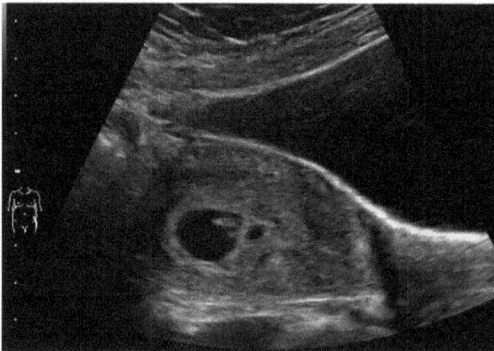

7.19a

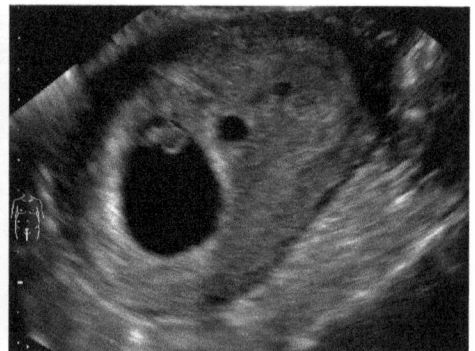

7.19b

Ultrasound Services in an Early Pregnancy and Acute Gynaecological Unit. Book 2

162

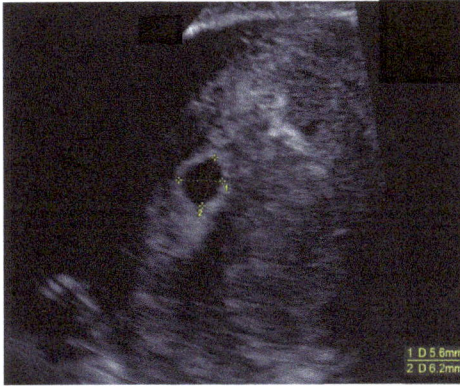

7.19c

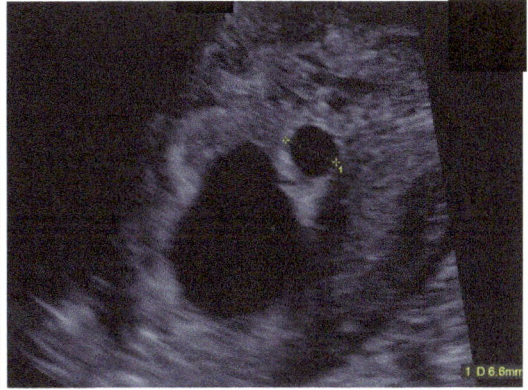

7.19d

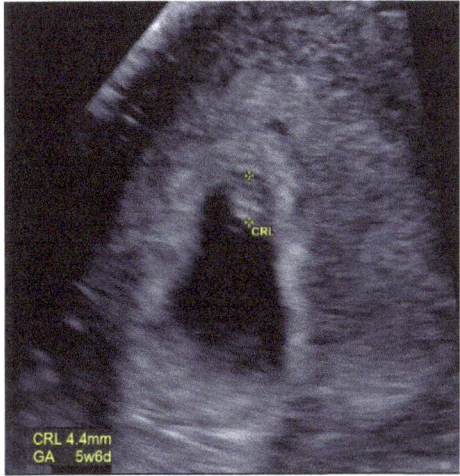

7.19e

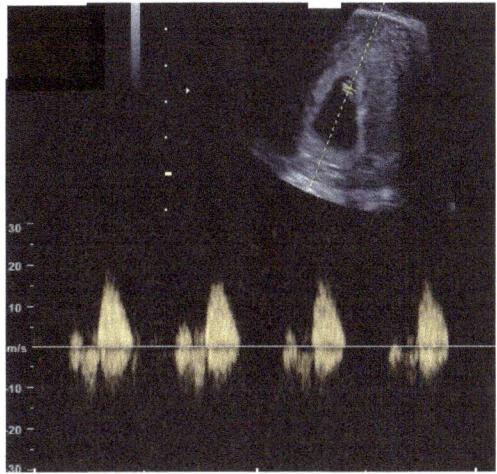

7.19f

a. Describe the ultrasound appearances.

b. Will you bring the woman back for another scan before the routine anomaly scan why or why not?

Ultrasound Services in an Early Pregnancy and Acute Gynaecological Unit. Book 2

163

20

This was discovered during a scan. No obvious abnormality was seen in the fetus.

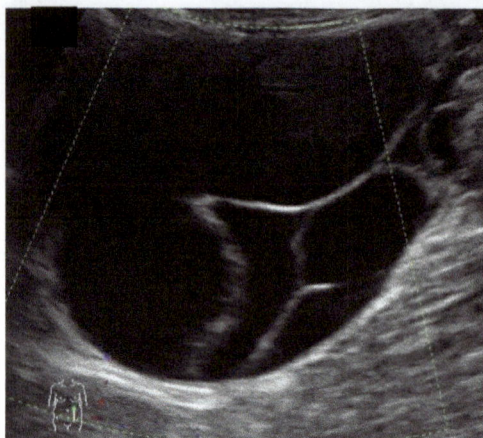

7.20a

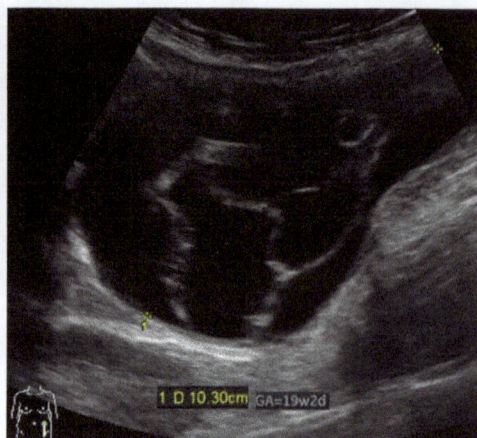

7.20b

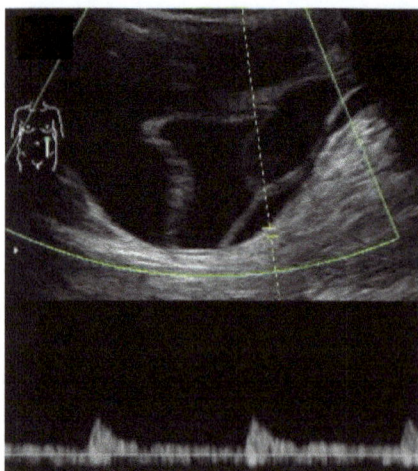

7.20c

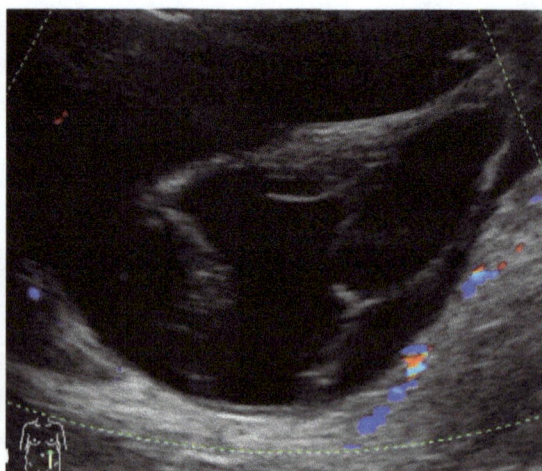

7.20d

Ultrasound Services in an Early Pregnancy and Acute Gynaecological Unit. Book 2

164

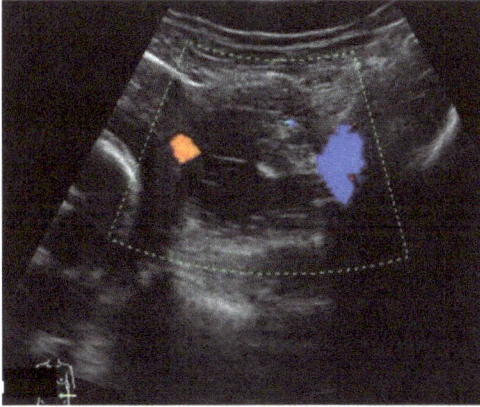

7.20e

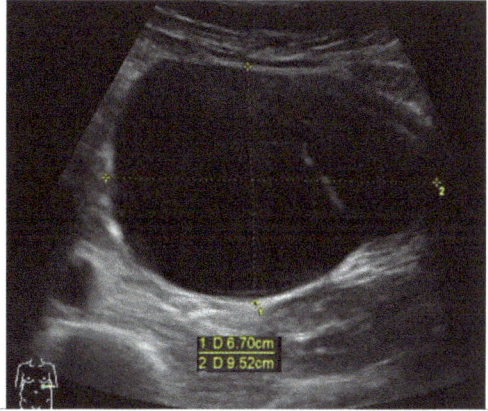

7.20f

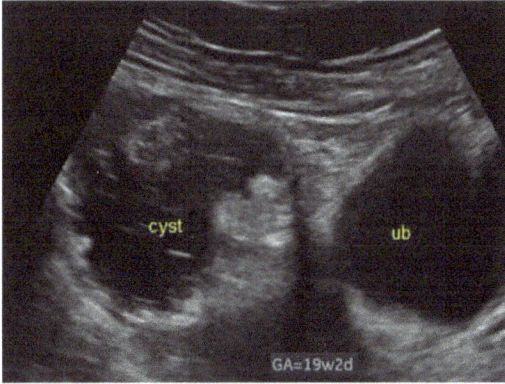

7.20g

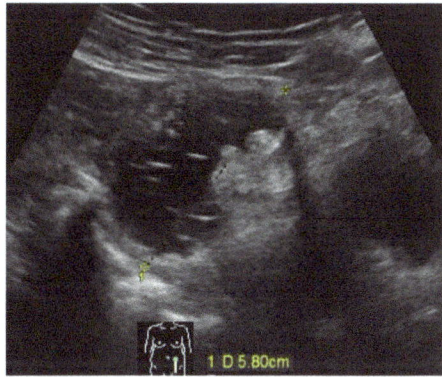

7.20h

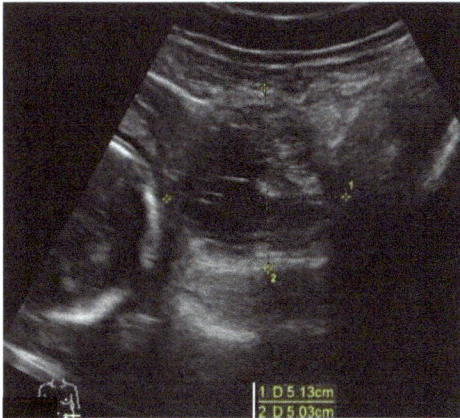

7.20i

a. Is there anything wrong?

b. What else should the sonographer examine and document?

Ultrasound Services in an Early Pregnancy and Acute Gynaecological Unit. Book 2

165

c.   Will this pregnancy require any referral and where to?

d.   Is there any implications to this finding in terms of the management of this pregnancy?

21

This woman was referred for a scan with a history of maternal anxiety. Both ovaries not shown here appeared sonographically normal.

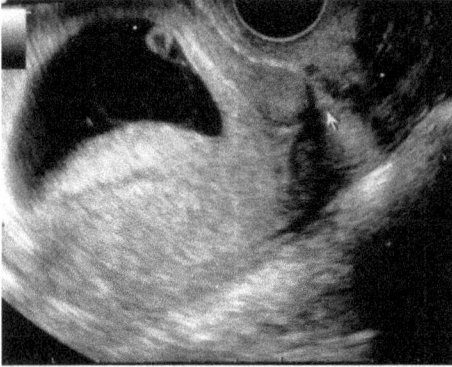

7.21a

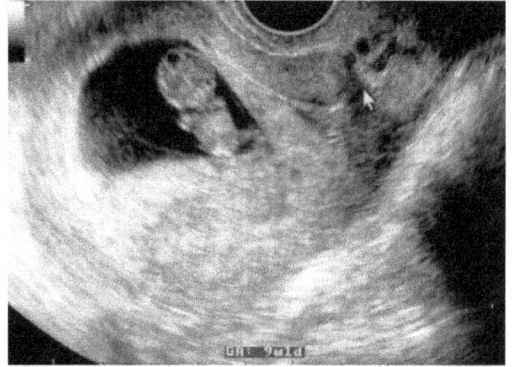

7.21

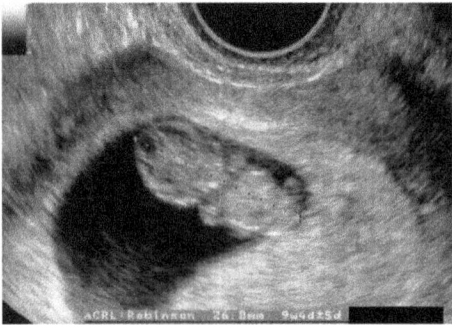

7.21c

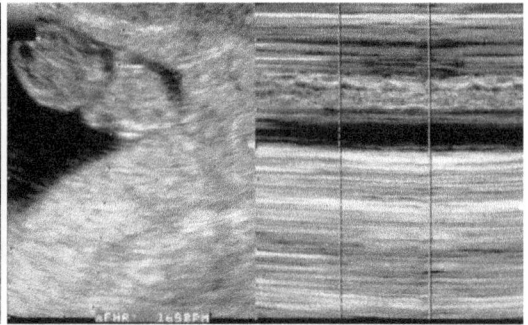

7.21d

a. Identify the arrow in 7.21a-b.

b. Write the ultrasound report.

Ultrasound Services in an Early Pregnancy and Acute Gynaecological Unit. Book 2

166

22

This is a follow up in a patient with a PUL. Left ovary not shown here appeared sonographically normal.

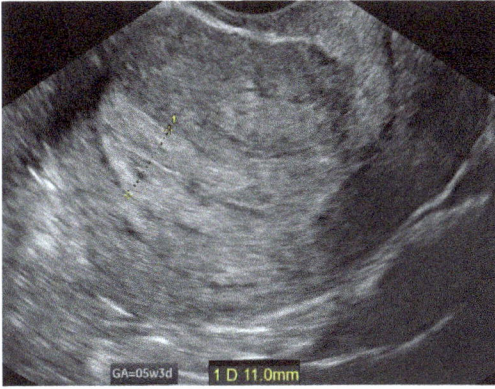

7.22a

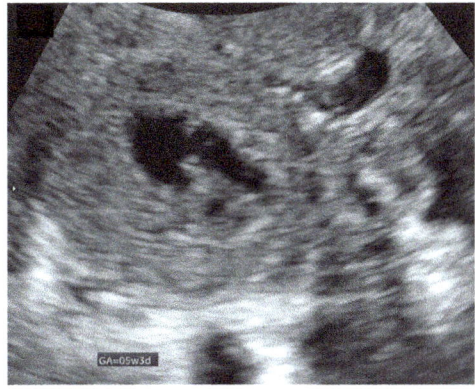

7.22b Right adnexa

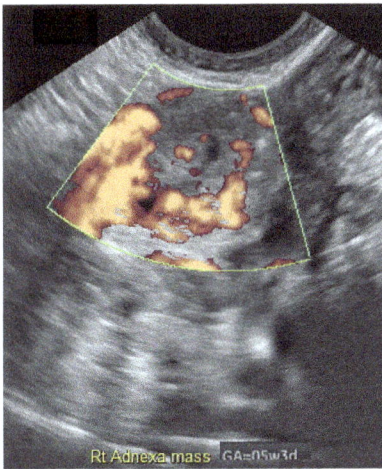

7.22c

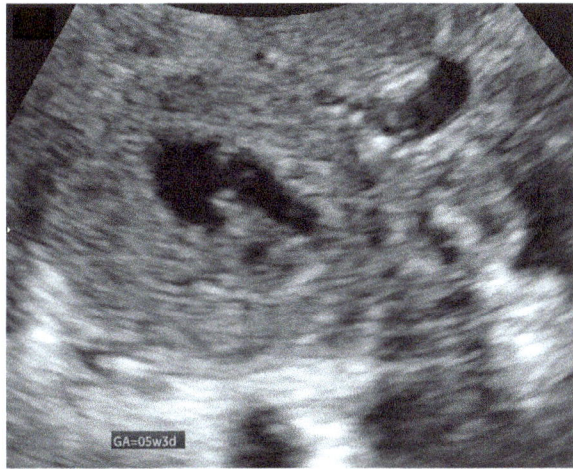

7.22d

Ultrasound Services in an Early Pregnancy and Acute Gynaecological Unit. Book 2

167

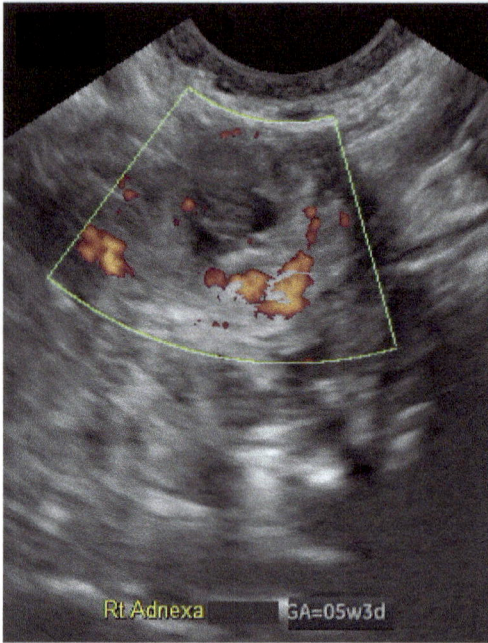

7.22e

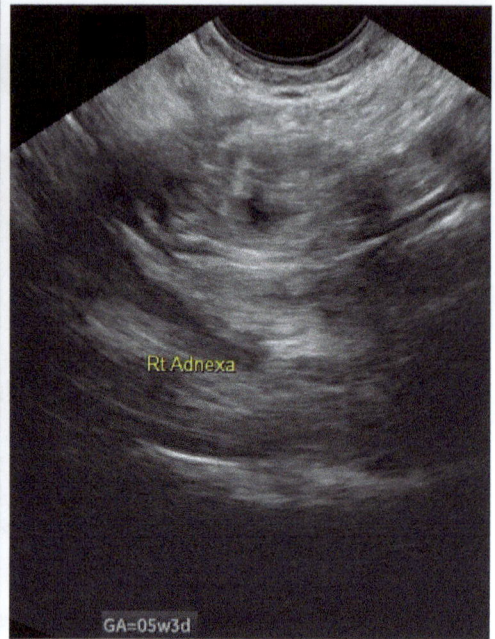

7.22f

Some minutes later:

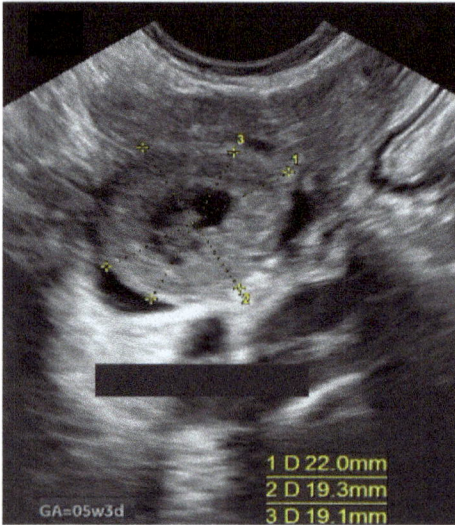

7.22g

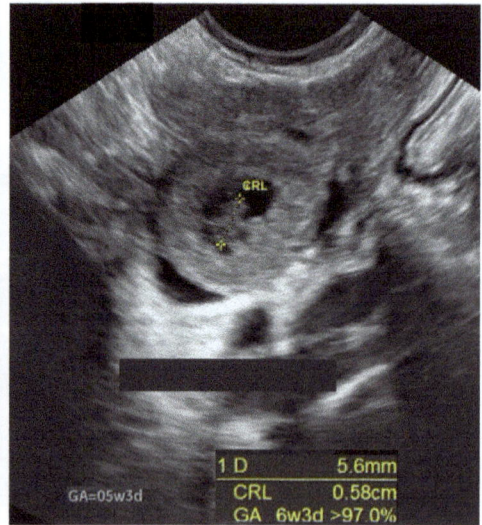

7.22h

a. Describe the ultrasound appearances in 22a-f

b. Is there any significant difference between the ultrasound images in 22a –f and images 22g – h

c. What is the possible ultrasound diagnosis of 22g – h?

Ultrasound Services in an Early Pregnancy and Acute Gynaecological Unit. Book 2

168

23

This woman was referred for a dating scan.

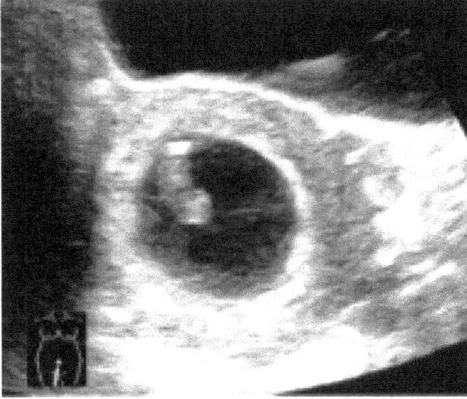
7.23a

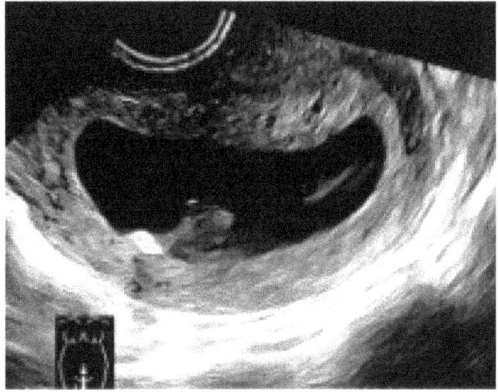
7.23B

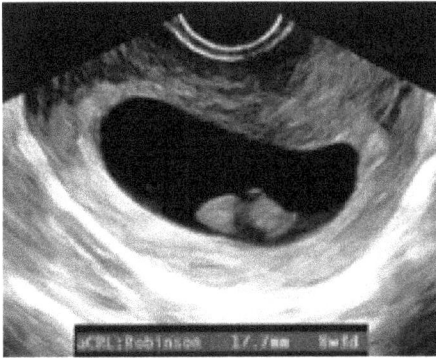
7.23c

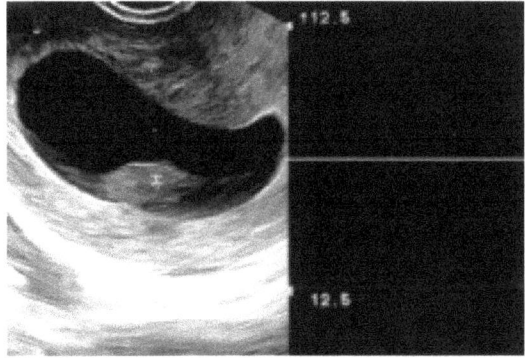
7.23d

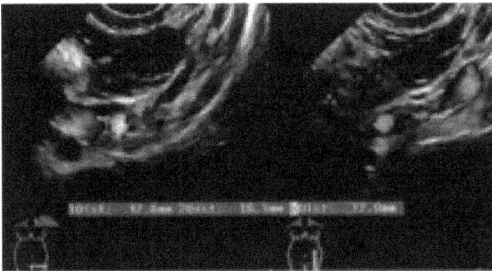
7.23e

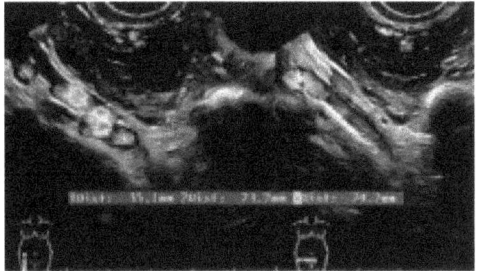
7.23f

a. Is there any abnormality shown in 7.23a-b?

b. Write the ultrasound report.

c. Which other ultrasound findings of the Yolk sac can be abnormal?

Ultrasound Services in an Early Pregnancy and Acute Gynaecological Unit. Book 2

169

24

This woman was referred with a history of 3/52 abdominal pain at 5+4/40. Natural conception.

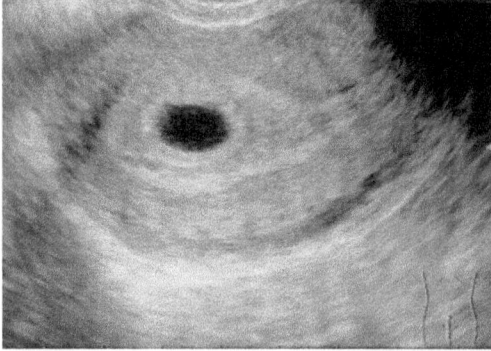
7.24a

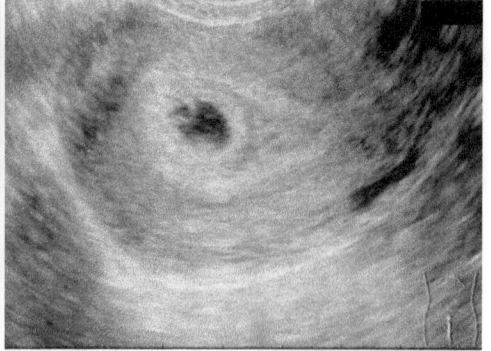
7.24b

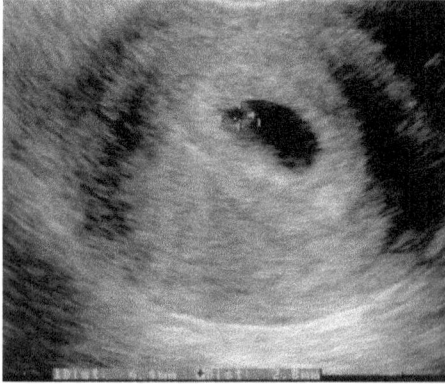
7.24c

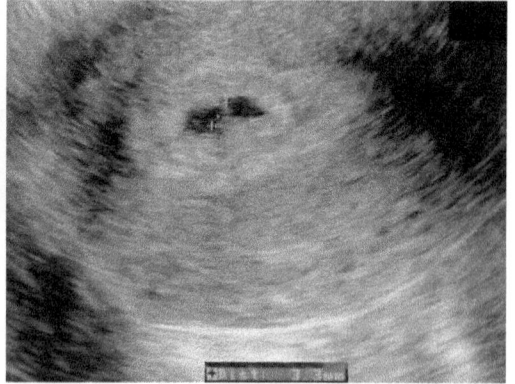
7.24d

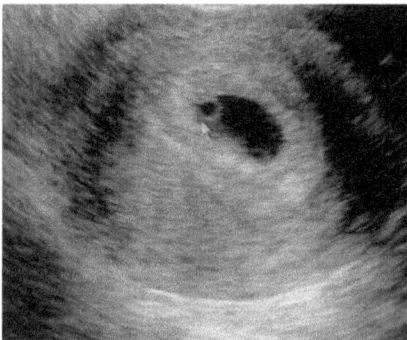
7.24e

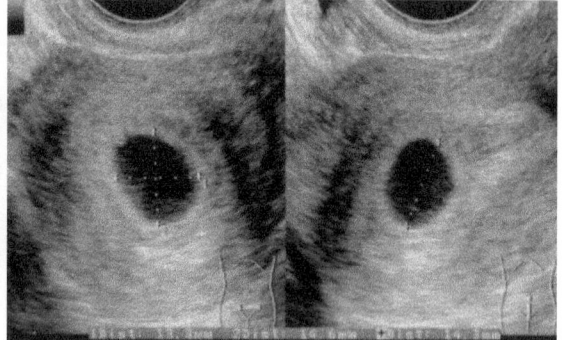
7.24f

Ultrasound Services in an Early Pregnancy and Acute Gynaecological Unit. Book 2

170

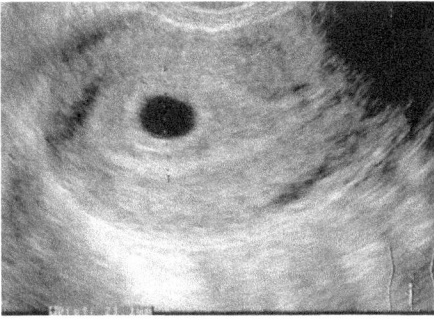

7.24g

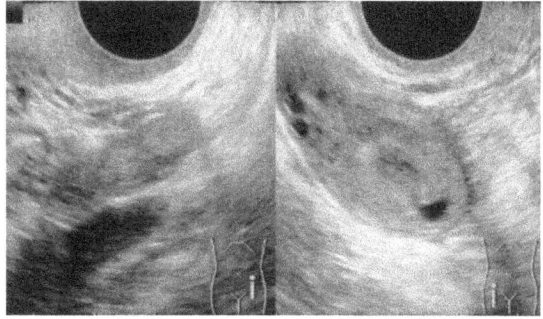

7.24h

a. Write the ultrasound report.
b. Will the sonographer have to bring this woman back, why or why not.

25

This woman was referred for a scan with a history of light pv. bleeding for some days before the scan.

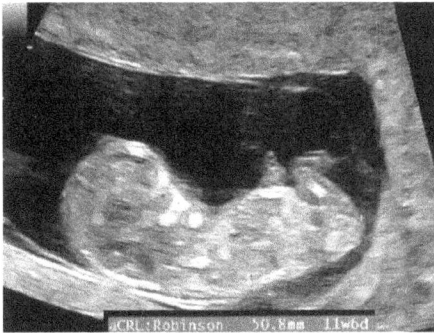

7.25a

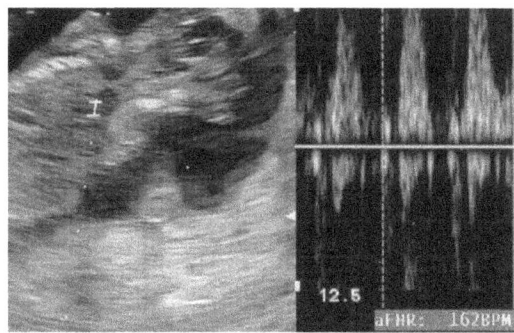

7.25b

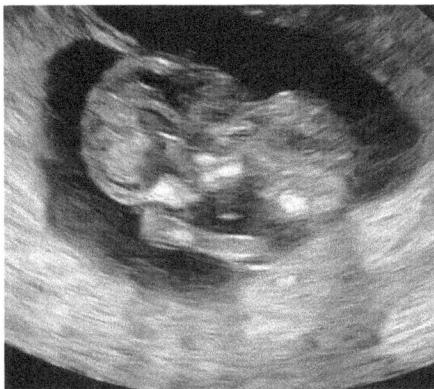

7.25c

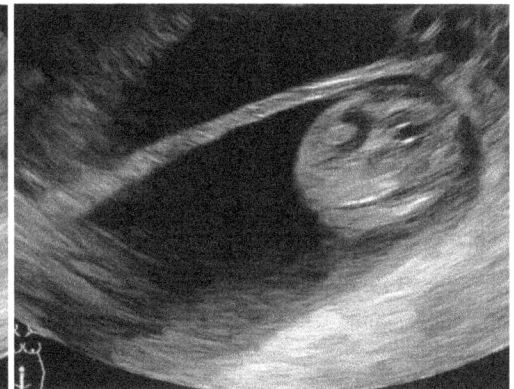

7.25d

Ultrasound Services in an Early Pregnancy and Acute Gynaecological Unit. Book 2

171

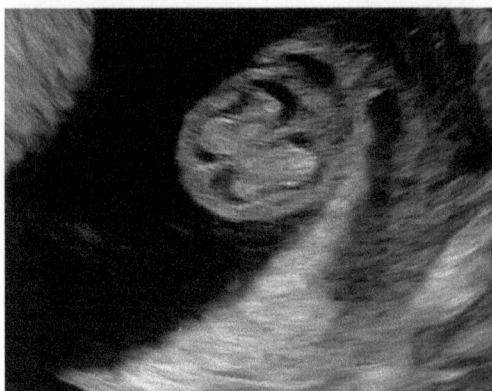
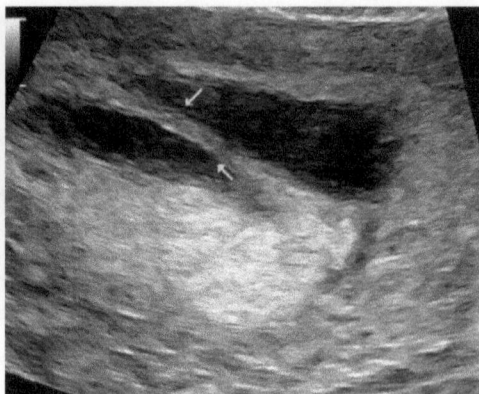

7.25e   7.25f

a. Is there any unusual findings?
b. Write an ultrasound report.
c. What is the significance of this findings?

26

This woman was referred for a scan with a history of pelvic pain around her mid cycle.

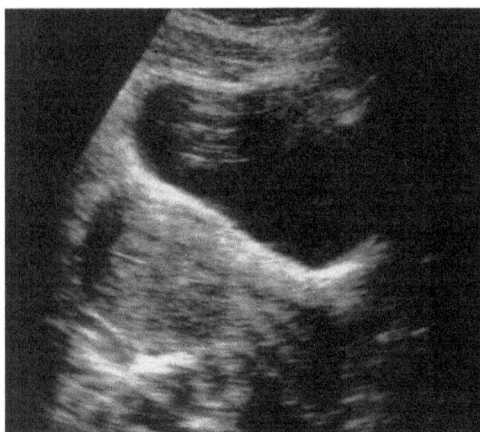
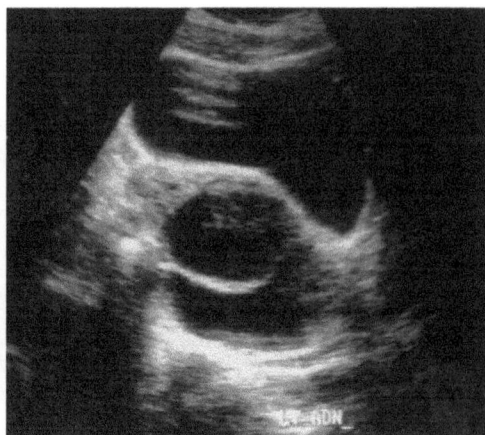

7.26a   7.26b

Ultrasound Services in an Early Pregnancy and Acute Gynaecological Unit. Book 2

172

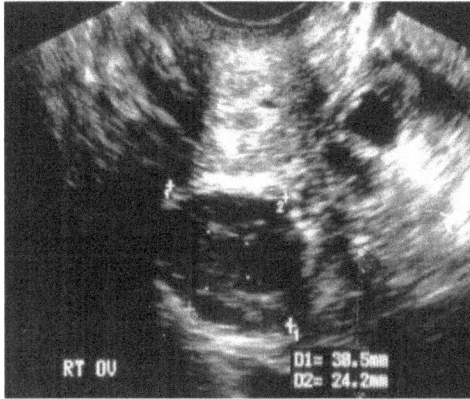

7.26c

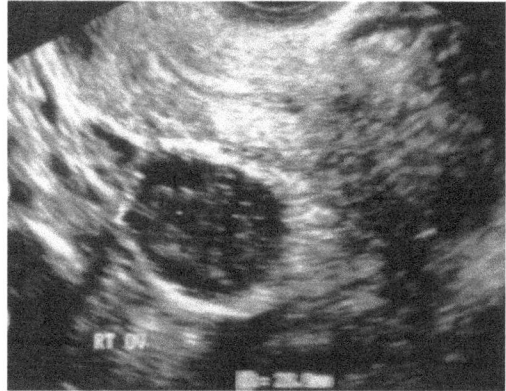

7.26d

Left adnexa 48 x 54 x 45mm.

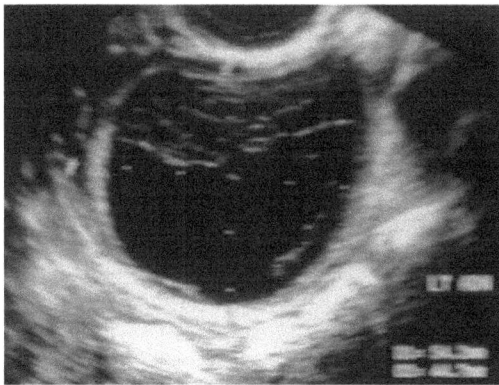

7.26e

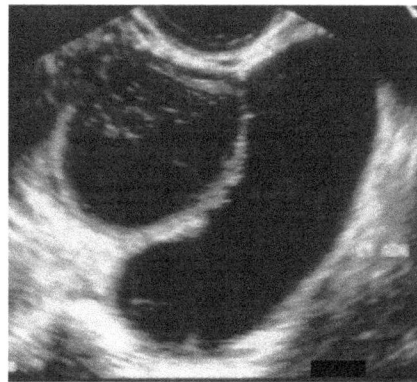

7.26f

a. Describe the ultrasound findings.

b. What else should the sonographer have done and why?

Ultrasound Services in an Early Pregnancy and Acute Gynaecological Unit. Book 2

173

27

This woman was referred with a history of pain following IUCD insertion.

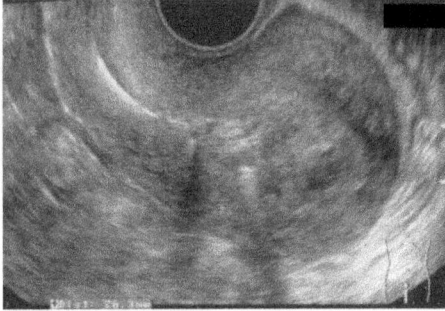

7.27a

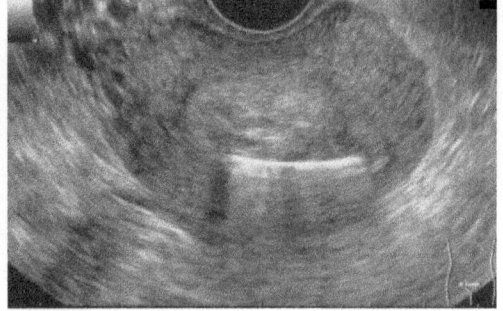

7.27b

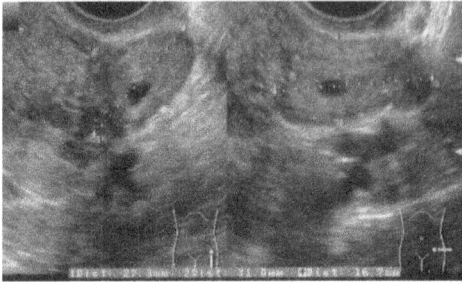

7.27c

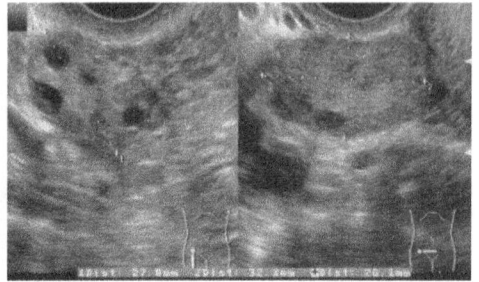

7.27d

a. Describe the ultrasound findings.

b. Identify any cause for the patient's pain.

Ultrasound Services in an Early Pregnancy and Acute Gynaecological Unit. Book 2

174

28

This woman was referred with a history of pelvic pain and vomiting.

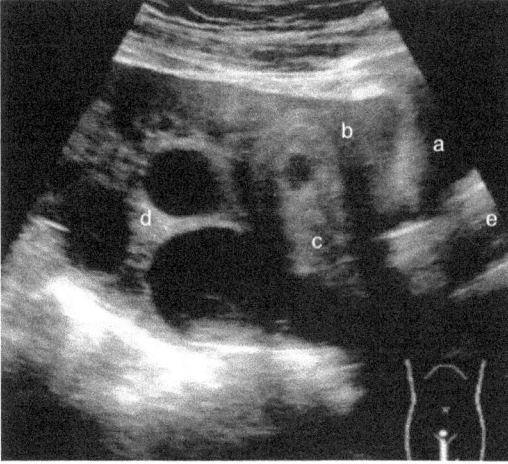

7.28a

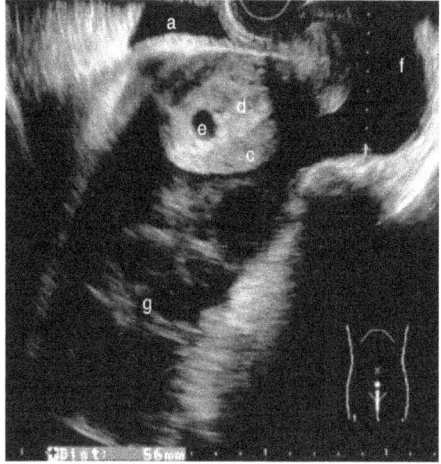

7,28b

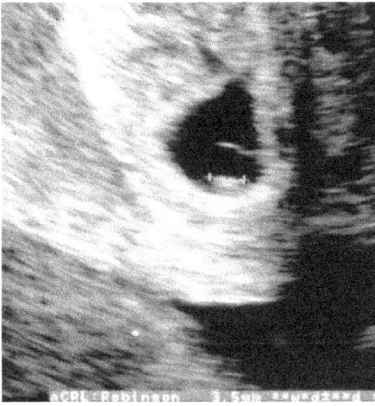

7.28c

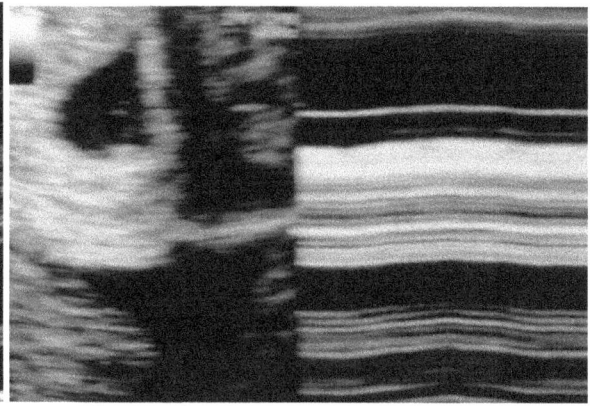

7.28d

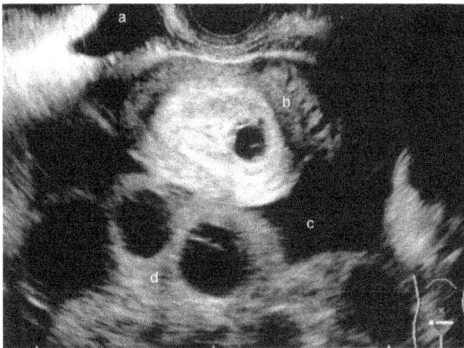

7.28e

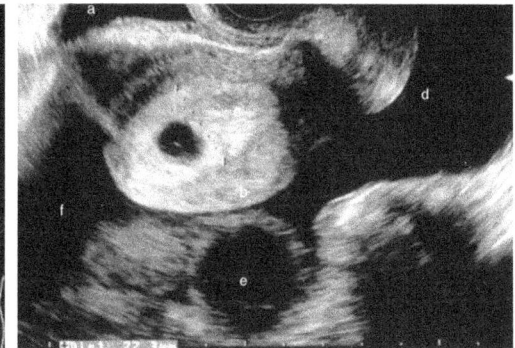

7.28f

Ultrasound Services in an Early Pregnancy and Acute Gynaecological Unit. Book 2

175

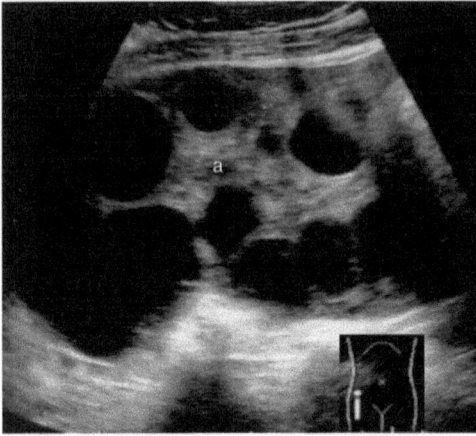

7.28g 124 x 84 x 81mm

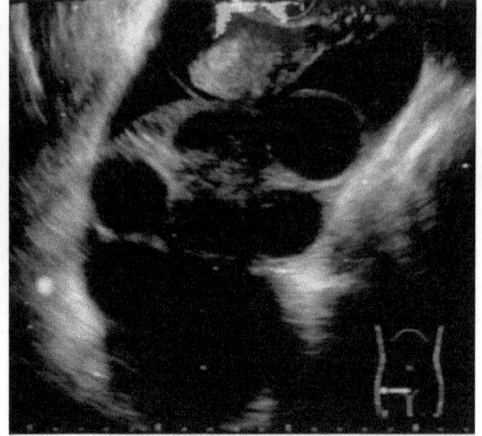

7.28h

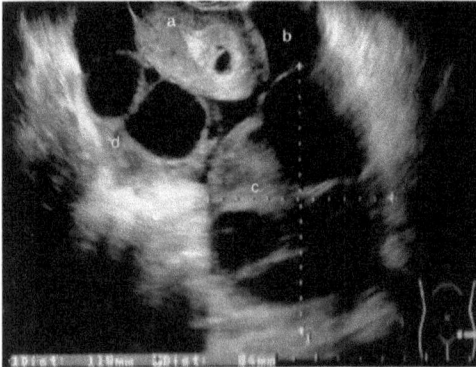

7.28i 121 x 118 x 84mm

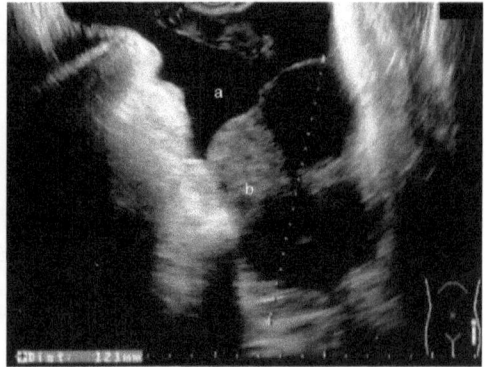

7.28j

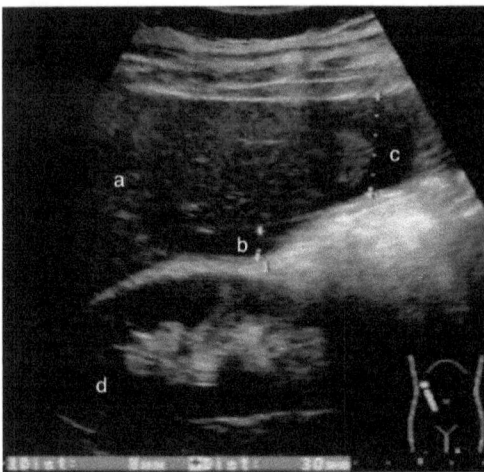

7.28k

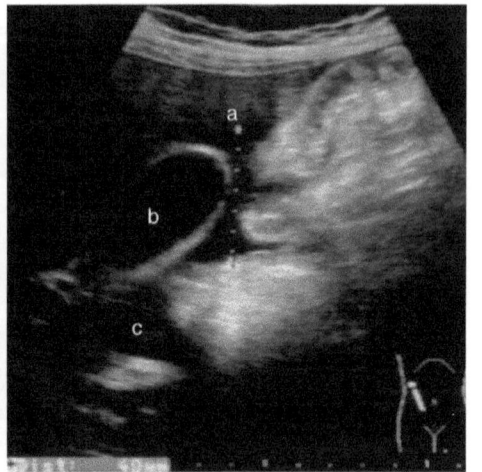

7.28l

Ultrasound Services in an Early Pregnancy and Acute Gynaecological Unit. Book 2

176

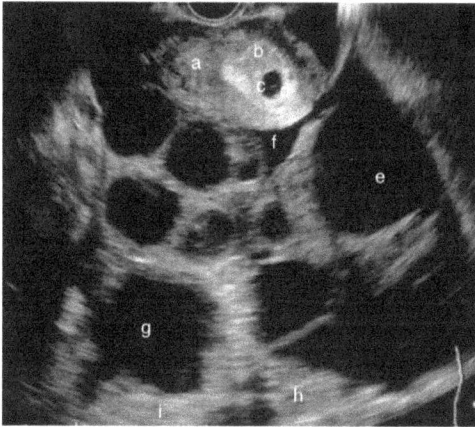

7.28m

a. Which question should the sonographer have asked the patient in order to interpret the ultrasound findings and why?

b. Label the parts identified in the above images

c. What is the difference between 7.28a and 7.28b?

d. Describe the ultrasound appearances.

e. What is role of ultrasound in the future management of this pregnancy?

f. Which 2 letter word cannot be used to describe the ovaries in 7.28m?

29

Patient should be 9/40 by her period date. She was referred with a history of irregular period, got pregnant immediately after discontinuing the pill.

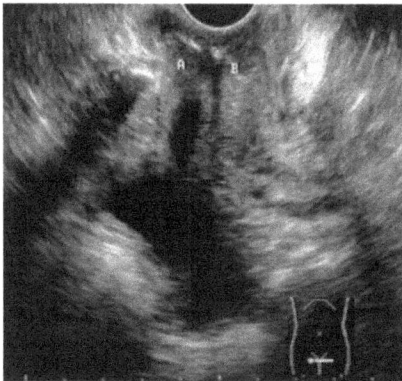

7.29a

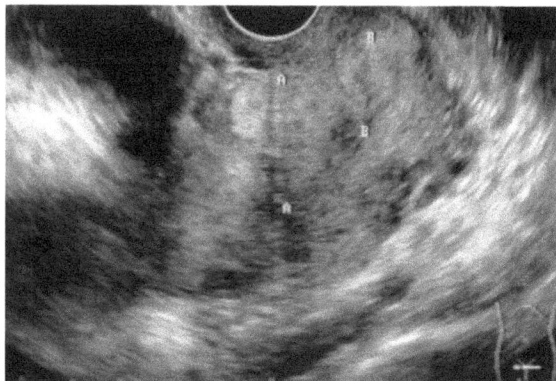

7.29b

Ultrasound Services in an Early Pregnancy and Acute Gynaecological Unit. Book 2

177

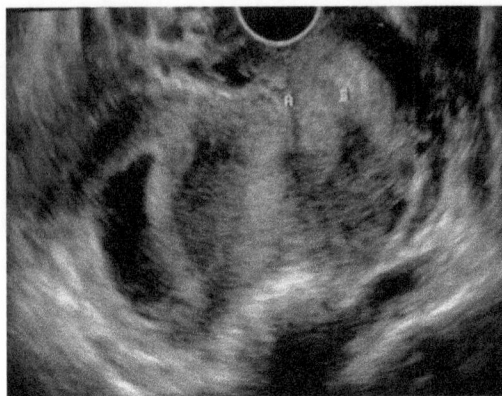

7.29c

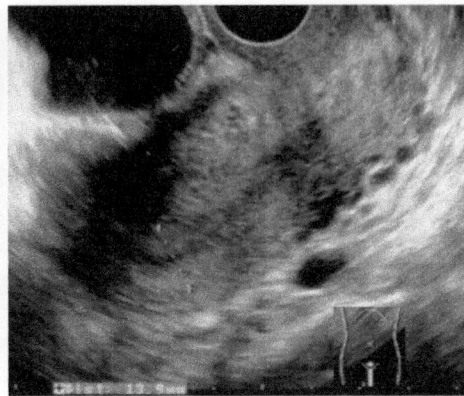

7.29d

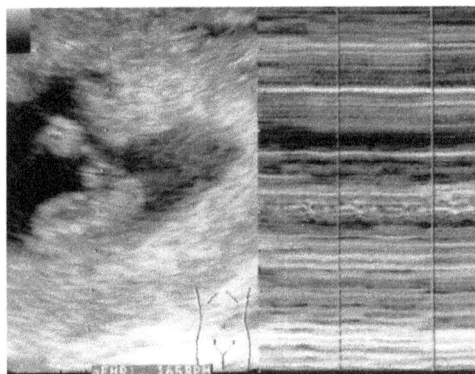

7.29 e
CRL = 26.5mm= 8+3/40

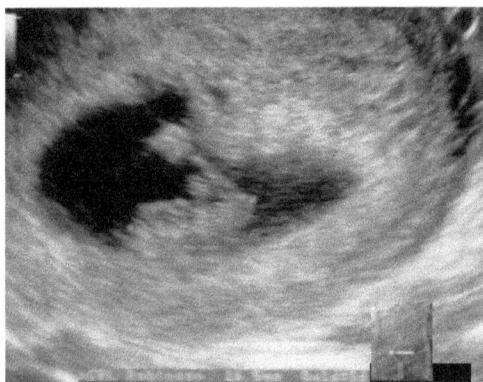

7.29f

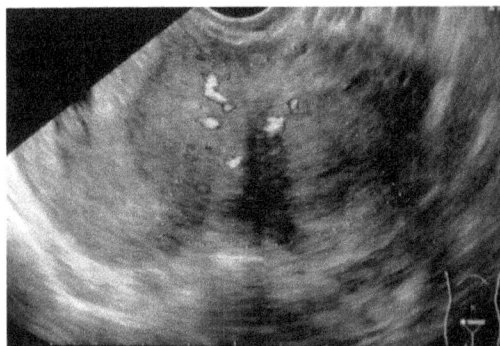

7.29g

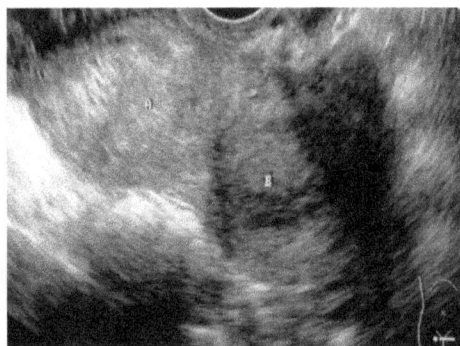

7.29h

Ultrasound Services in an Early Pregnancy and Acute Gynaecological Unit. Book 2

178

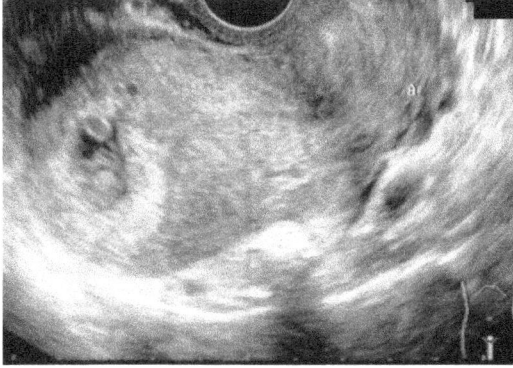

7. 29i

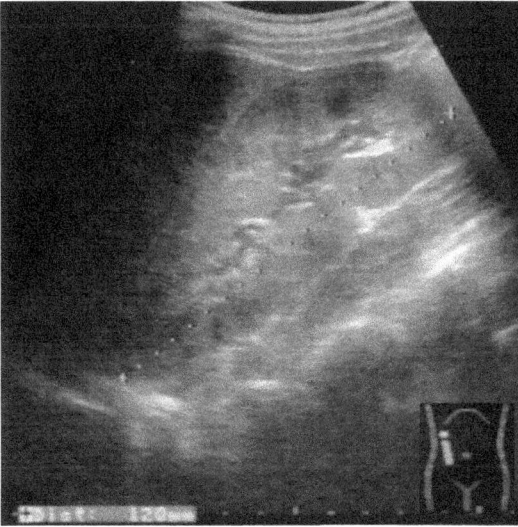

7.29j

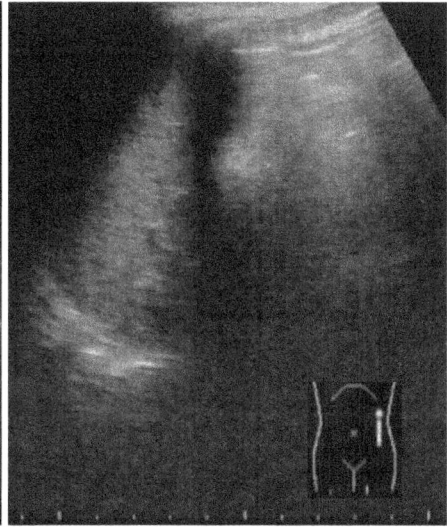

7.29k

a.   Describe the ultrasound findings in images a-k.

b.   Is there any unusual finding?

c.   Describe the ultrasound findings

d.   What implication could this unusual finding have on the pregnancy.

30

This woman was referred with a history of anxiety in pregnancy and brownish discharge for 2/7. Below are ultrasound findings in utero. Yolk sac and left ovary not shown here appeared sonographically normal.

Ultrasound Services in an Early Pregnancy and Acute Gynaecological Unit. Book 2

179

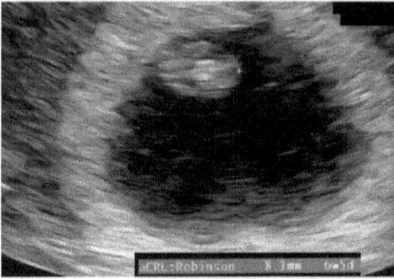
7.30a

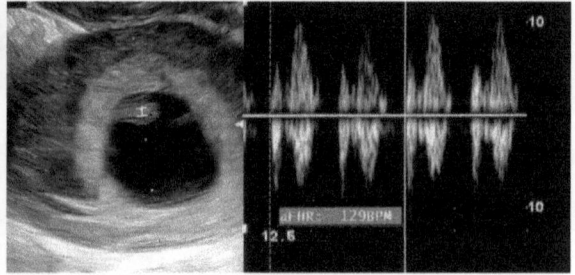
7.30b

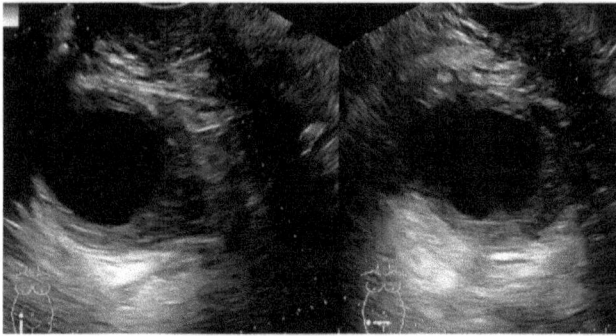
7.30c

a. Write the ultrasound report.

b. Is the EHB normal?

31. This woman was referred with a history of 3/7 light bleeding and maternal anxiety. GA by previous scan = 12+2/40.

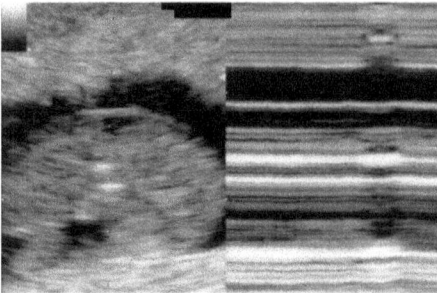
7.31a

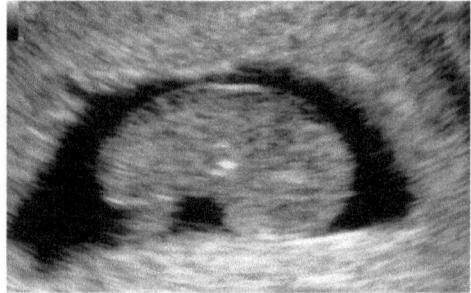
7.31b

Ultrasound Services in an Early Pregnancy and Acute Gynaecological Unit. Book 2

180

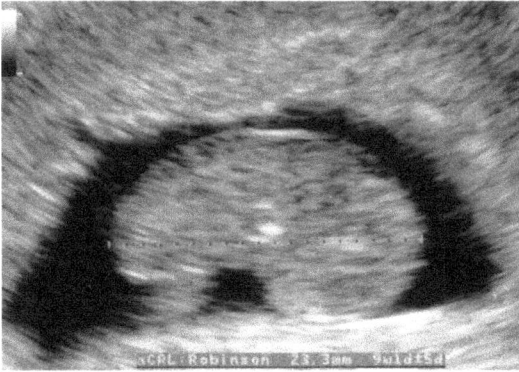

7.31c

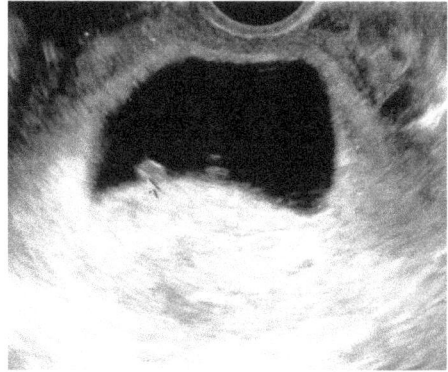

7.31d

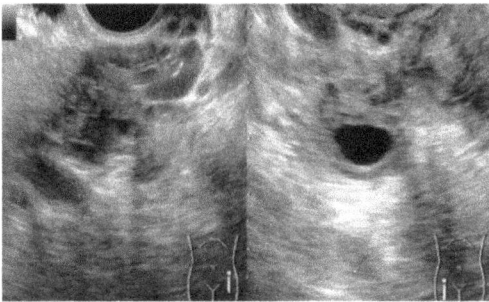

7.31e

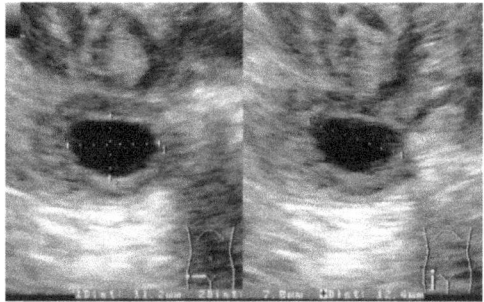

7.31f

a. Describe the ultrasound appearances.

b. What is the ultrasound diagnosis?

32

This woman was referred with a history of natural conception, positive pregnancy test result. LIF pain. GA by LMP = 5/40. GSV = 0.4ml.

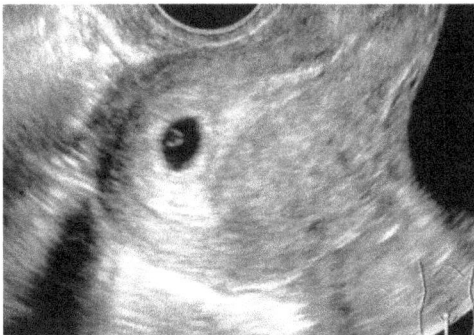

7.32a

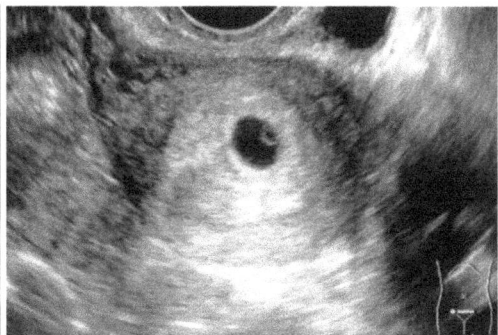

7.32b

Ultrasound Services in an Early Pregnancy and Acute Gynaecological Unit. Book 2

181

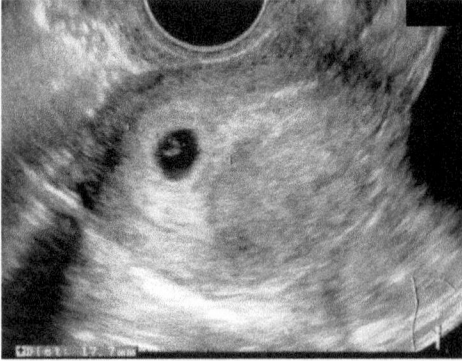

7.32c

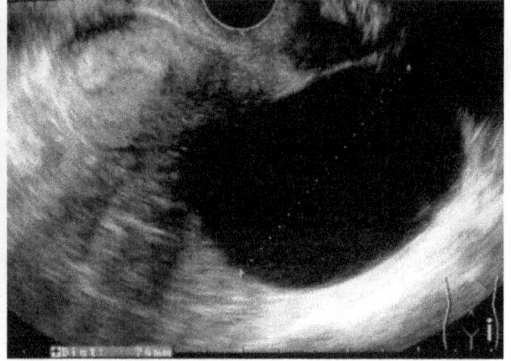

7.32d

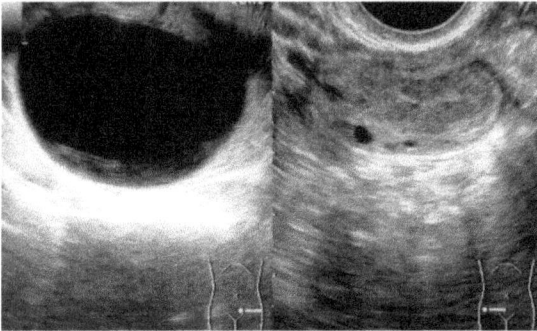

7.32e

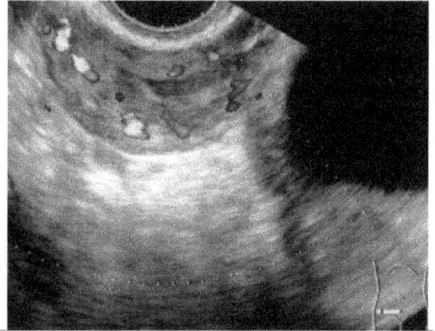

7.32f

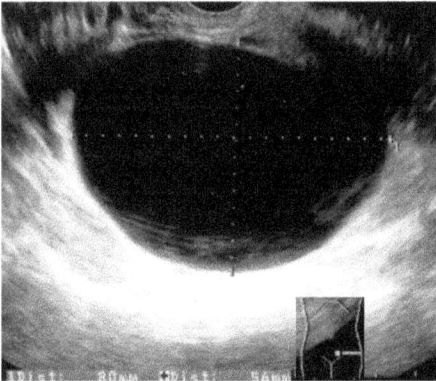

7.32g

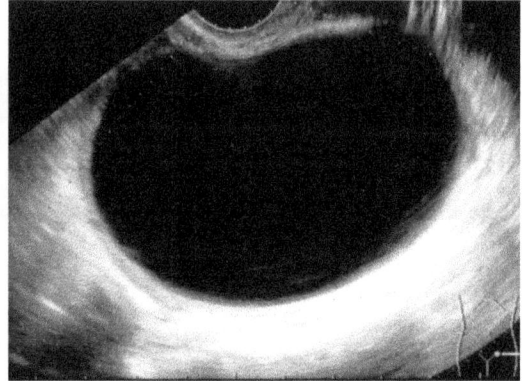

7.32h

a. What is the difference between the cysts?

b. Is there any ultrasound explanation for her pain?

c. Which painful condition will the Sonographer need to exclude?

d. What are the ultrasound signs of an ovarian torsion.

Ultrasound Services in an Early Pregnancy and Acute Gynaecological Unit. Book 2

182

e. Write the ultrasound report.

f. How would ultrasound be used in the management of this woman.

33

This woman was referred with a history of 5/7 abdominal pain and light bleeding for 3/52. GA by LMP = 6/40.

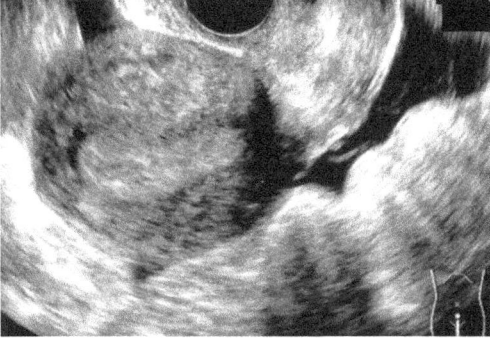
7.33a

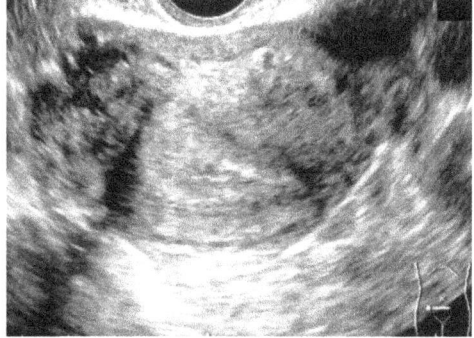
7.33b

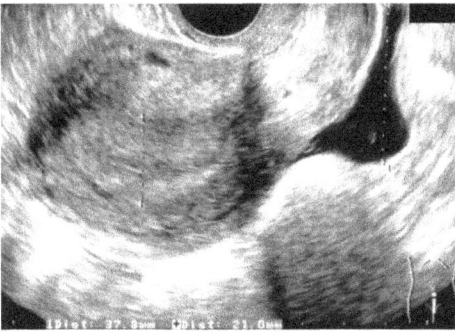
7.33c

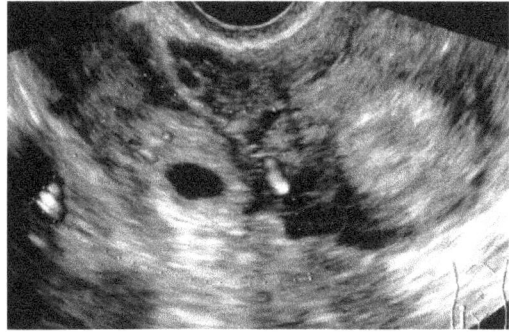
7.33d

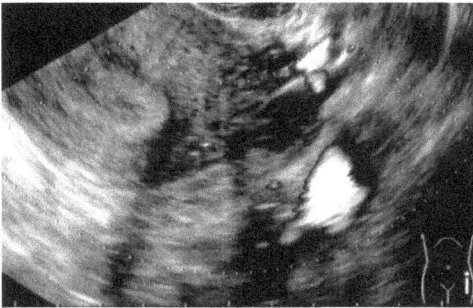
7.33e

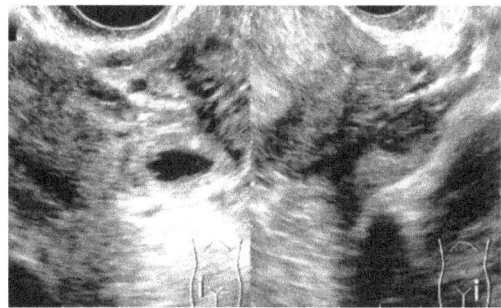
7.33f

Ultrasound Services in an Early Pregnancy and Acute Gynaecological Unit. Book 2

183

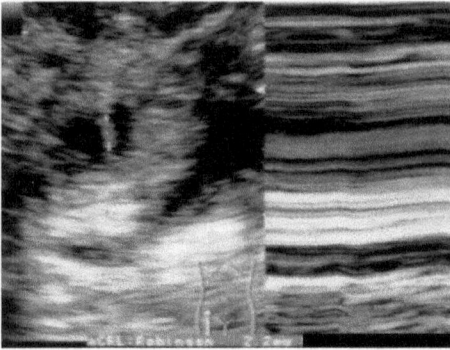

7.33g

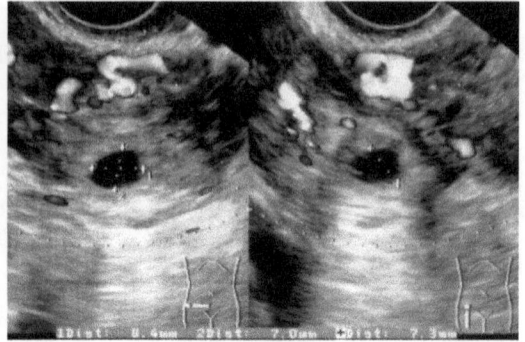

7.33h

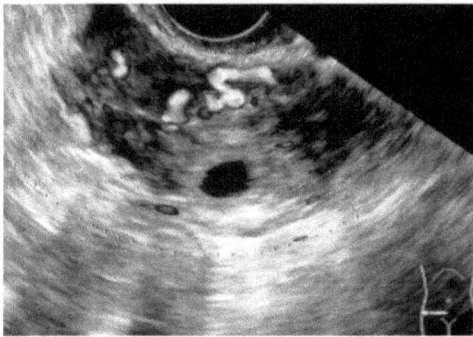

7.33i

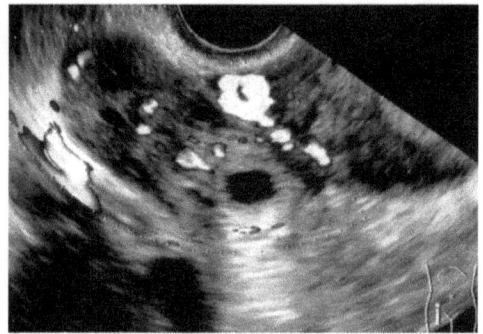

7.33i

a. Describe the ultrasound findings

b. What is the ultrasound diagnosis?

34

This woman was referred with a history of light bleeding. GA by LMP = 9+2/40.

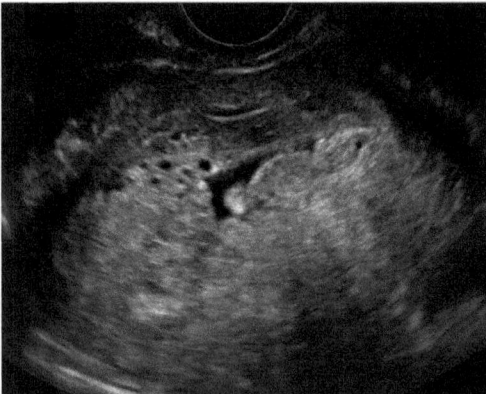

7.34a

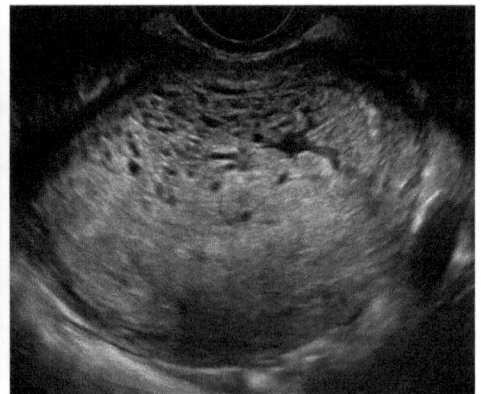

7.34b

Ultrasound Services in an Early Pregnancy and Acute Gynaecological Unit. Book 2

184

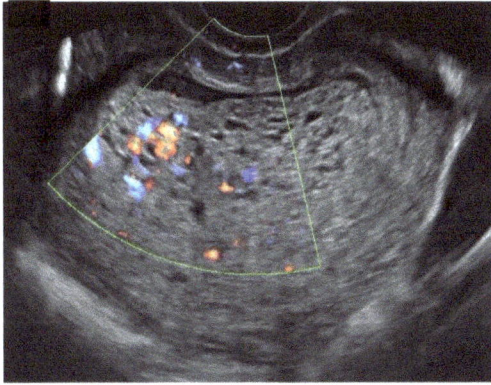

7.34c

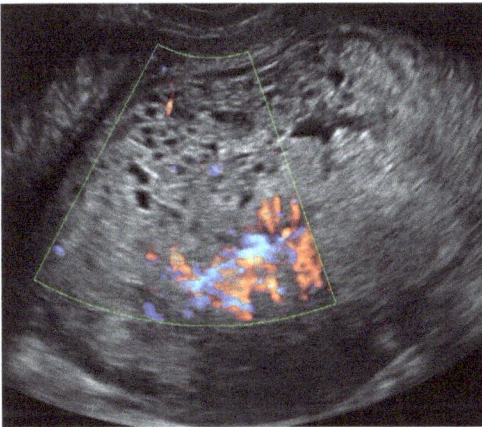

7.34d

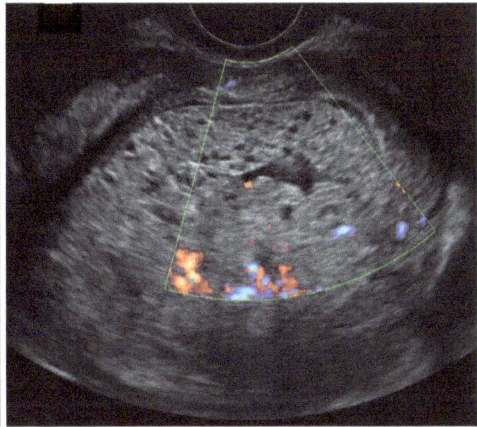

7.34e

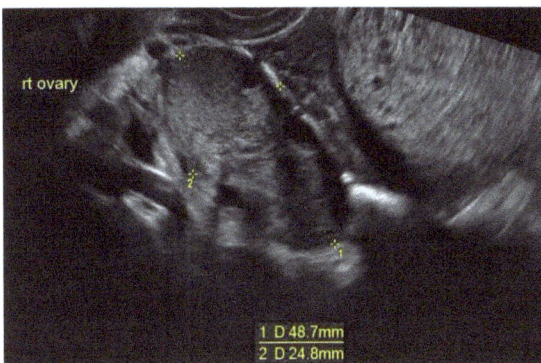

7.34f

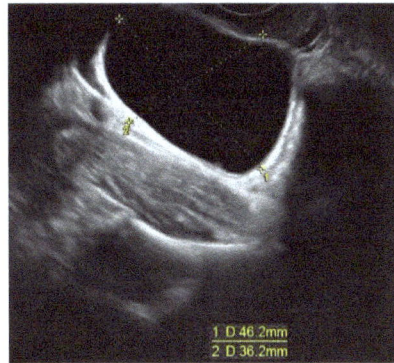

7.34g left ovary

a Describe the ultrasound findings

b. What is the ultrasound diagnosis

Ultrasound Services in an Early Pregnancy and Acute Gynaecological Unit. Book 2

185

7.35

This woman was referred with a history of maternal anxiety and previous ectopic pregnancy. Natural conception. GA by LMP = 5+6/40 no flow or peristaltic movements are seen in the hypoechoic tubular structures.

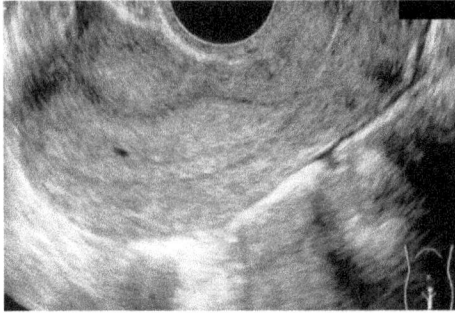

7.35a   4 x 2 x 3mm

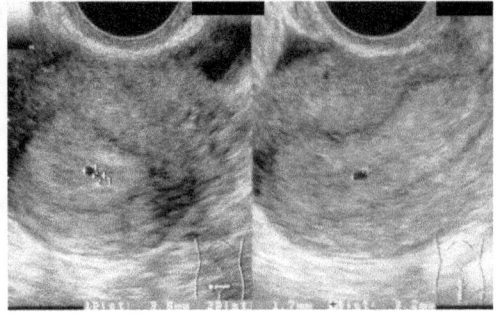

7.35b

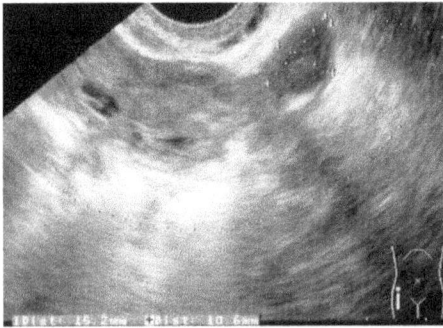

7.35c

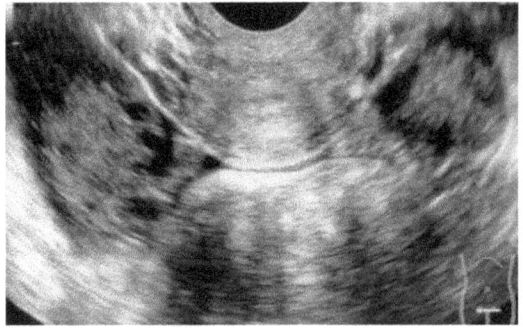

7.35d

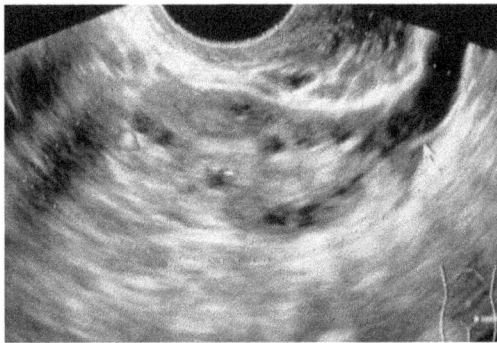

7.35e

a. Is this woman pregnant or not?

b. Is there any abnormal findings on the images?

c. Describe the ultrasound findings

Ultrasound Services in an Early Pregnancy and Acute Gynaecological Unit. Book 2

186

d. Describe the ultrasound findings in 7.35d.

e. Will this woman need another scan and how soon?

36

This woman was referred with a history of light pvb for1/7 at 6+6/40. Right ovary was seen and appeared sonographically normal but the left ovary was not visualized.

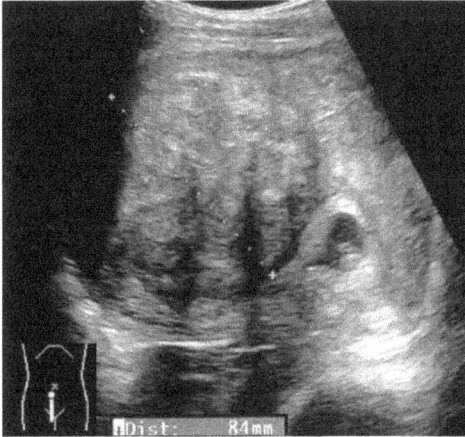
7.36a

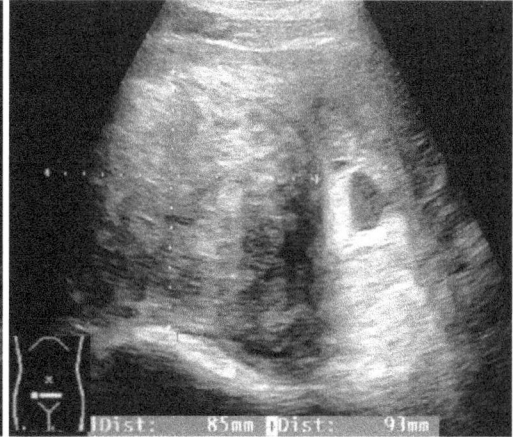
7.36b

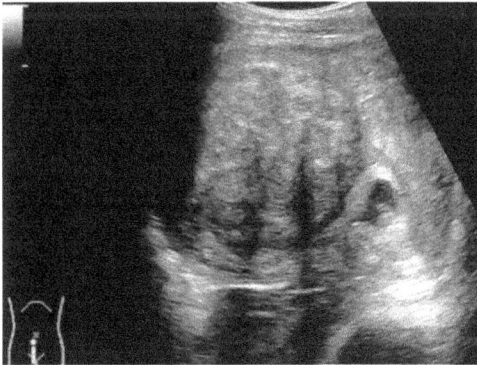
7.36c

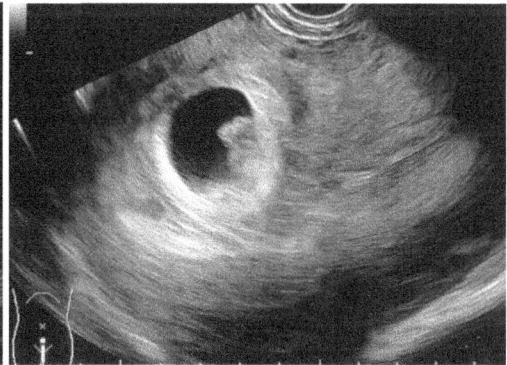
7.36d

Ultrasound Services in an Early Pregnancy and Acute Gynaecological Unit. Book 2

187

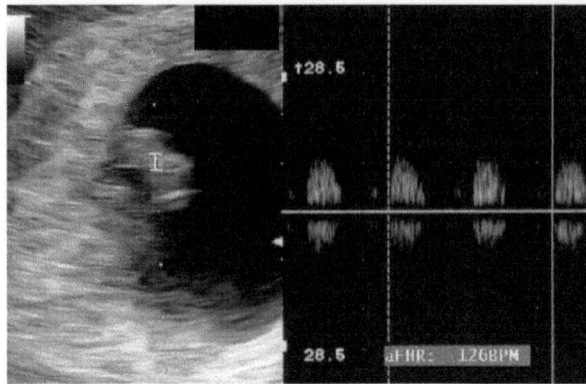

7.36e

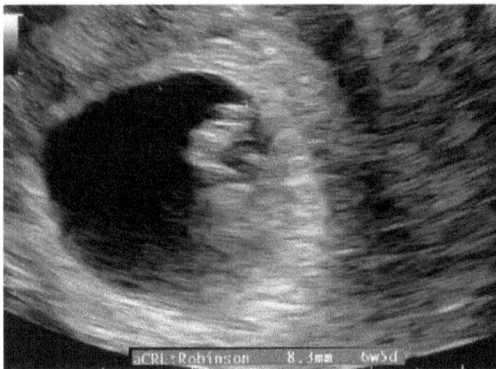

7.36f

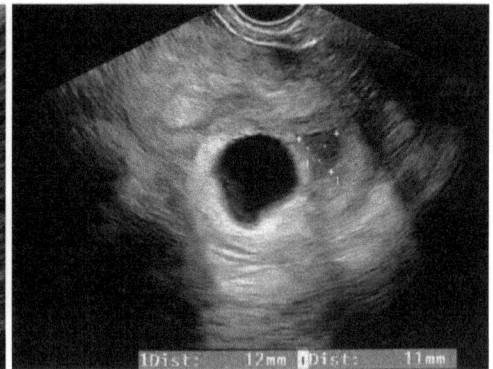

7.36g

a. How was this woman scanned?

b. Is there any evidence of this woman's pvb?

c. Describe the ultrasound findings

d. In which ways may ultrasound be useful in the management of this pregnancy?

37

This woman was referred for a scan with a history of maternal anxiety at 8+5 /40 and pv spotting. Both ovaries not shown appeared sonographically normal.

Ultrasound Services in an Early Pregnancy and Acute Gynaecological Unit. Book 2

188

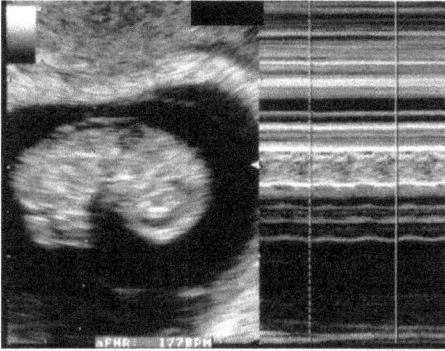

7.37a

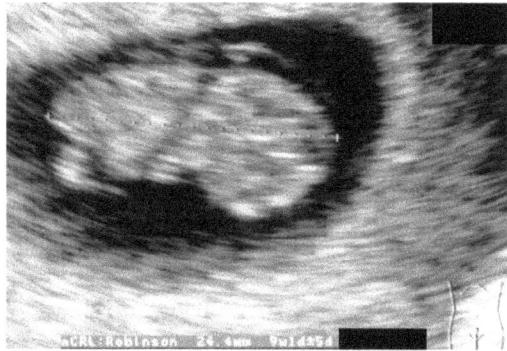

7.37b

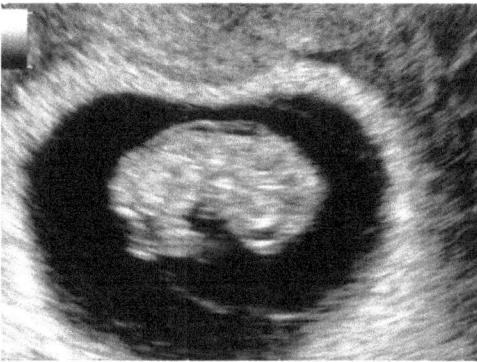

7.37c

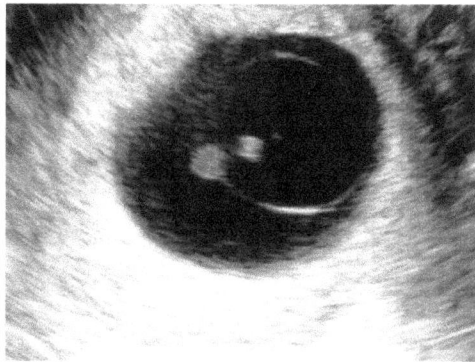

7.37d

a. Is there any ultrasound cause for pv spotting shown.
b. Identify as many anatomical parts as you can in 7.37c-d
c. Write an ultrasound report.
d. What is your clinical diagnosis?

38
This woman had clomid treatment and was referred for a scan at 6+5/40.
beta hCG a week earlier was over 22000 mIU/ml.

Ultrasound Services in an Early Pregnancy and Acute Gynaecological Unit. Book 2

189

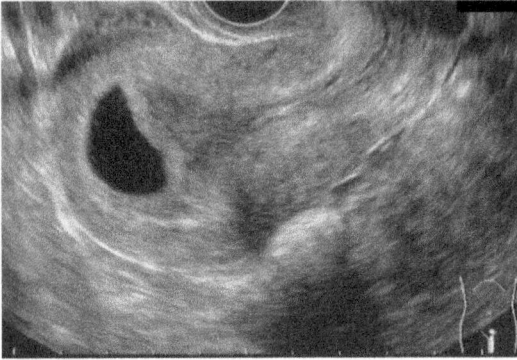

7.38a

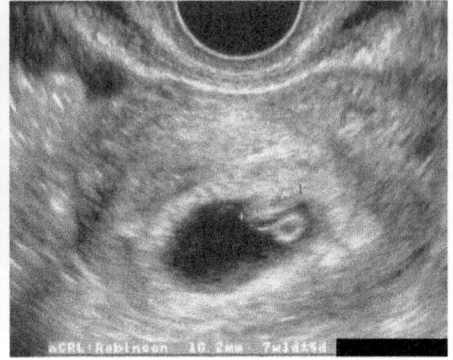

7.38b

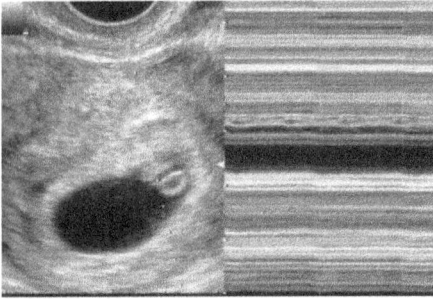

7.38c

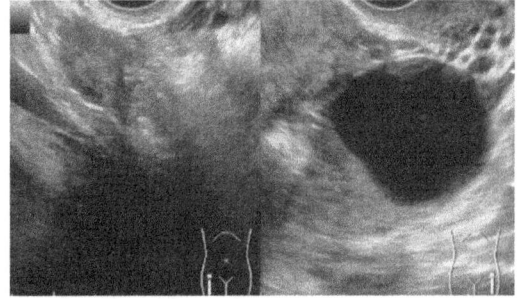

7.38d

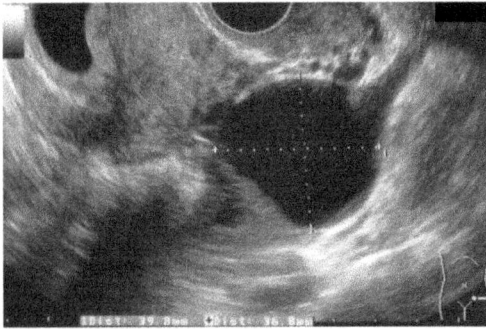

7.38e

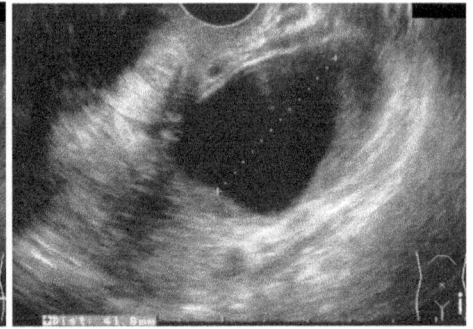

7.38f

a. What is clomid treatment?
b. Which patients are suitable for clomid treatment.
c. How is clomid treatment different from IVF?
d. Write an ultrasound report
e. What is the role of ultrasound in the future management of this pregnancy?

Ultrasound Services in an Early Pregnancy and Acute Gynaecological Unit. Book 2

190

7.39

This woman was referred for a dating scan with a history of unknown LMP.

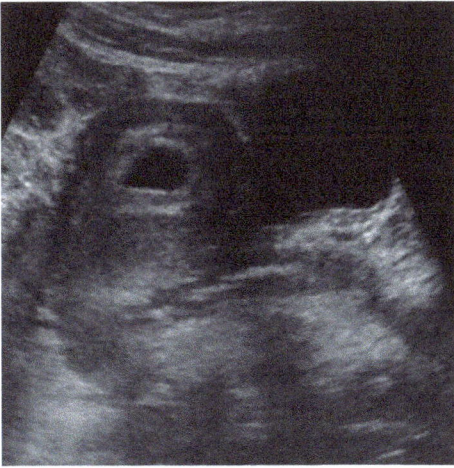

7.39a

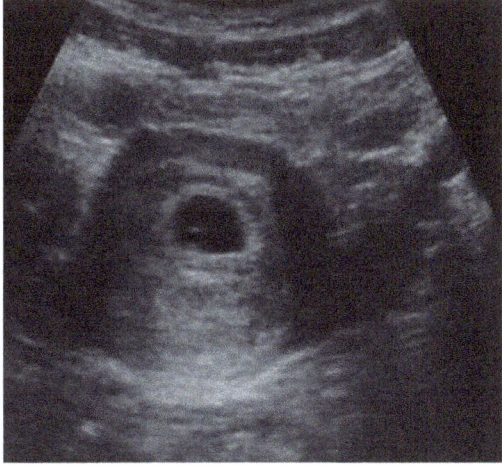

7.39b

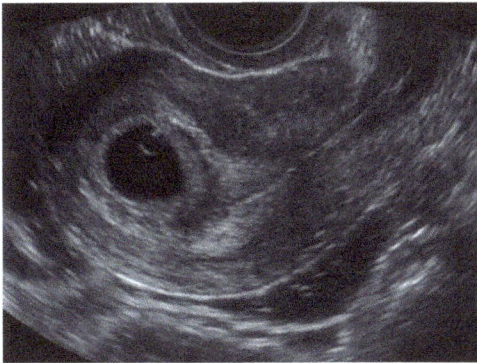

7.39c

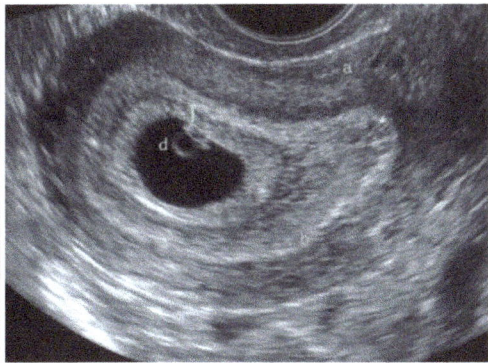

7.39d

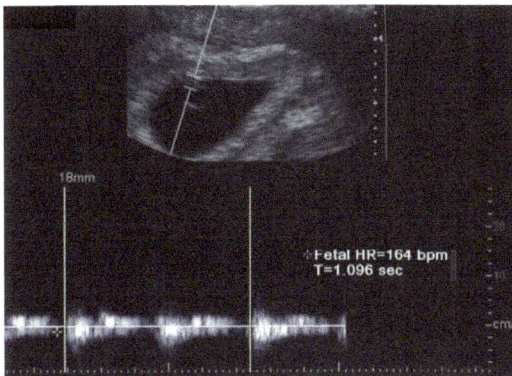

7.39e

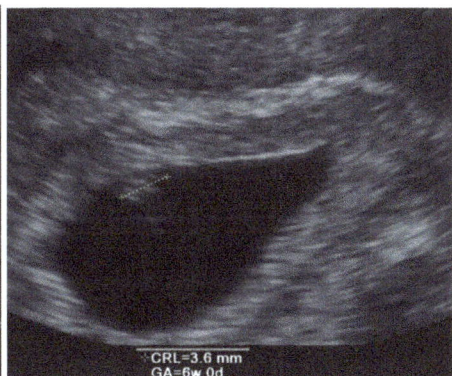

7.39f

Ultrasound Services in an Early Pregnancy and Acute Gynaecological Unit. Book 2

191

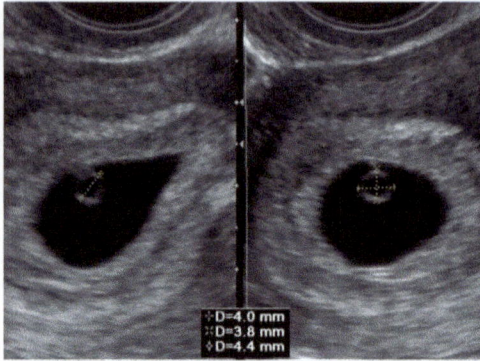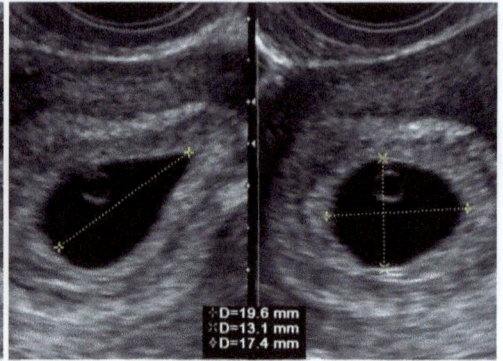

7.39g   **7.39h**

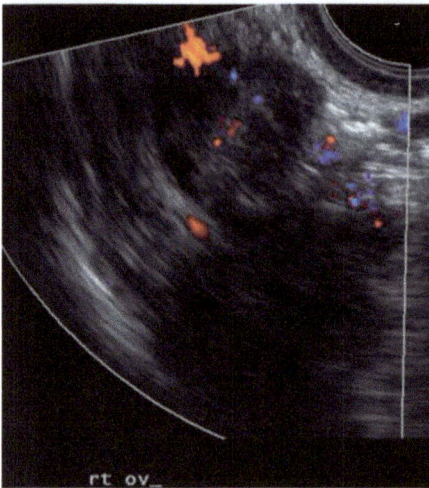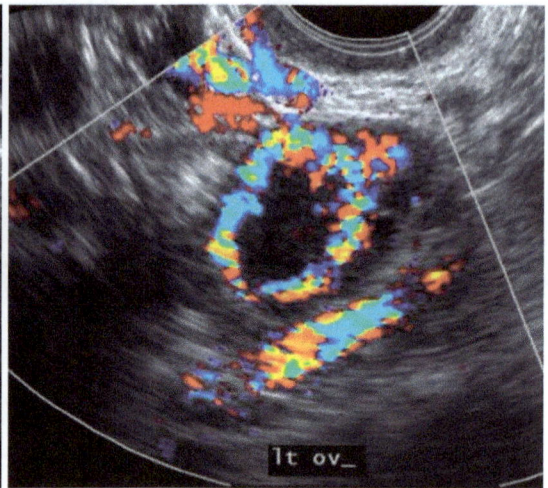

7.39i   **7.39j**

a. How was this woman scanned?

b. Identify a-d & l in 7.39f

c. Which measurements were done

d. Write the ultrasound report

e. Will this woman need another scan? Why or why not?

f. What are some of the reasons for unknown LMP

Ultrasound Services in an Early Pregnancy and Acute Gynaecological Unit. Book 2

192

40

Below are images from four women

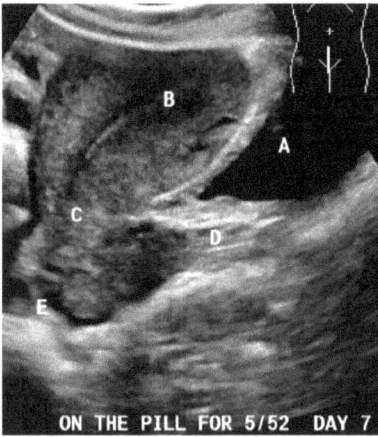

7.40a

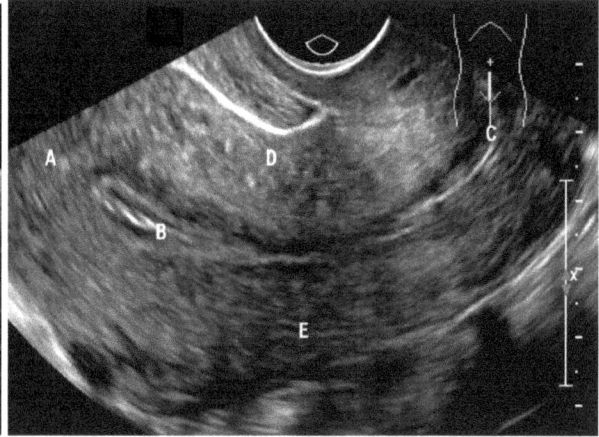

7.40b

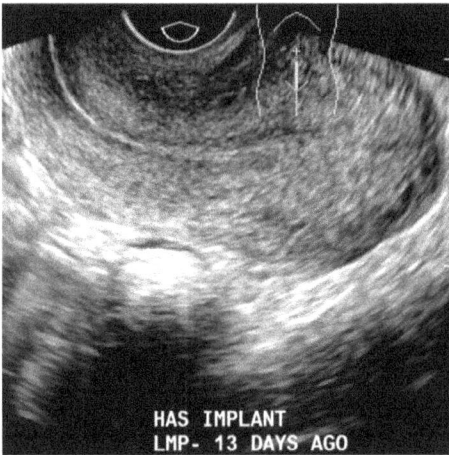

7.40c

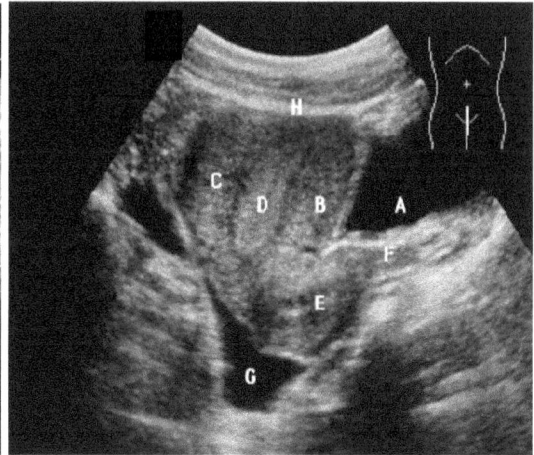

7.40d

a. Identify the labeling in 7.40 a -b and d

b. How were these women scanned?

c. What is the difference between 7.40b and c?

d. What is the difference between 7.40a and d?

e. How does the contraceptive pill works?

f. How does the contraceptive implant work?

g. What is the difference between a contraceptive pill and a contraceptive implant?

Ultrasound Services in an Early Pregnancy and Acute Gynaecological Unit. Book 2

193

41

This woman was referred with a history of pvb at 14+1/40.

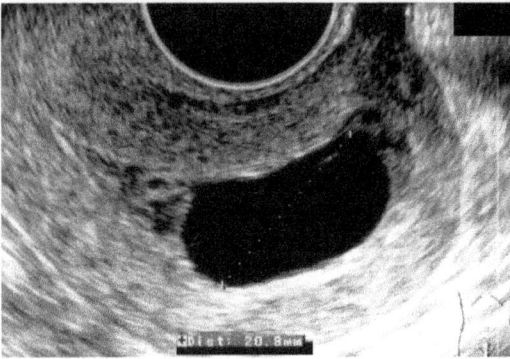

7.41a

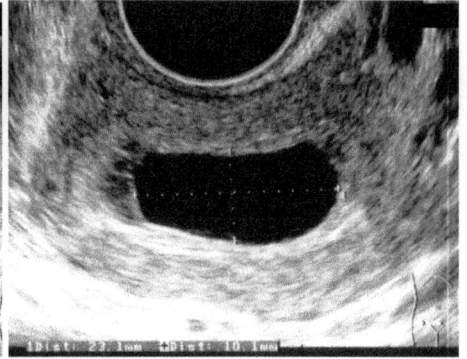

7.41 b

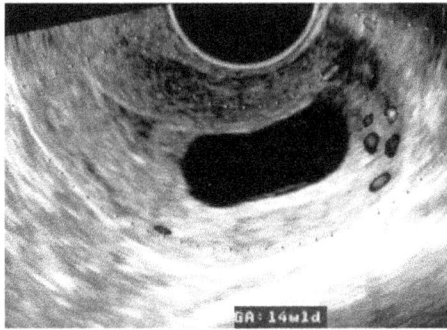

7.41c

a. Describe the ultrasound findings of the uterus

b. What is the diagnosis?

c. How is this condition different from missed miscarriage or abortion?

d. What is the future role of ultrasound in the management of this pregnancy?

Ultrasound Services in an Early Pregnancy and Acute Gynaecological Unit. Book 2

194

42

This woman was referred with a history of ?SROM in pregnancy.

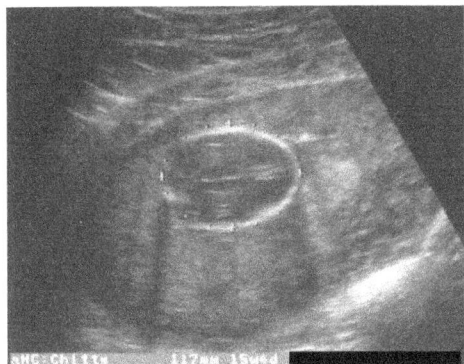
7.42a

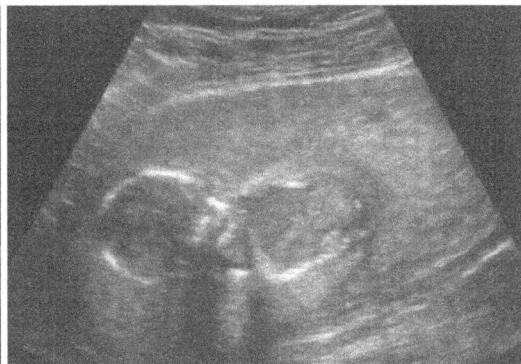
7.42b

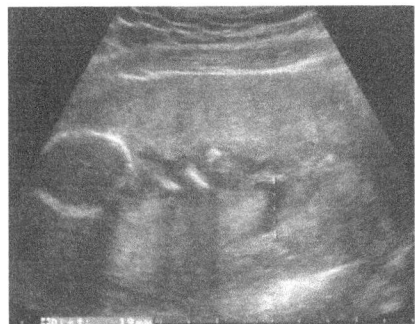
7.42c

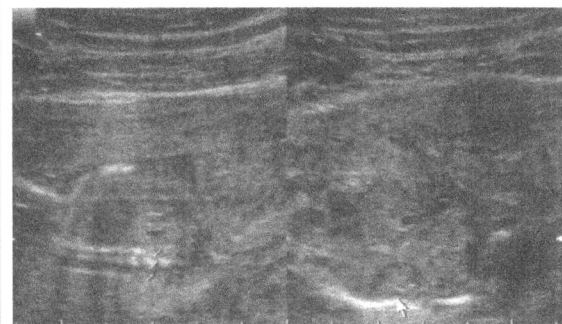
7.42d

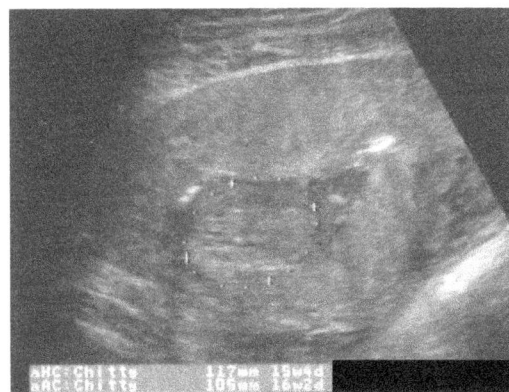
7.42e

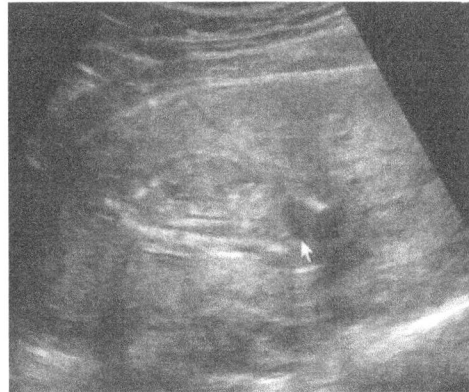
7.42 f

Ultrasound Services in an Early Pregnancy and Acute Gynaecological Unit. Book 2

195

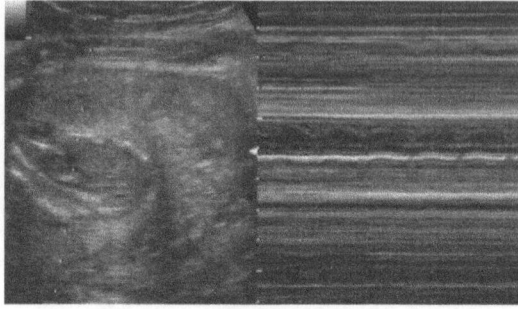

7.42g

a. Is there any factor that can make this examination challenging for the sonographer.
b. Identify the arrows and /// in the above.
c. What measurement is the 19mm measurement in 7.42c only measurement obtainable.
d. Which medical condition has been excluded and why or how?
e. Write the ultrasound report.

43

This woman was referred with a history of lost coil and string. Please locate and exclude pelvic pathology.

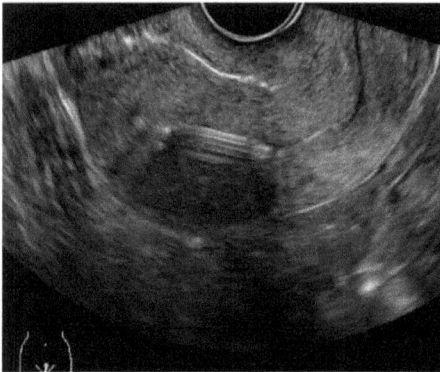

43a

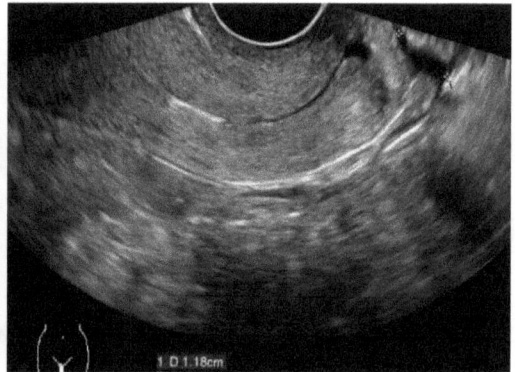

43b

Ultrasound Services in an Early Pregnancy and Acute Gynaecological Unit. Book 2

196

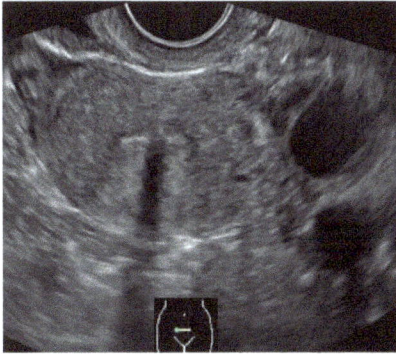
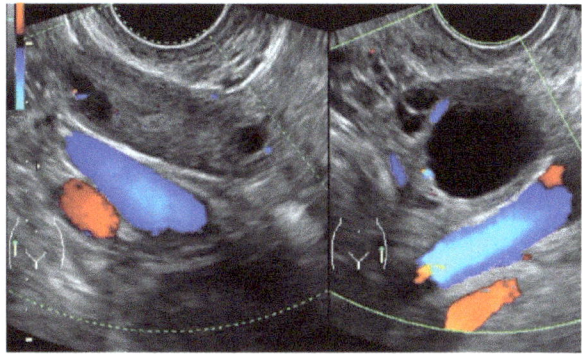

43c   **43d**

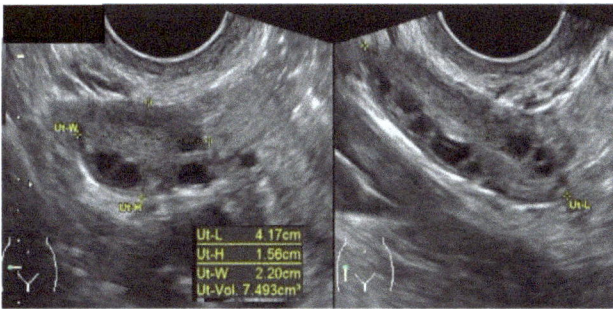

43e

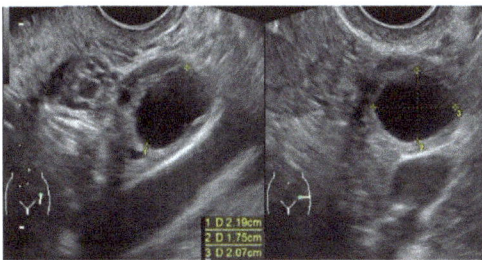
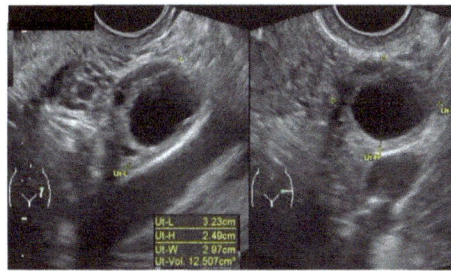

43f   **43g**

a. Is there an IUCD and string in the above images?

b. What type of IUCD is shown?.

c. Write the ultrasound report

d. Is it normal for a person with IUCD to have a corpus luteum or functional cyst?

Ultrasound Services in an Early Pregnancy and Acute Gynaecological Unit. Book 2

197

44

This woman was referred with a history of pvb at 10+4/40. Both ovaries were not identified.

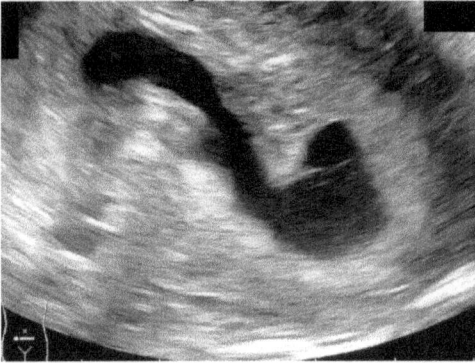

7.744a

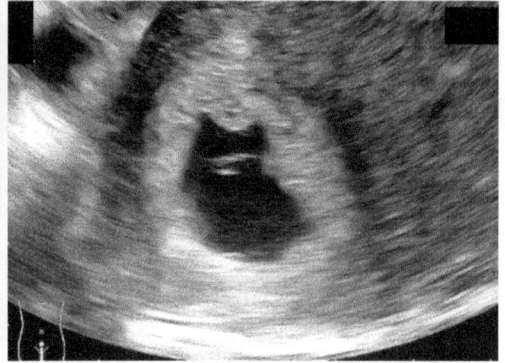

7.44b

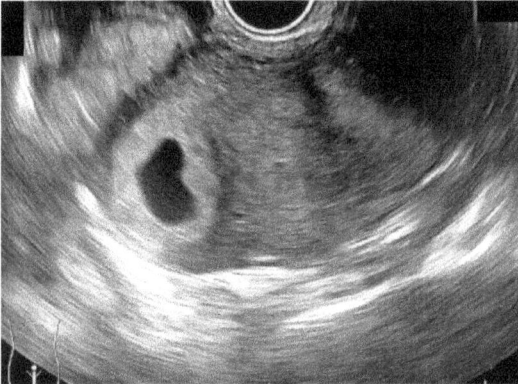

7.44c

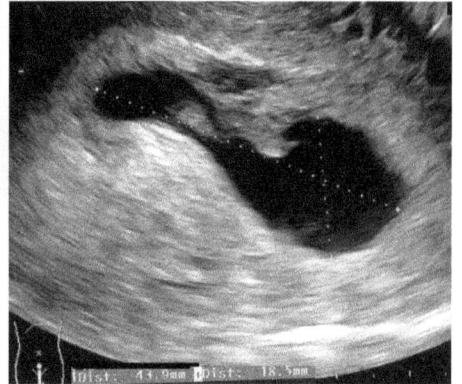

7.44d

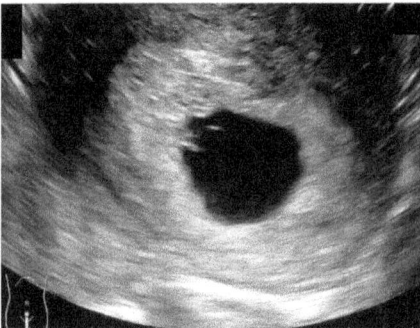

7.44e

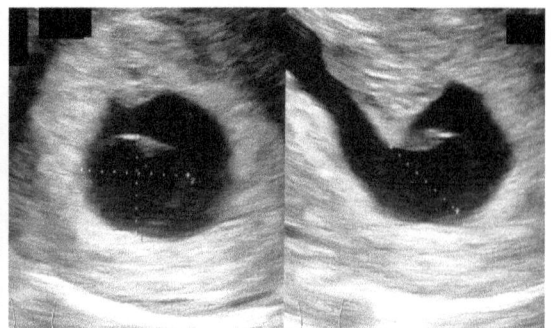

7.44f   ++12 x 12 x 13mm

Ultrasound Services in an Early Pregnancy and Acute Gynaecological Unit. Book 2

198

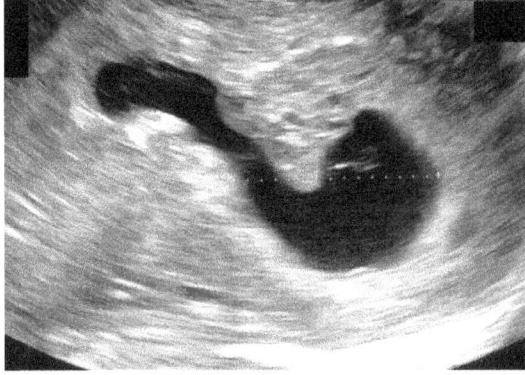

7.44g   ++22mm

a. Describe the ultrasound findings.

b. What is the diagnosis?

c. Is there any ultrasound reason for this woman's pv bleeding.

45

This woman was referred with a history of RIF pain, previous appendicectomy and known Irritable bowel syndrome (IBS). GA at the time of the scan by LMP = 7+1/40. EHB not shown here was seen.

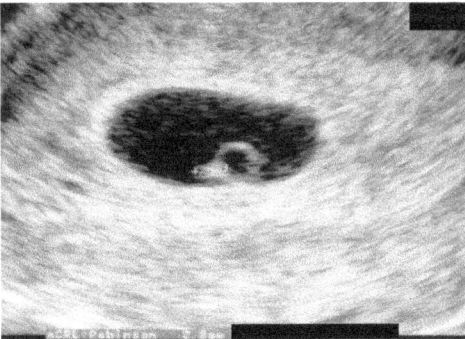

7.45a

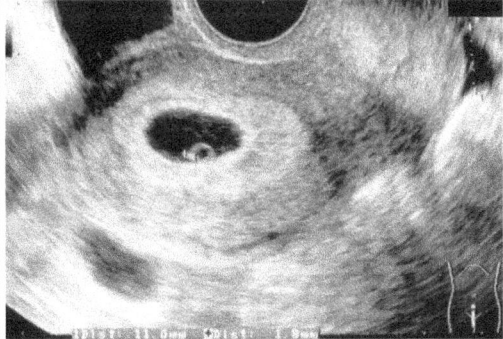

7.45b

Ultrasound Services in an Early Pregnancy and Acute Gynaecological Unit. Book 2

199

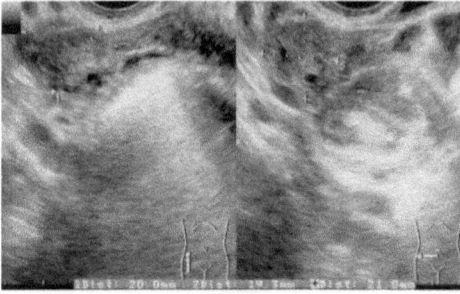

7.45c

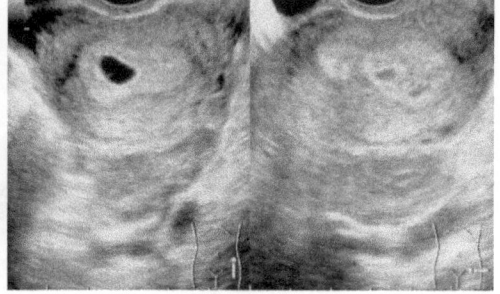

7.45d

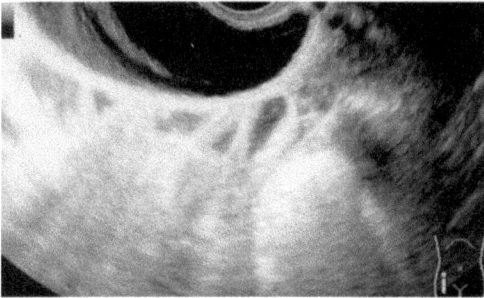

7.45e

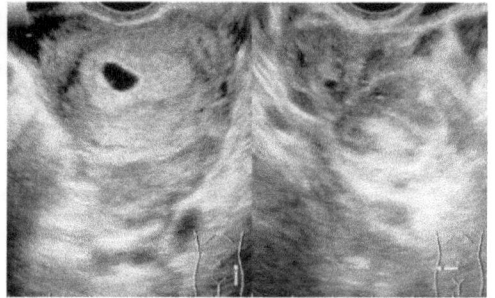

7.45f

a. Is there any ultrasound cause for the woman's RIF pain?

b. Will you bring the woman back? Why or why not

c. Write the ultrasound report.

46

This woman was referred with a history of IMB for some months. She has no other relevant past medical history. She has a regular monthly cycle and below are the images of her scan examination.

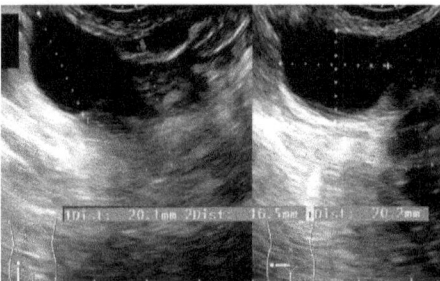

7.46a

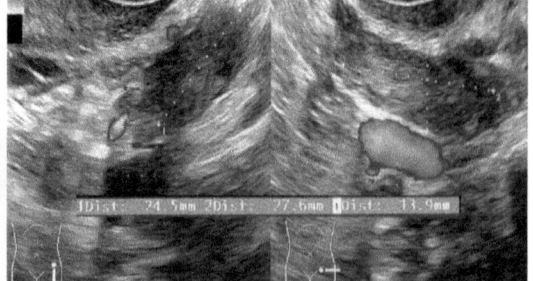

7.46b

Ultrasound Services in an Early Pregnancy and Acute Gynaecological Unit. Book 2

200

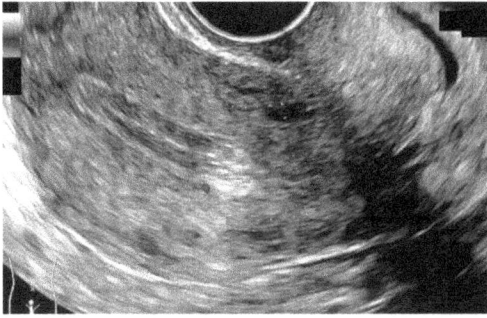

7.46c

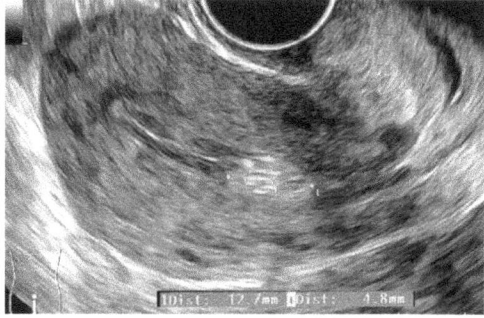

7.46d

a. Where about is this woman in her menstrual cycle and which ultrasound images confirms this?
b. Is there any ultrasound cause for this woman's IMB?
c. Write the ultrasound report.

47

This woman was referred for the follow up scan. FHB and movements were seen not shown here. Not all the fetal measurements have been included.

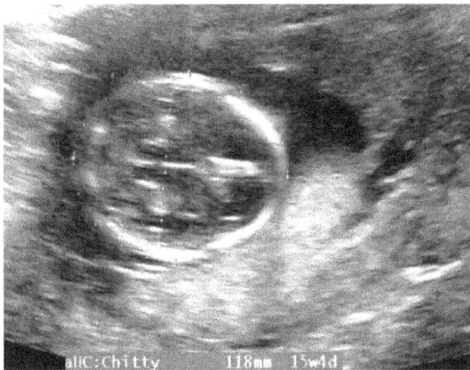

7.47a.

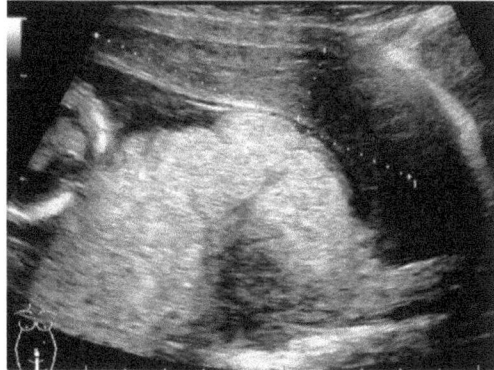

7.47b. ++86.7mm, 17.8mm

Ultrasound Services in an Early Pregnancy and Acute Gynaecological Unit. Book 2

201

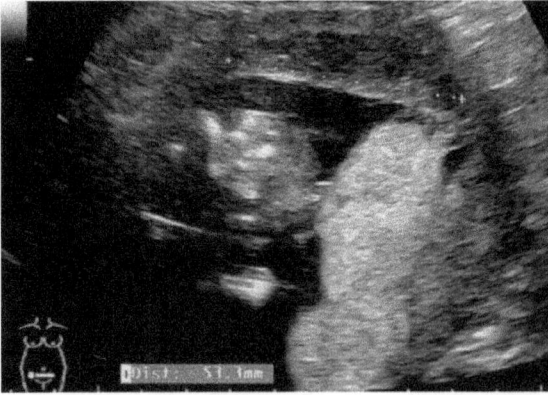

7.47c.

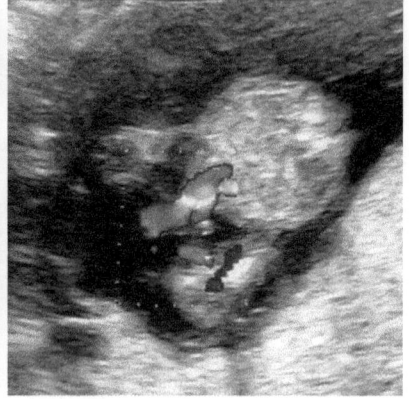

7.47d.

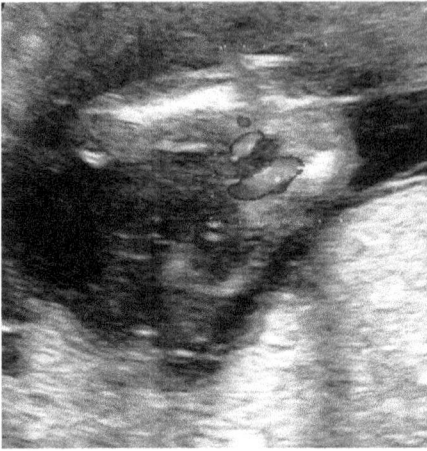

7.47e.

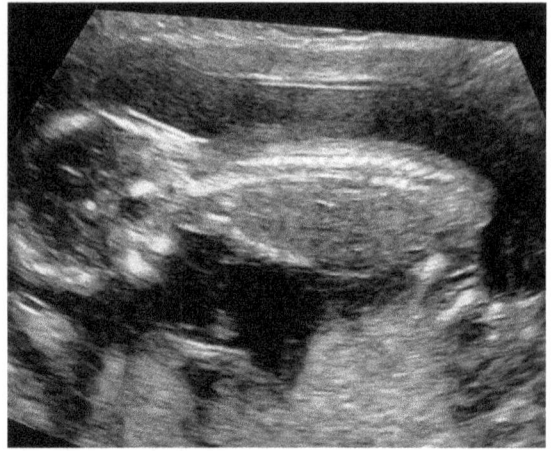

7.47 f

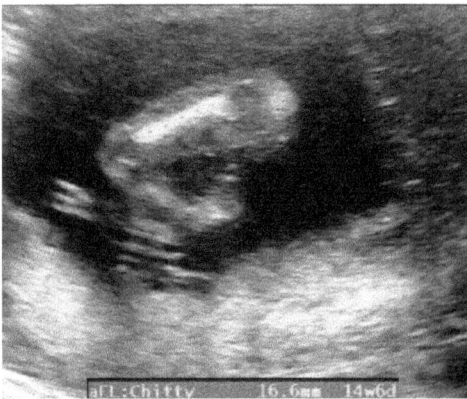

7.47g.

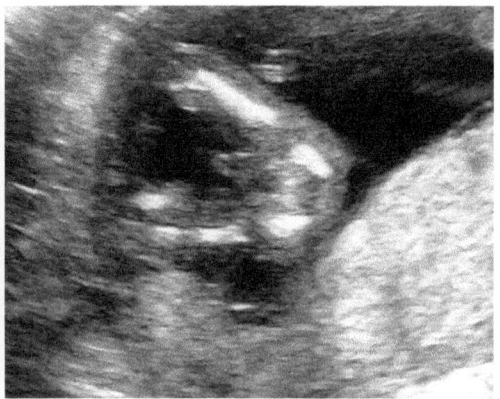

7.47h.

Ultrasound Services in an Early Pregnancy and Acute Gynaecological Unit. Book 2

202

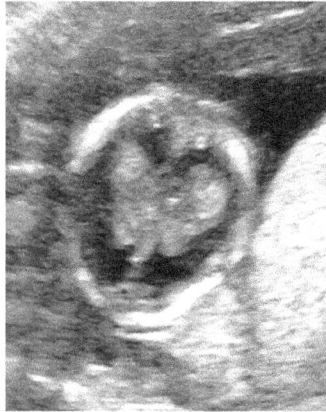

7.47 i.

a.   Identify as many views and the fetal anatomy as possible in the images a. –i.
b.   Should the sonographer be concerned about the placenta position now? Why or why not?
c.   Though not the aim of the examination, what is the fetal gender (7.47h)?
d.   Write the ultrasound report.

48
This woman was referred for a dating scan at 7+4/40.

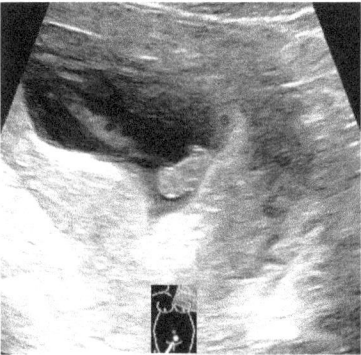

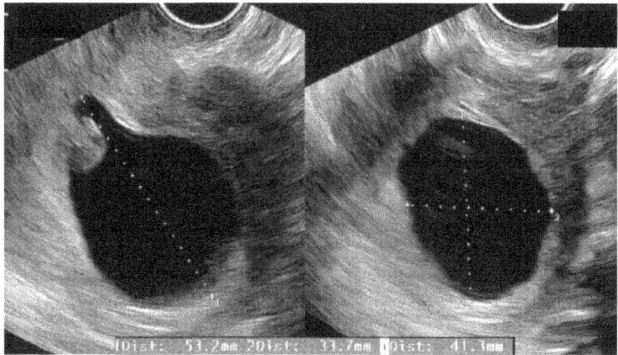

7.48a.   **7.48 b.**

Ultrasound Services in an Early Pregnancy and Acute Gynaecological Unit. Book 2

203

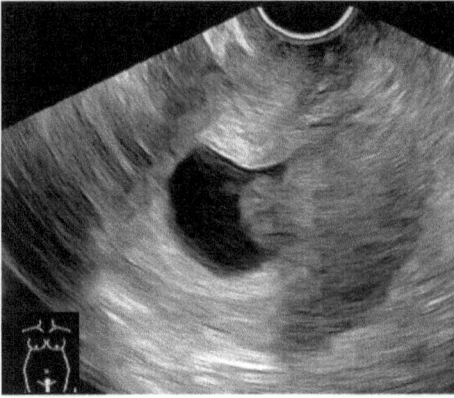 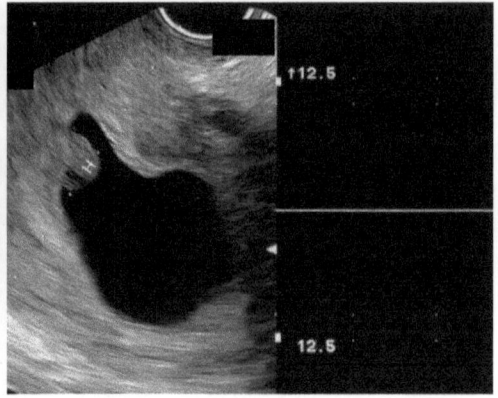

7.48c.   **7.48d.**

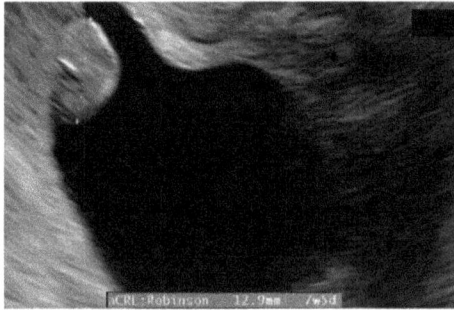

7.48e

a. What is your diagnosis and which images supports your diagnosis?

b. Why is image d. important?

c. How was this woman scanned?

Ultrasound Services in an Early Pregnancy and Acute Gynaecological Unit. Book 2

204

49

The next four images are from the same patient.

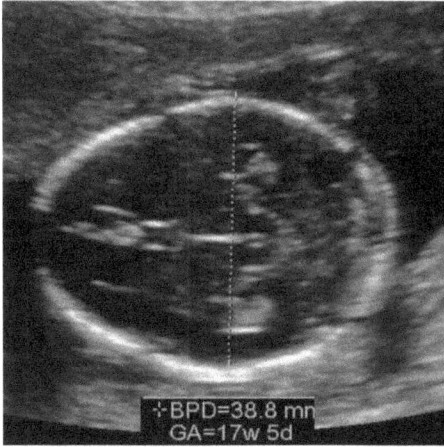

7.49a

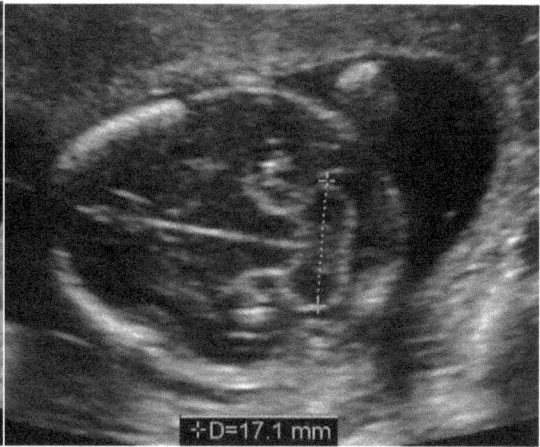

7.49b

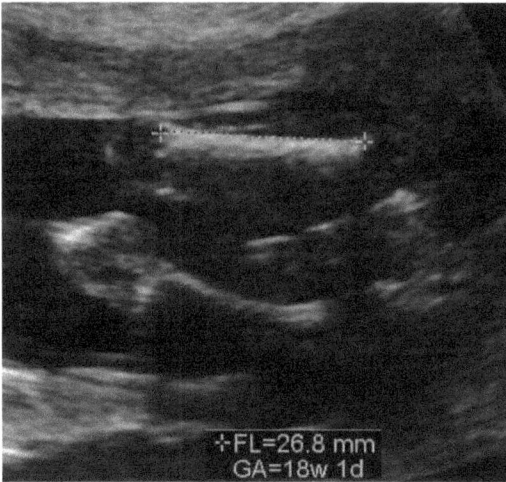

7.49c.

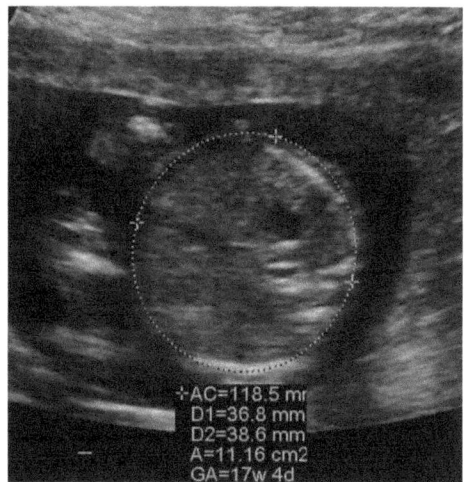

7.49d.

a. Please identify the sections and as many fetal anatomy as possible in images 7.49a-d

b. What is the difference between 7.49a and b?

c. Approximately how old is this fetus and which image supports this?

Ultrasound Services in an Early Pregnancy and Acute Gynaecological Unit. Book 2

205

50

This woman was referred with a history of LIF pain and positive pregnancy test result.

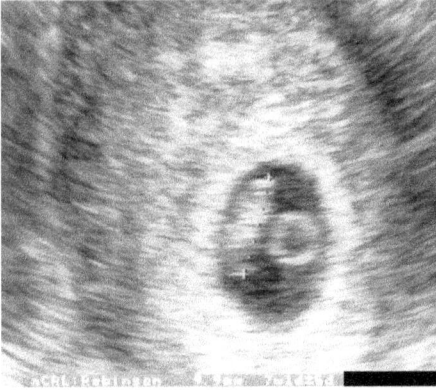
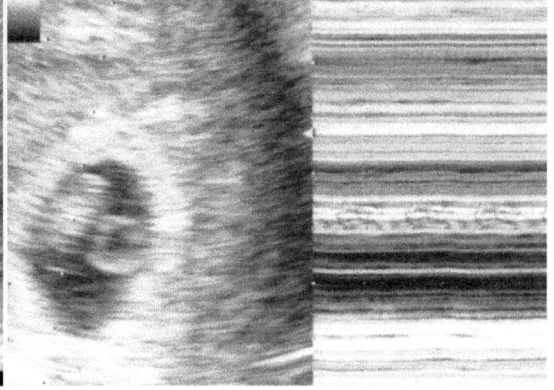

7.50a   7.50b

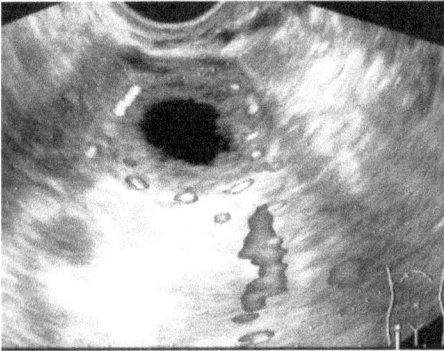
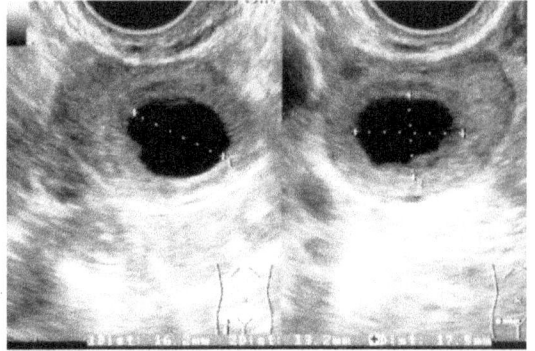

7.50c   7.50d

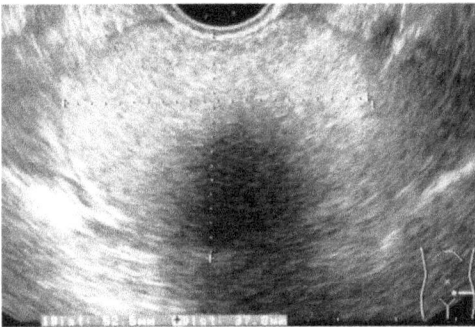
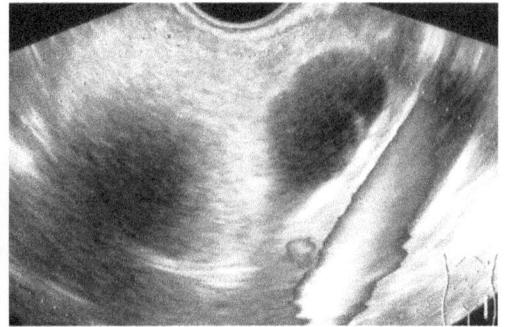

7.50e   7.50f

Ultrasound Services in an Early Pregnancy and Acute Gynaecological Unit. Book 2

206

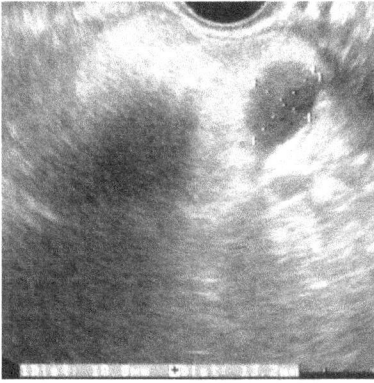

7.50g

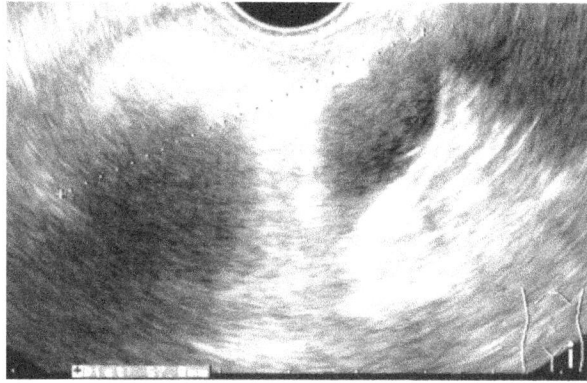

7.50h

a. Is there any ultrasound identifiable reason for this woman's pain?
b. How are 7.50c-d different from 7.50 e-h?
c. Write the ultrasound report.

51
These are from two different patients. Both pregnancies are ongoing.

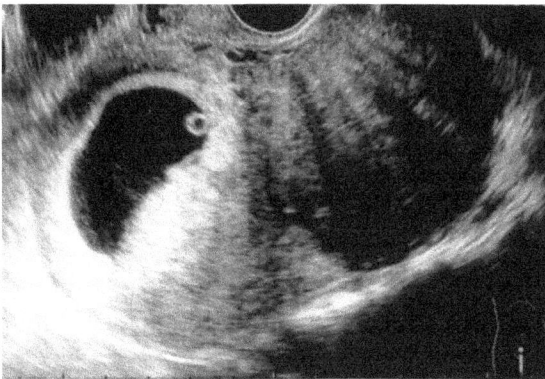

7.51a.

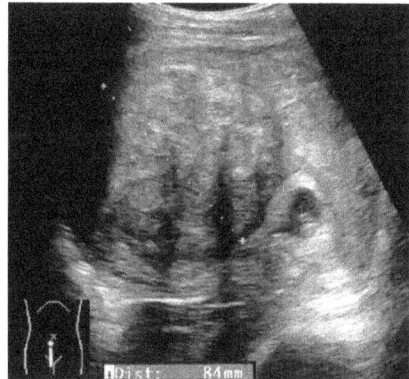

7.51b.

a. What is the similarity in 7.51a. and b.
b. What is the difference in 7.51a. and b.
c. In what ways could the common finding affect the pregnancies?

Ultrasound Services in an Early Pregnancy and Acute Gynaecological Unit. Book 2

207

52

This woman was referred with a PMH of 2 ectopic pregnancies. Currently having pain and tenderness in the RIF. Below were the images of her scan on day 21.

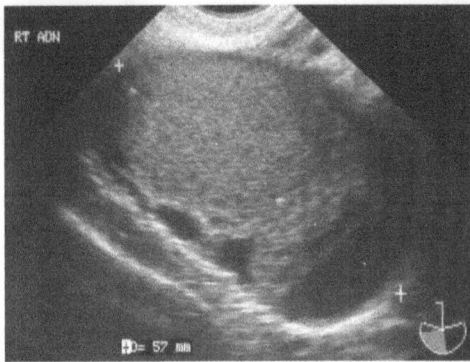

7.52a

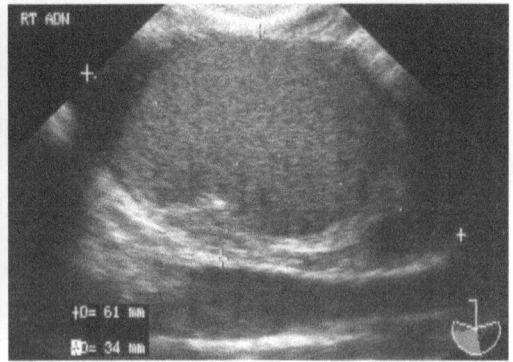

7.52b

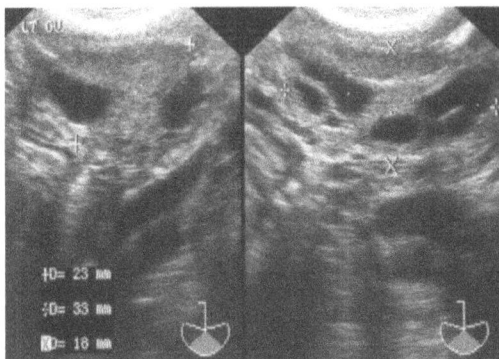

7.52c

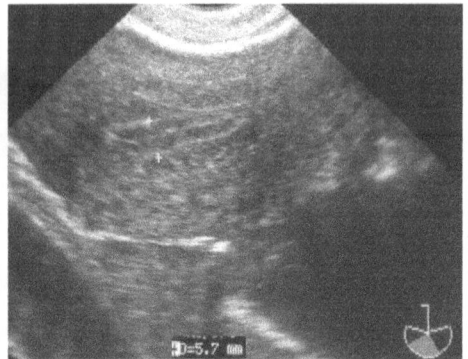

7.52d

a.   Is there anything that may explain the pain and tenderness in the RIF?

b.   Write an ultrasound report.

c.   What is the ultrasound diagnosis.

Ultrasound Services in an Early Pregnancy and Acute Gynaecological Unit. Book 2

208

53
This woman was referred with a history of ovarian cyst.

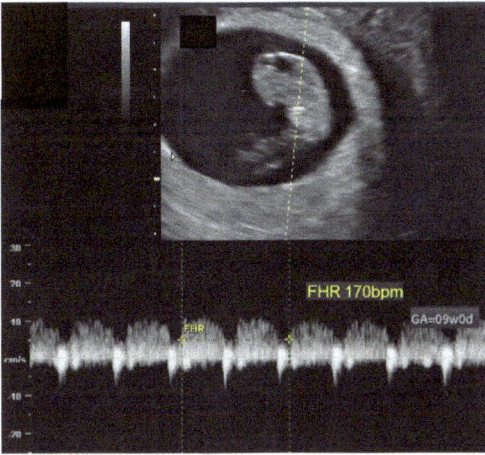

53a

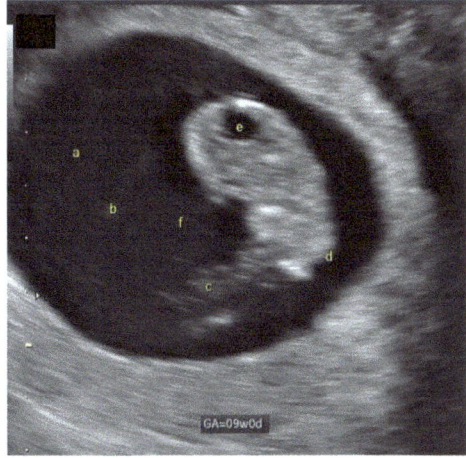

53b

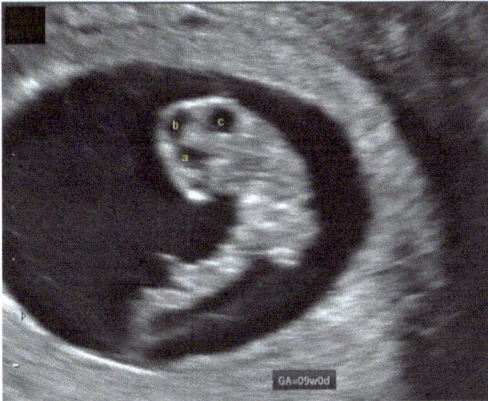

53c

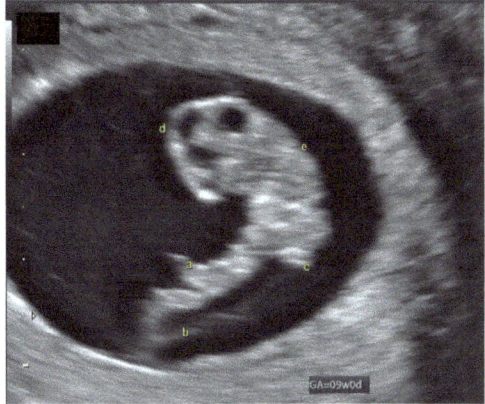

53d

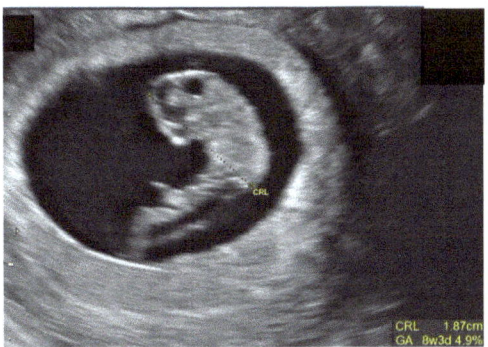

53e

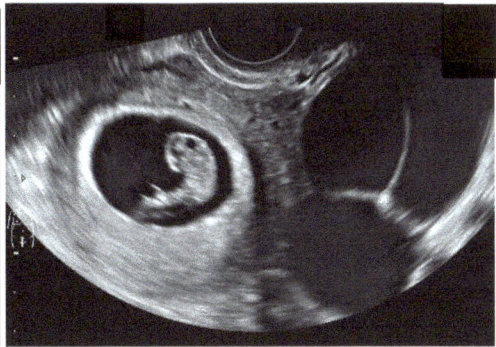

53f

Ultrasound Services in an Early Pregnancy and Acute Gynaecological Unit. Book 2

209

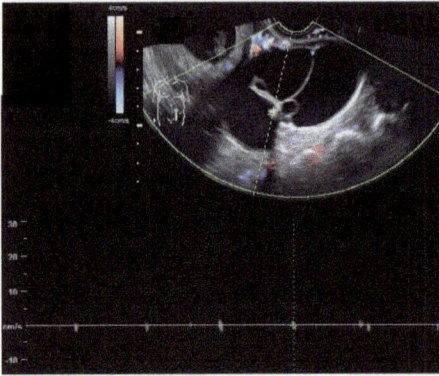
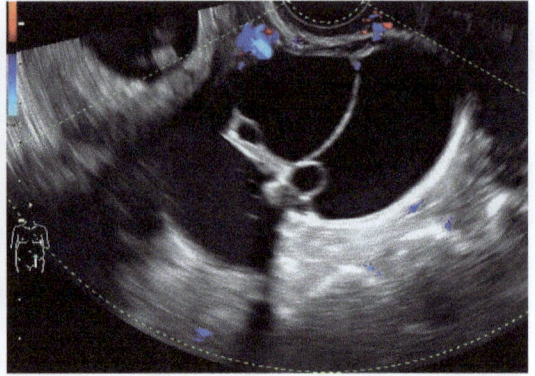

53g   **53h**

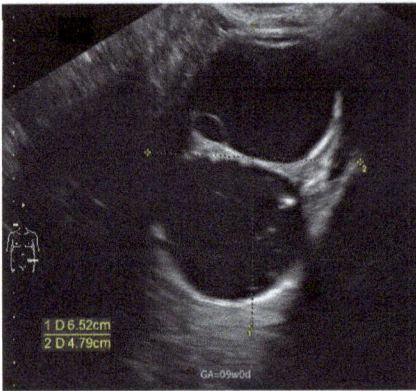
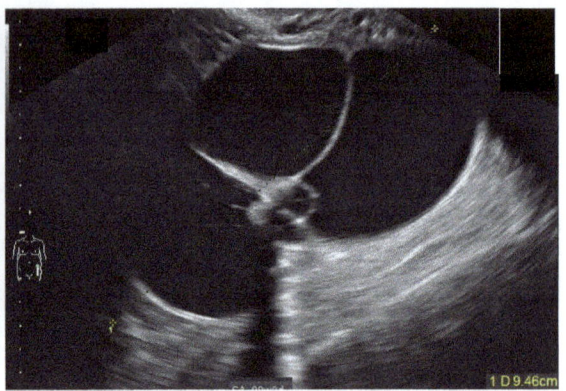

53i   **53j**

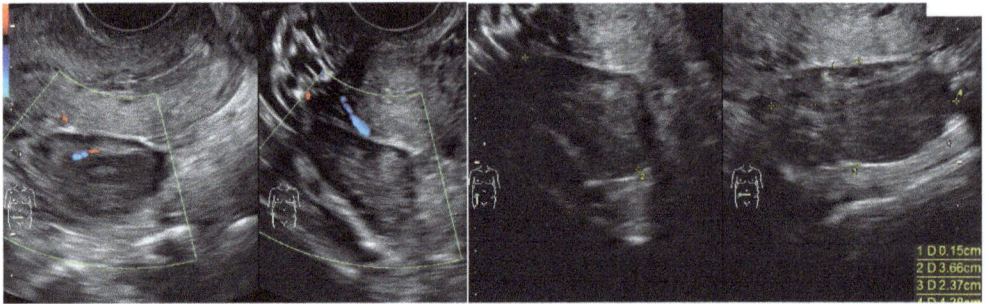

53k   **53l** 37 x 24 x 43mm

Ultrasound Services in an Early Pregnancy and Acute Gynaecological Unit. Book 2

210

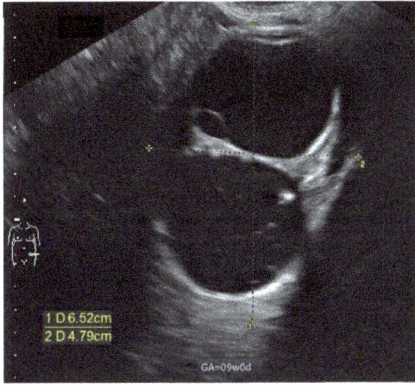

53k

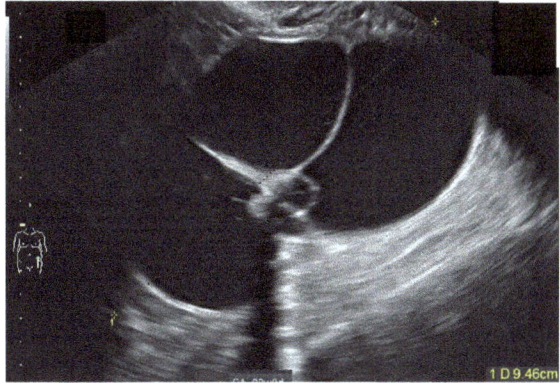

53l

a. Identify the labeled parts in 53b-d
b. Is the heart rate normal in 53a?
c. Would she require any other investigation why or why not and what or which investigation?
d. Write the ultrasound report

54

This woman was referred with a history of abdominal and pelvic pain for 3/7, heavy pv. bleeding. PMH TOP a month ago. Right ovary was not visualized.

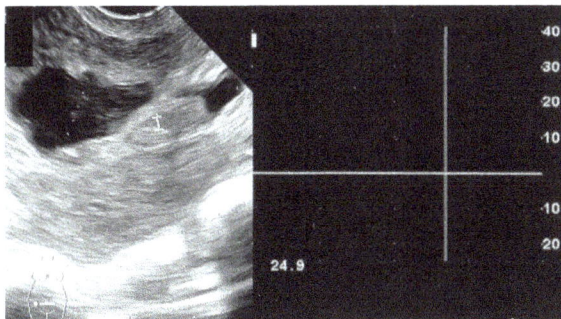

54a

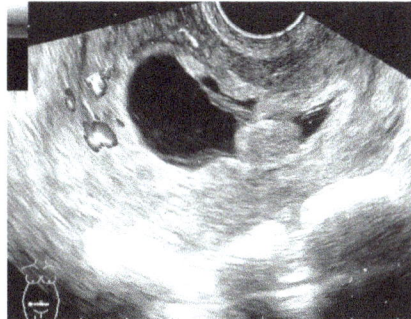

54b

Ultrasound Services in an Early Pregnancy and Acute Gynaecological Unit. Book 2

211

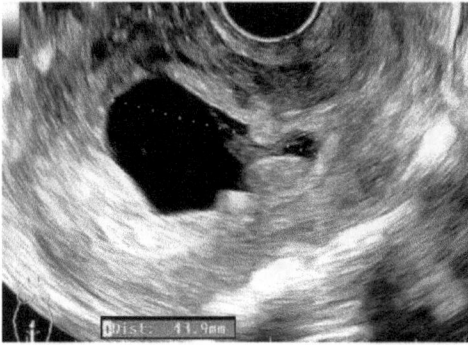

54c

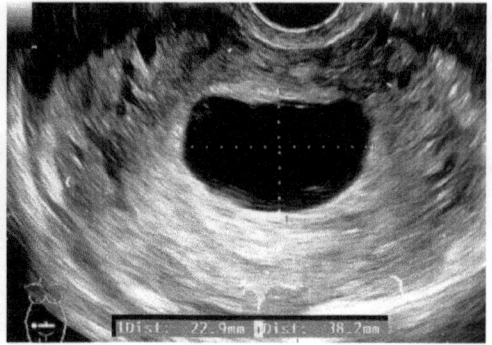

54d

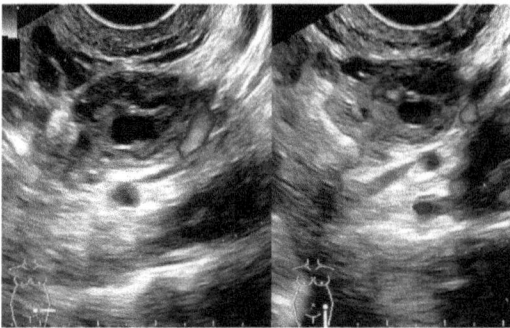

54e

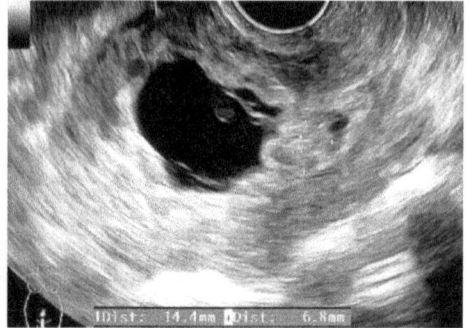

54f

e. Is there any ultrasound findings that explains the heavy pv. bleeding?
f. Write an ultrasound report.
g. What is the clinical impression?

Ultrasound Services in an Early Pregnancy and Acute Gynaecological Unit. Book 2

212

55

This woman was referred for a scan at 18+/40 with a history of 1/7 pv bleed. Measurements obtainable were equal to date, FHB and movements not shown were noted. No previous maternal abdominal surgery.

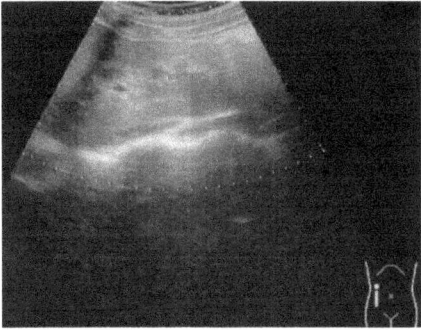

55a

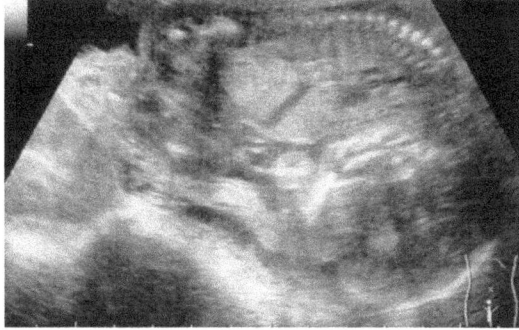

55b

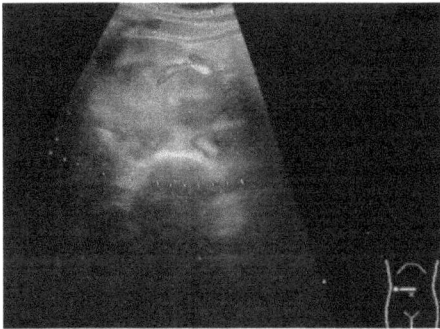

55c

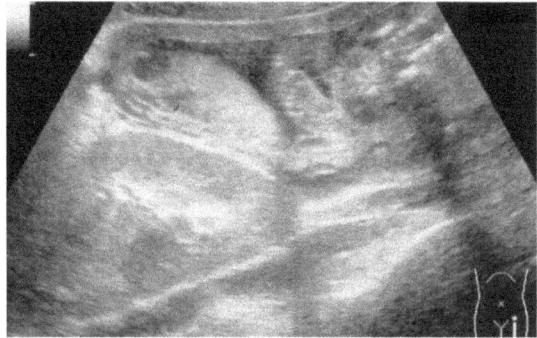

55d

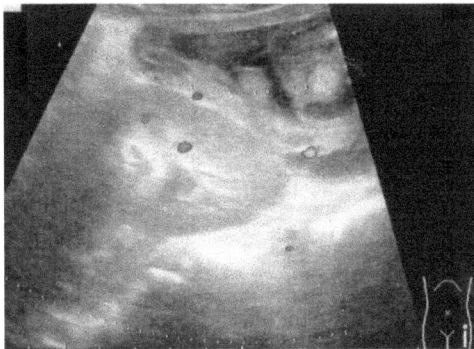

55e

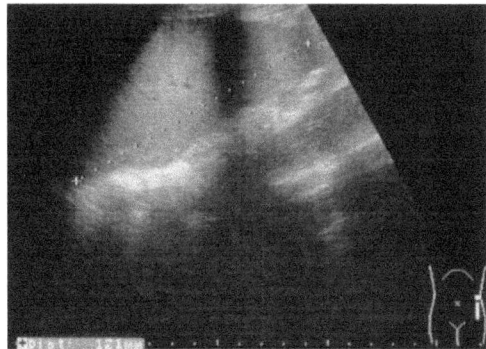

55f

a.   Can you identify anything that may make the examination difficult or measurements un obtainable?

Ultrasound Services in an Early Pregnancy and Acute Gynaecological Unit. Book 2

213

b.   b. What is the accidental finding in this case?

56

This woman was referred with a history of 4/7 pv bleeding at 16+5 /40. Below are the ultrasound findings. Fetal measurements = dates. FHB and movements were noted.

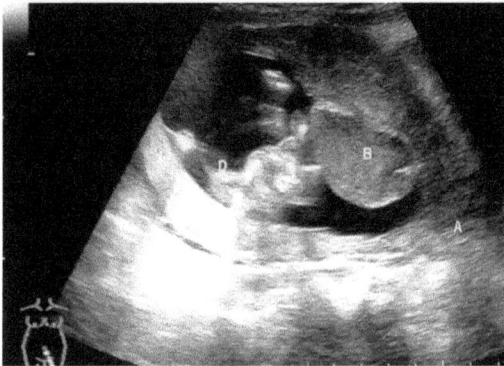

56a

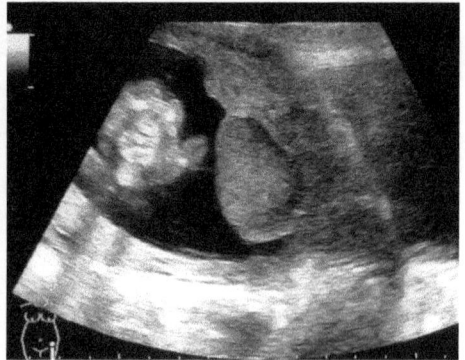

56b

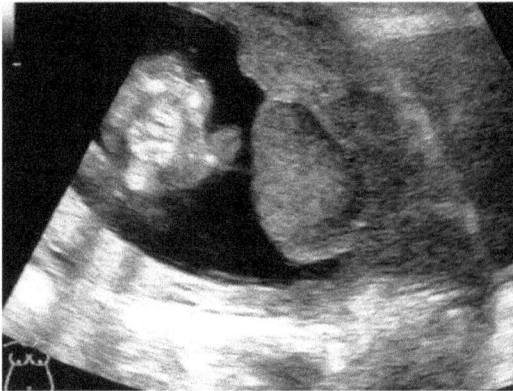

56c

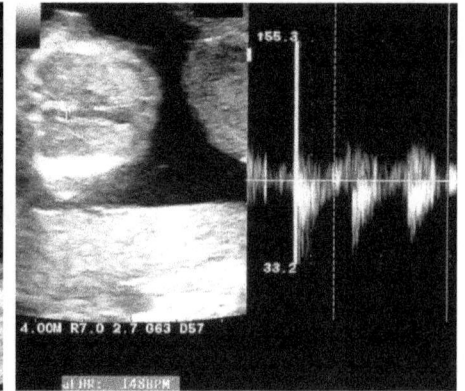

56d

Ultrasound Services in an Early Pregnancy and Acute Gynaecological Unit. Book 2

214

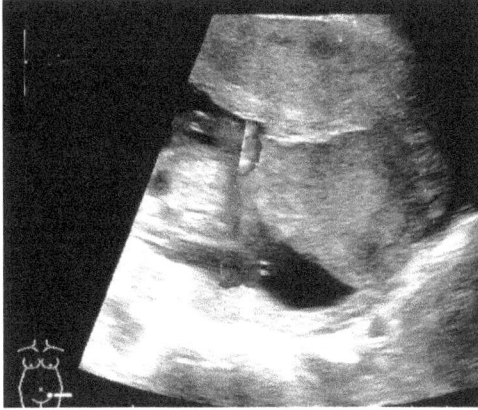
56e

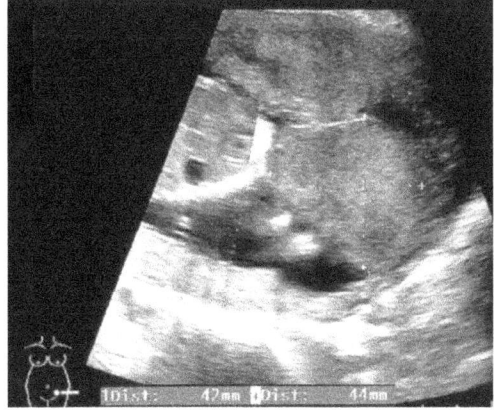
56f

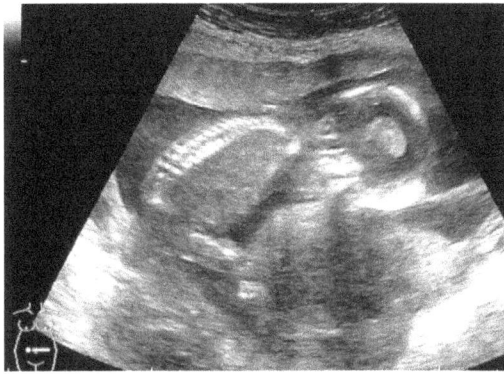
56g

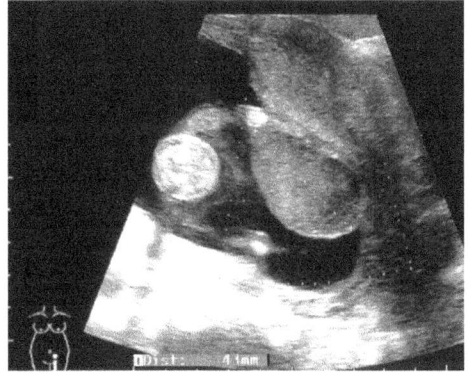
58h

a. Identify a-d in the 56a

b. Is there any evidence or cause for pv bleed identified?

c. What is the significance of this finding?

57

This woman was referred following fertility treatment with a history of maternal anxiety and heavy pv bleeding. Multiple corpus luteal cysts were noted.

Ultrasound Services in an Early Pregnancy and Acute Gynaecological Unit. Book 2

215

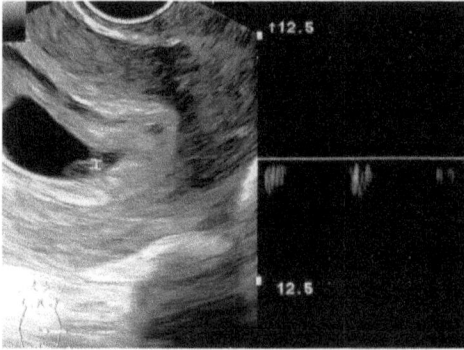

57a

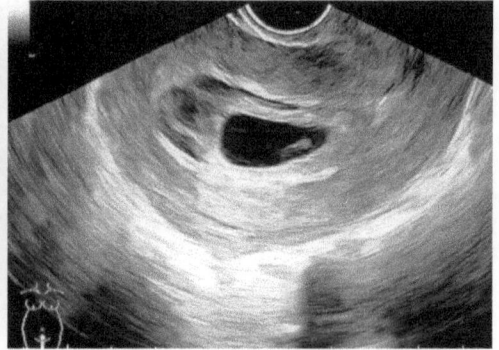

57b

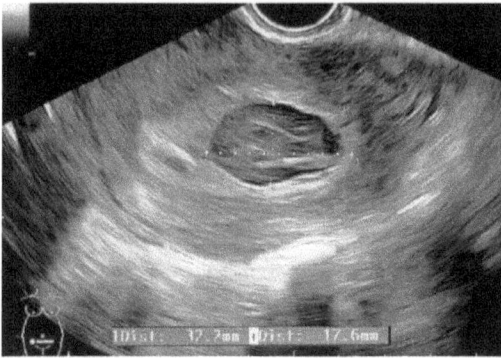

57c

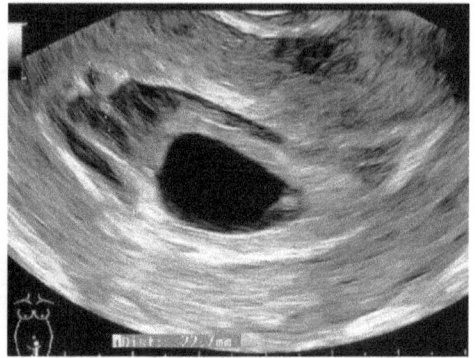

57d

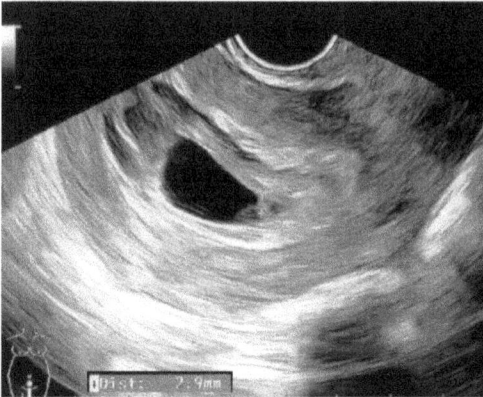

57e

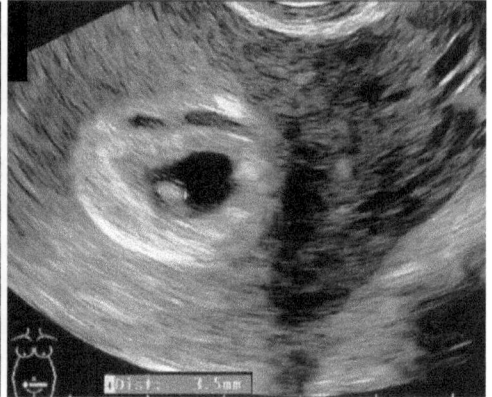

57f

a. What other information's does the sonographer needs and why?
b. Is there any ultrasound identifiable cause for pv bleeding seen?
c. What else may the sonographer be able or not able to exclude?
d. Write an ultrasound report.

Ultrasound Services in an Early Pregnancy and Acute Gynaecological Unit. Book 2

216

58

This woman was referred for a scan with a history of abdominal pain, positive pregnancy test result and unsure LMP.

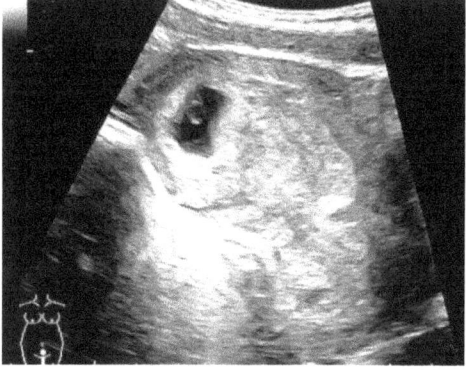

58a   CRL =3.8mm

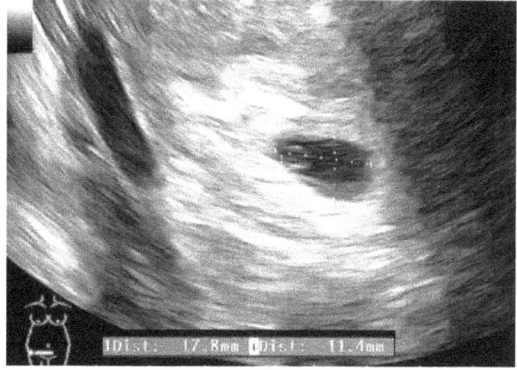

58b

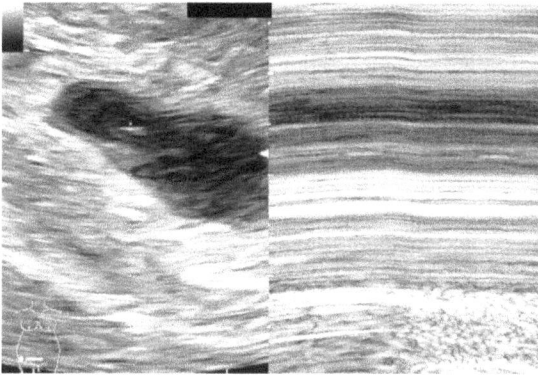

58c

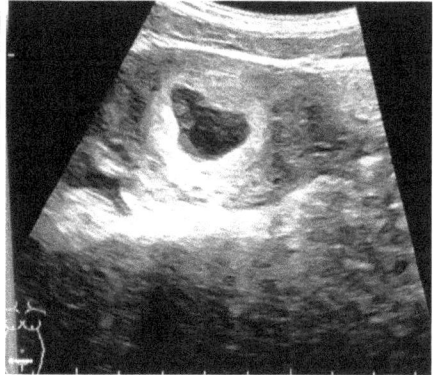

58d

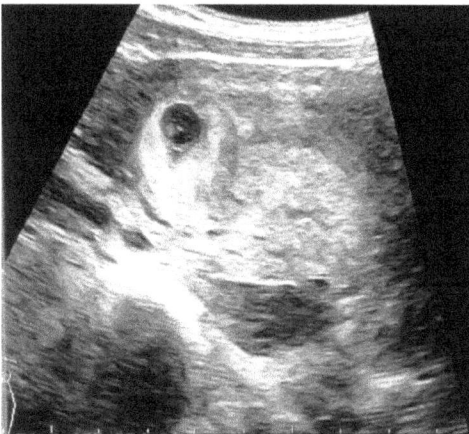

58e

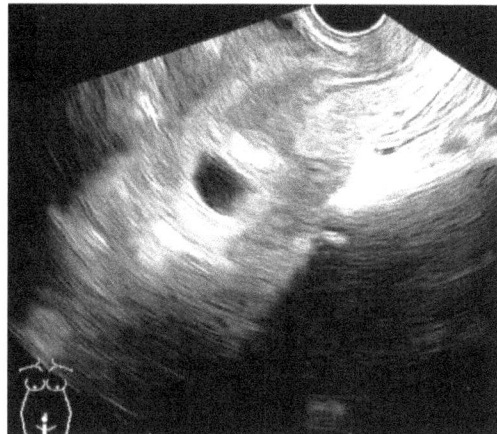

58f

Ultrasound Services in an Early Pregnancy and Acute Gynaecological Unit. Book 2

217

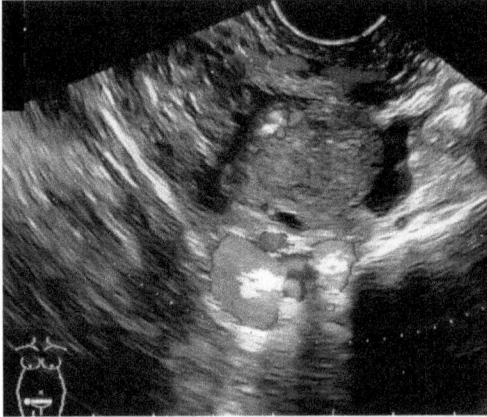

58g

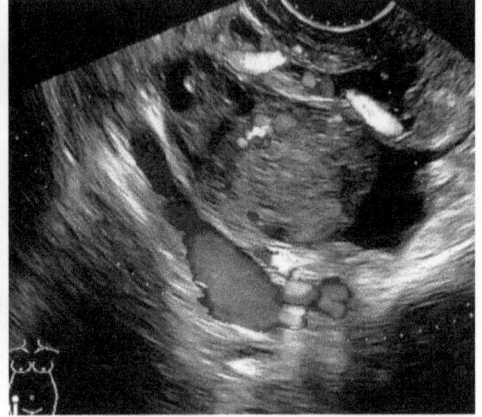

58h

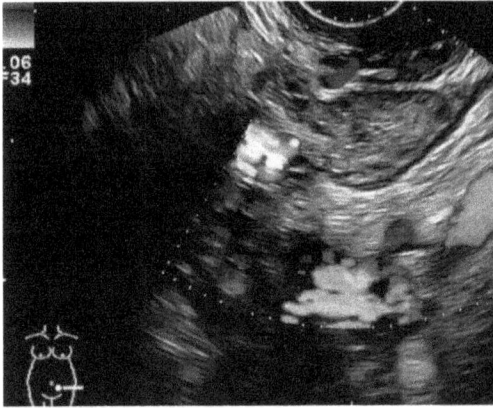

58i

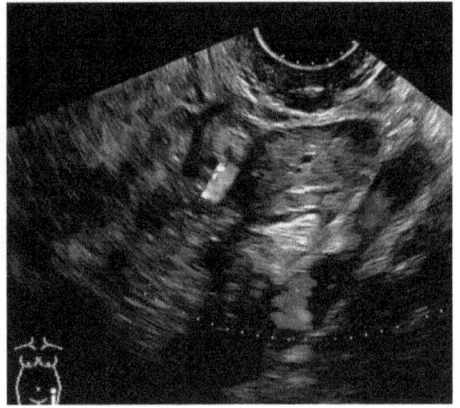

58j

a. Describe the ultrasound findings.

b. Which clinical or ultrasound condition is shown above?

Ultrasound Services in an Early Pregnancy and Acute Gynaecological Unit. Book 2

218

59

This woman was referred for a follow up scan at 10+/40.

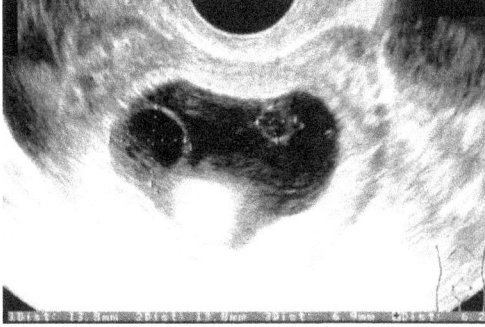

59a

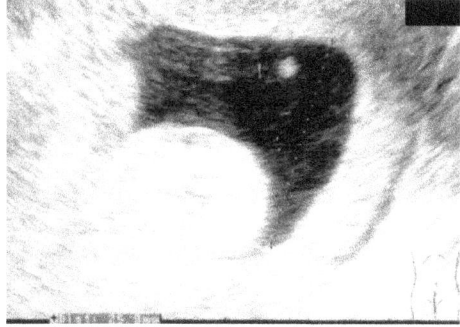

59b

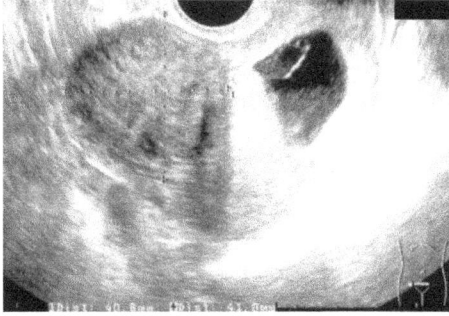

59c

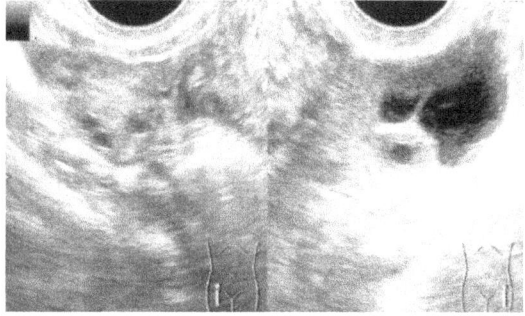

59d

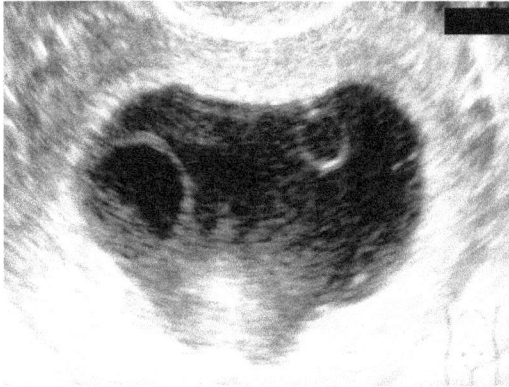

59e

a. Describe the ultrasound findings
b. What is the likely condition seen above?

Ultrasound Services in an Early Pregnancy and Acute Gynaecological Unit. Book 2

219

60

This woman was referred with a history of previous 4cm right intermitted torted cyst. LMP was about two weeks before this examination and she was not in any pain at the time of the examination. 1st examination in the unit. Previous ultrasound images or report was not available.

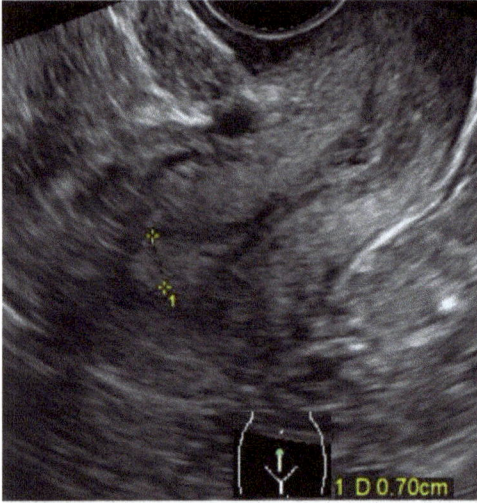

60a

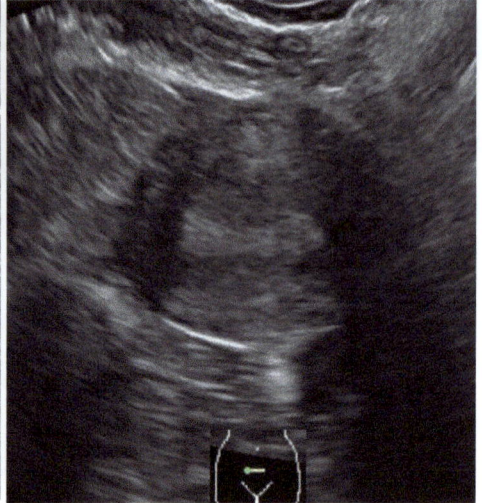

60b

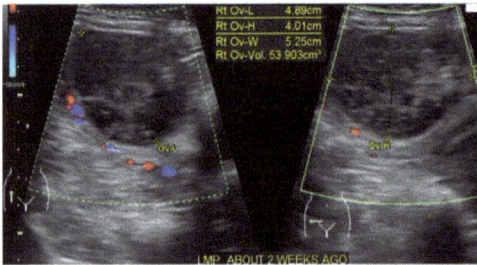

60c

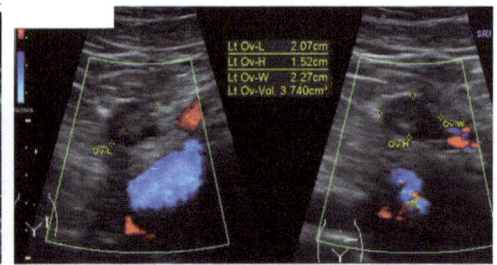

60d

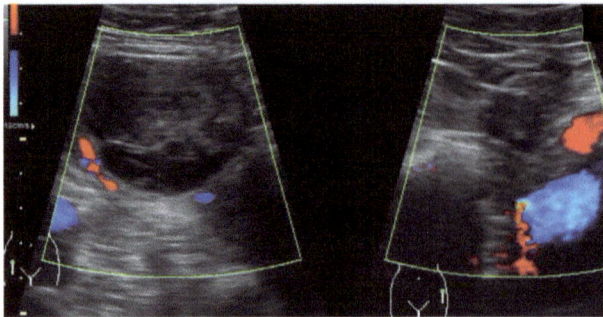

60e

Ultrasound Services in an Early Pregnancy and Acute Gynaecological Unit. Book 2

220

a. Is there any worrying feature?
b. Write an ultrasound report?
c. What are the ultrasound features or signs of an ovarian torsion
d. What other imaging techniques might be helpful?

61

This woman in her late fifties was referred for a scan with a history of pmb. She has never been on HRT. Menopause over ten years earlier.

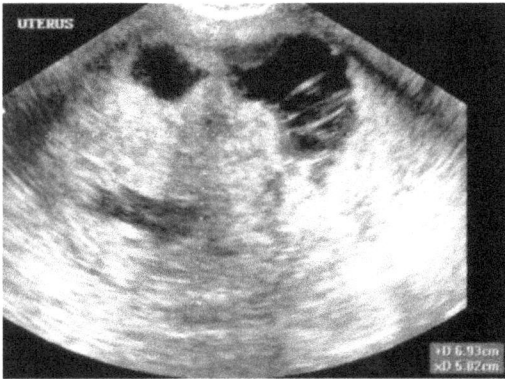

61a

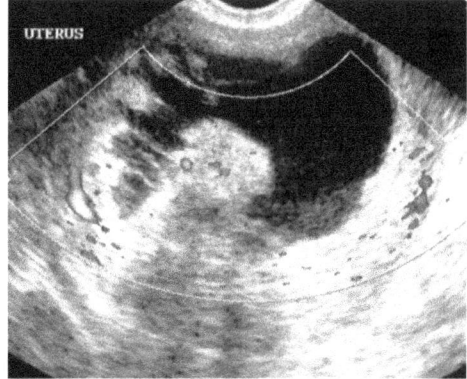

61b

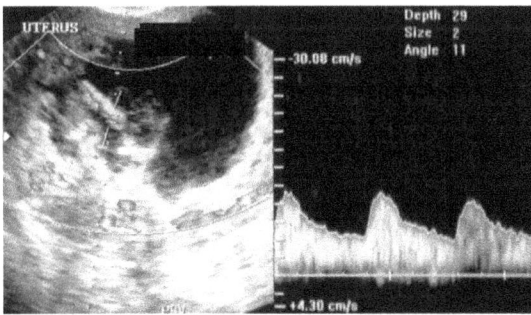

61c

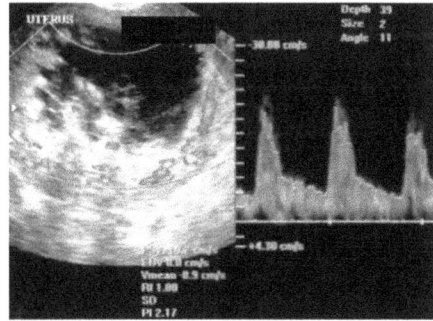

61d

Ultrasound Services in an Early Pregnancy and Acute Gynaecological Unit. Book 2

221

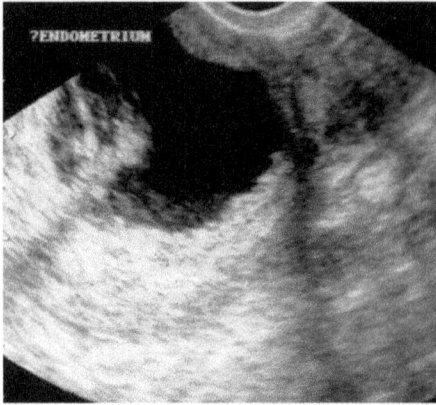

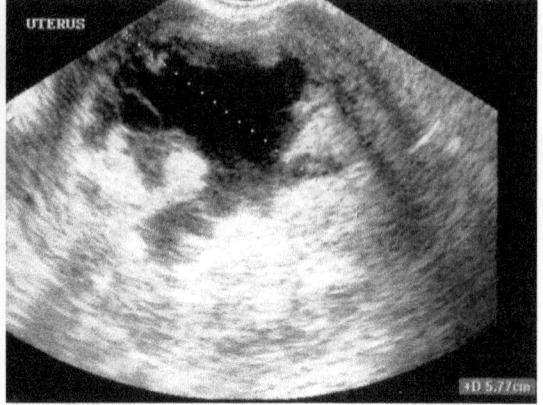

61.e + + = 0.68 mm   **61f**

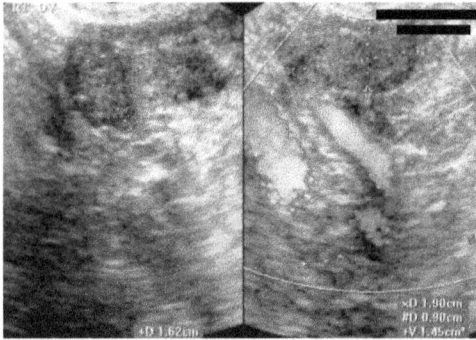

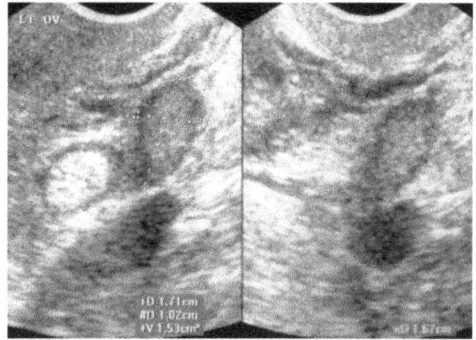

61g   **61h**

a. Describe the ultrasound findings.

b. Would this woman need any follow up, why or why not?

Ultrasound Services in an Early Pregnancy and Acute Gynaecological Unit. Book 2

222

62

This woman was referred with a 2/7 history of pv bleed.

Background history IVF/ovum donation (OD). GA at the time of the scan 8+5/40.

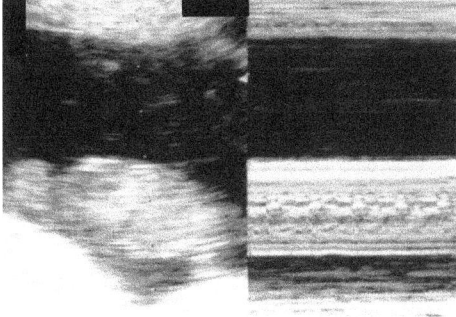
62a

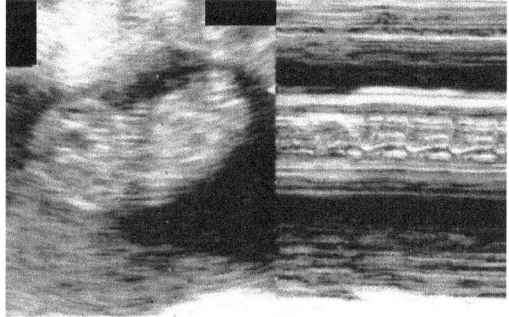
62b

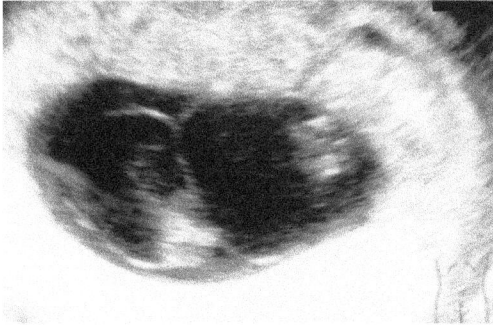
62c

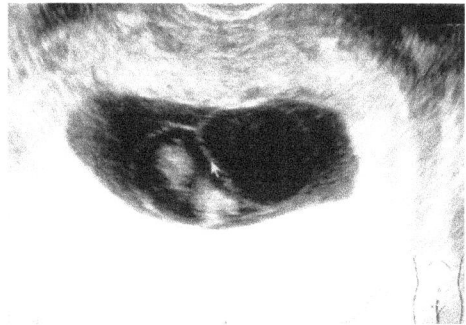
62d

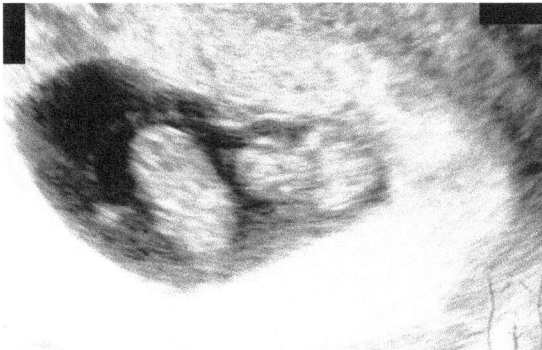
62e

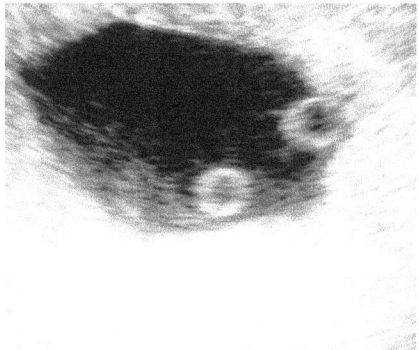
62f

Ultrasound Services in an Early Pregnancy and Acute Gynaecological Unit. Book 2

223

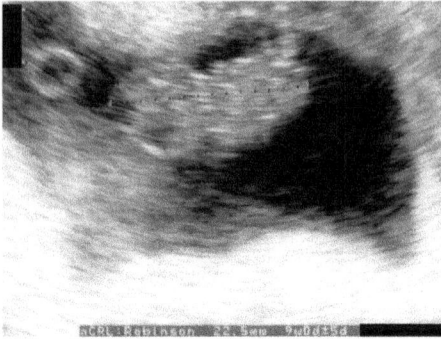

62g

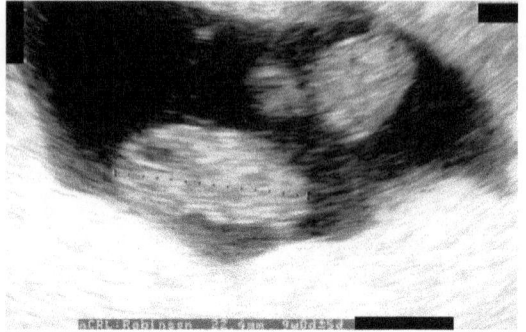

62 h

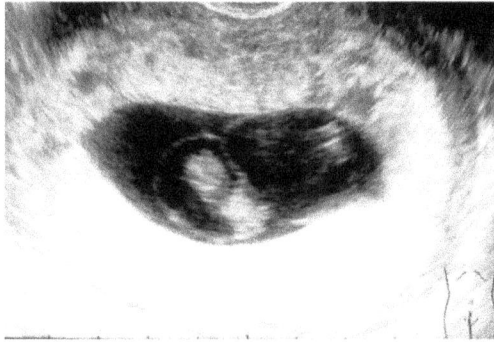

62i.

a. In what ways may or how will her background history affect her ovaries?
b. Which type of pregnancy is this?
c. Write an ultrasound report.
d. What is the role of ultrasound in the future management of this pregnancy?

Ultrasound Services in an Early Pregnancy and Acute Gynaecological Unit. Book 2

224

63

This woman was referred at 11/40 with a history of maternal anxiety and not feeling pregnant again.

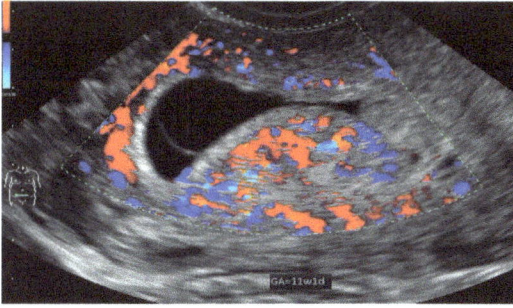

63.a

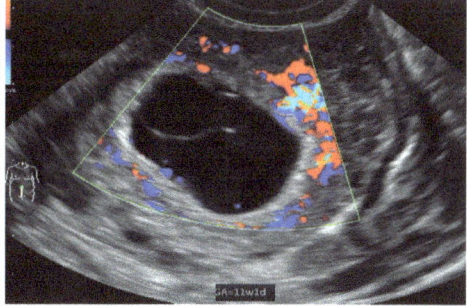

63.b

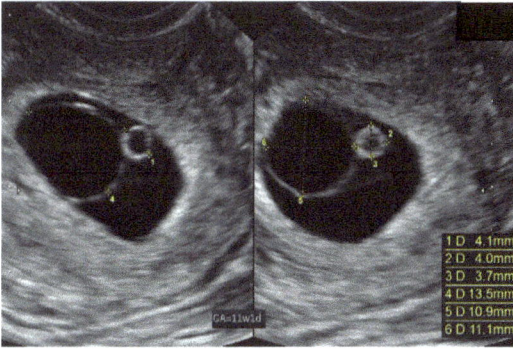

63c

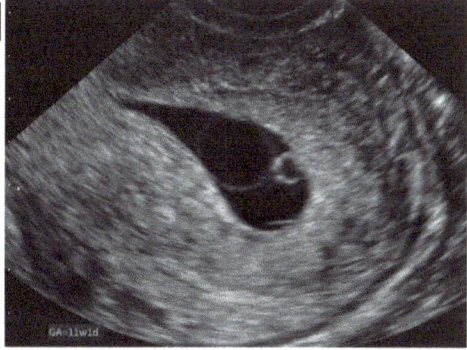

63d

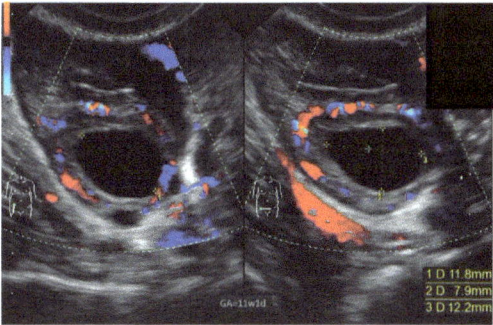

63e

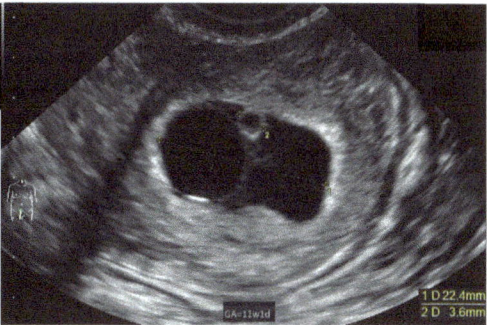

63f

Ultrasound Services in an Early Pregnancy and Acute Gynaecological Unit. Book 2

225

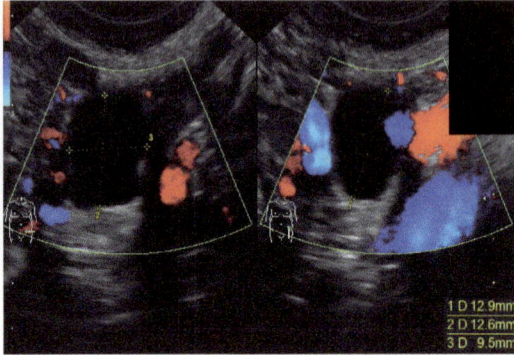

63g

a. Is this patient pregnant or not?

b. Write the ultrasound report

c. What is an empty amnion sign?

64

This woman was referred by the GP with a history of light bleeding for 4/7 at 5+6/40.

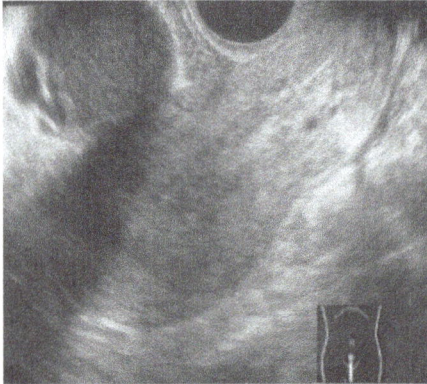

64a

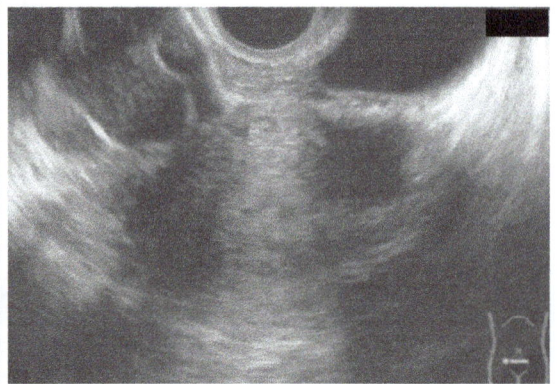

64b

Ultrasound Services in an Early Pregnancy and Acute Gynaecological Unit. Book 2

226

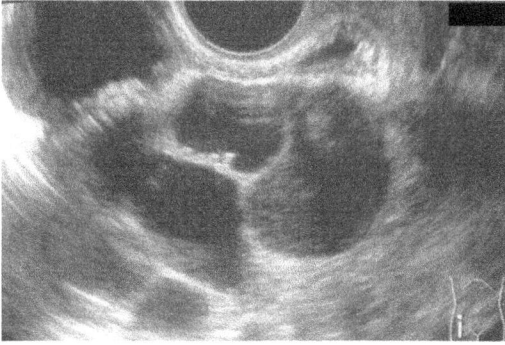

64c

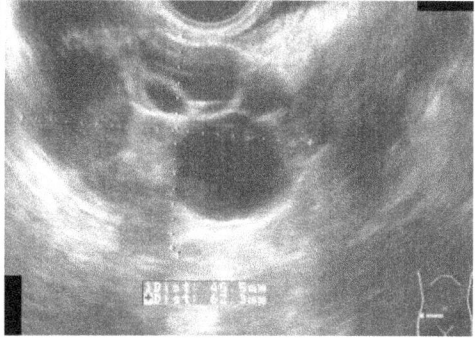

64d

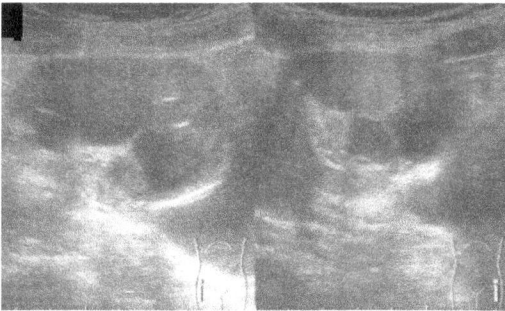

64e

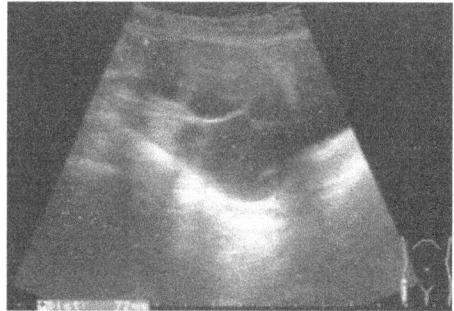

64f

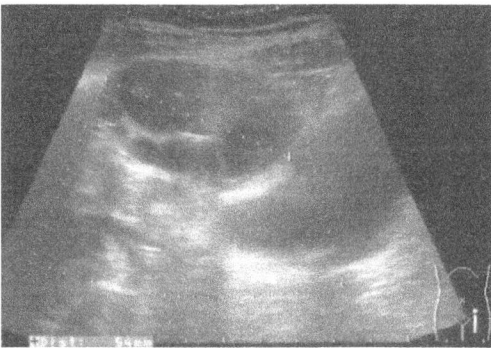

64g

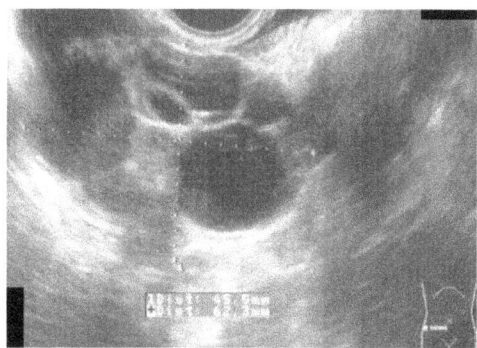

64h

a. Is there any ultrasound identifiable pregnancy?

b. What challenges may the Sonographer experience performing this scan?

c. Which other test should be done to help to confirm the pregnancy or otherwise?

d. Write the ultrasound report

Ultrasound Services in an Early Pregnancy and Acute Gynaecological Unit. Book 2

227

65

This woman was referred with a history of total hysterectomy 3 weeks before and pelvic pain. No peristalsis was seen in 65.a and b.

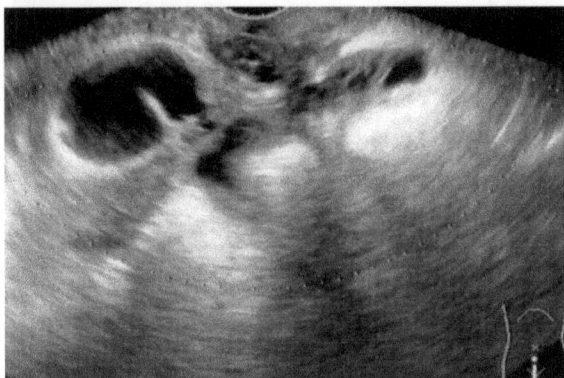

65a

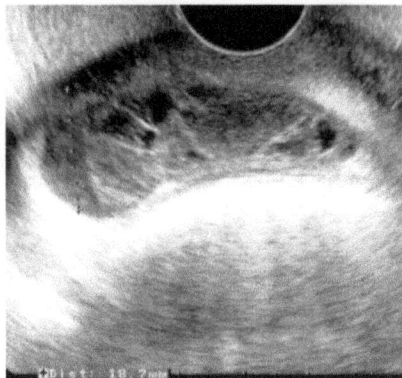

65b

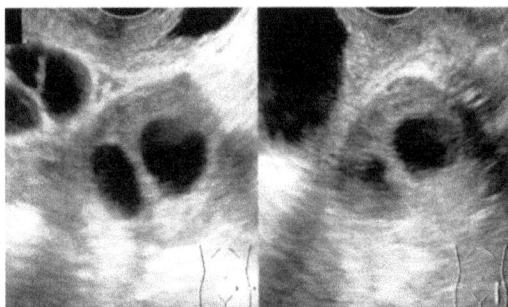

65c

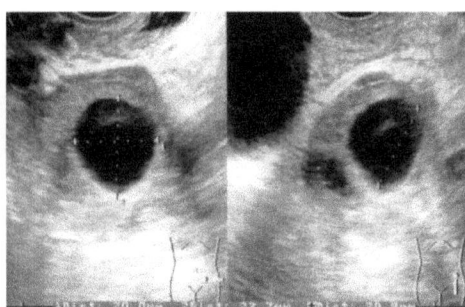

65d

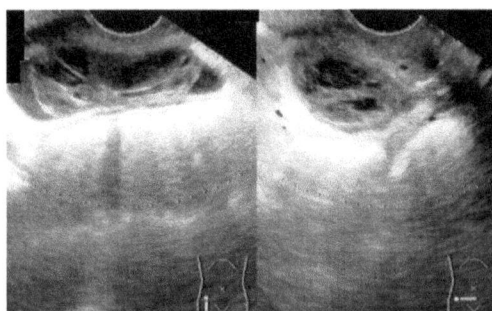

65e

a. What could make the examination challenging for the Sonographer?

b. Describe the ultrasound findings.

c. What is a hydrosalpinx?

d. What causes hydrosalpinx?

e. What are the ultrasound features of a hydrosalpinx?

Ultrasound Services in an Early Pregnancy and Acute Gynaecological Unit. Book 2

228

f. What is the clinical presentation of hydrosalpinx?

g. What is the difference between a hydrosalpinx and a pyosalpinx?

66

This woman was referred with a history of pain and pvb in pregnancy. GA by LMP – 8+1/40. During the examination, the patient was tender in the RIF.

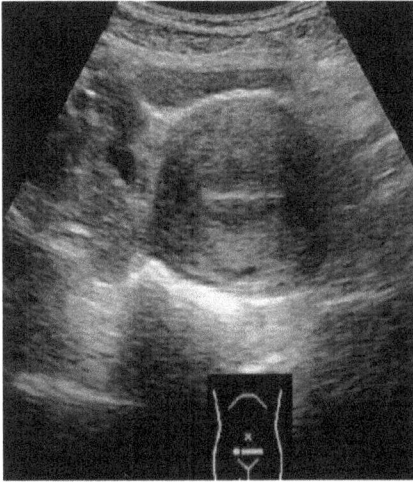

66a

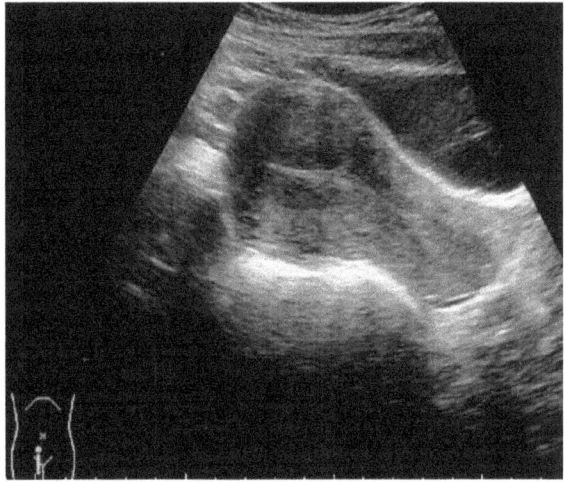

66b

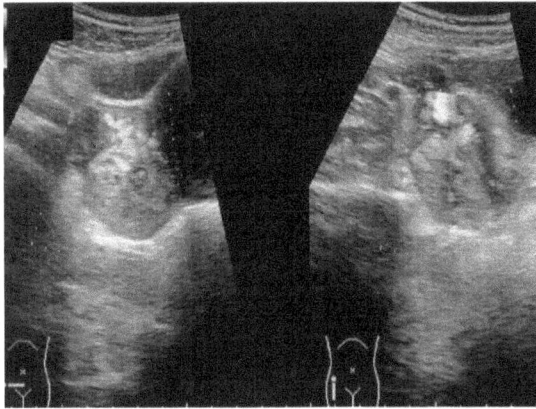

66c

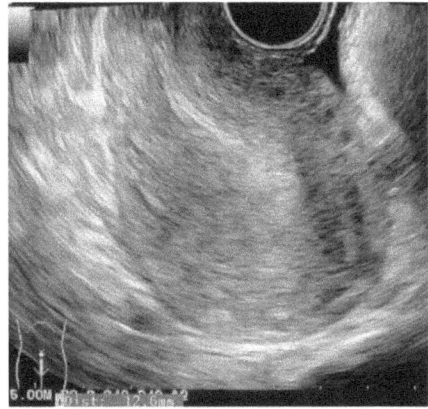

66d

Ultrasound Services in an Early Pregnancy and Acute Gynaecological Unit. Book 2

229

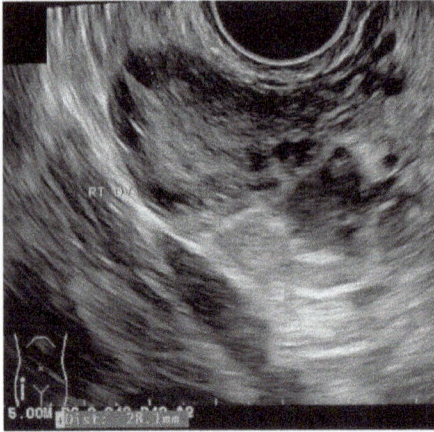

66e

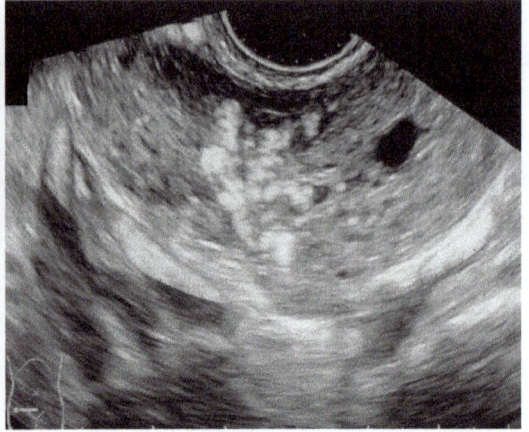

66f

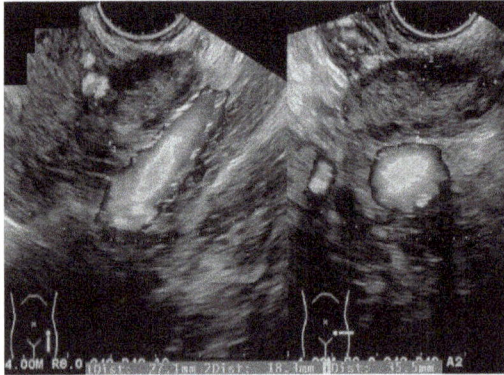

66g

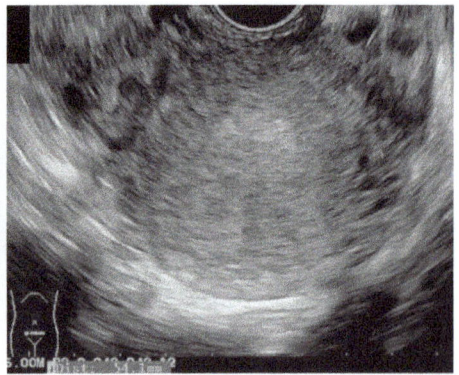

66h

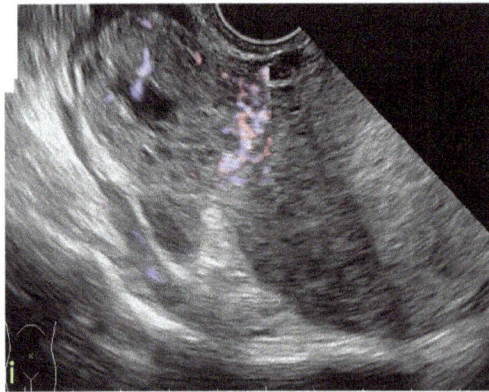

66i

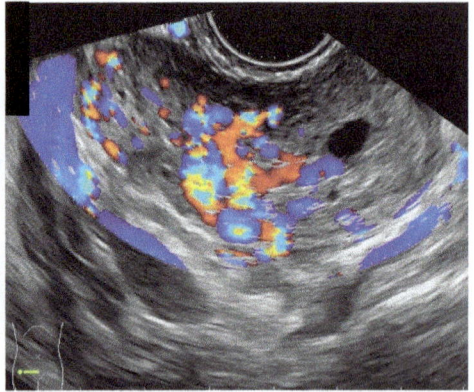

66j

Ultrasound Services in an Early Pregnancy and Acute Gynaecological Unit. Book 2

230

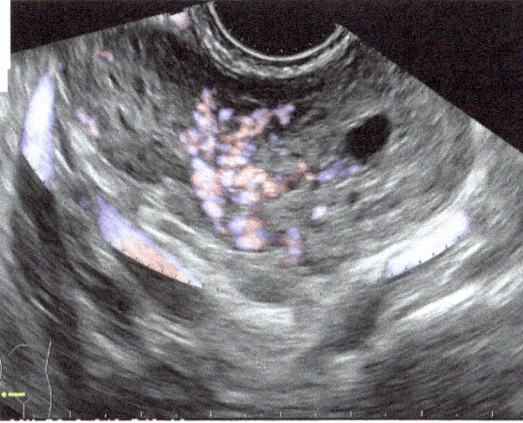

66j

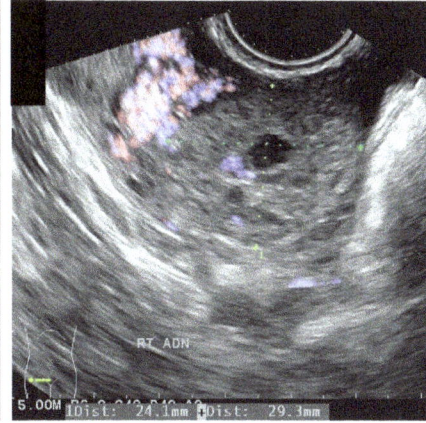

66k.

66

a. Write the ultrasound report.

b. What is a doughnut or bagel's sign?

c. How common is this finding?

67

This woman was referred because of anxiety. GA by LMP = 7/40.

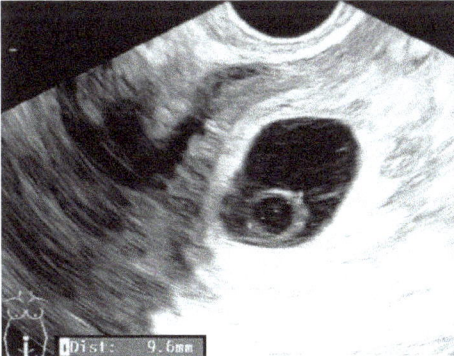

67a

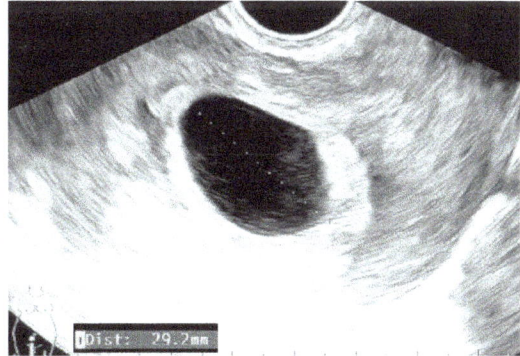

67b

Ultrasound Services in an Early Pregnancy and Acute Gynaecological Unit. Book 2

231

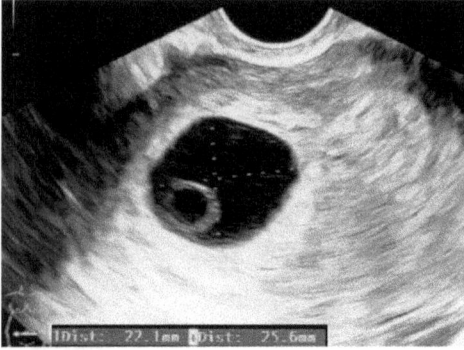

67c

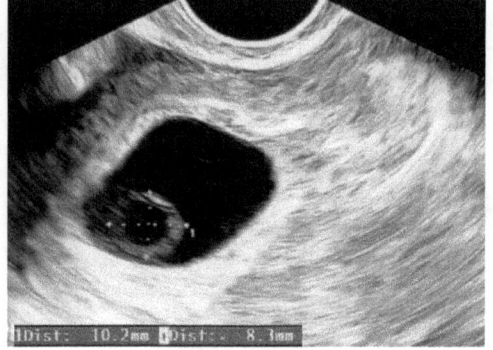

67d

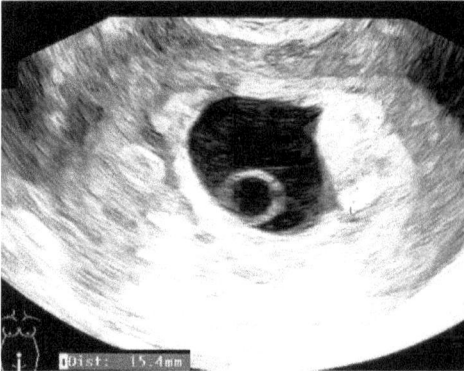

67e

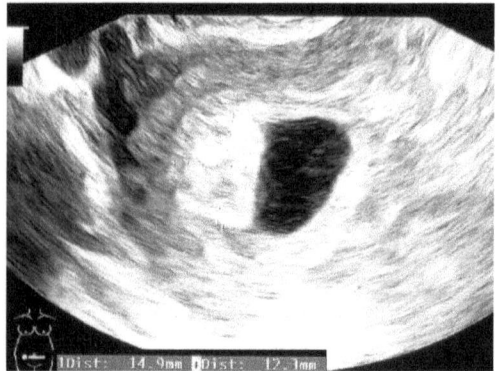

67f

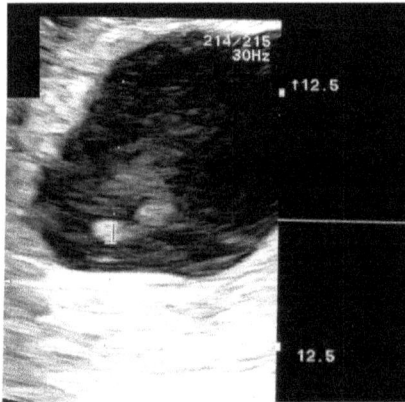

67g

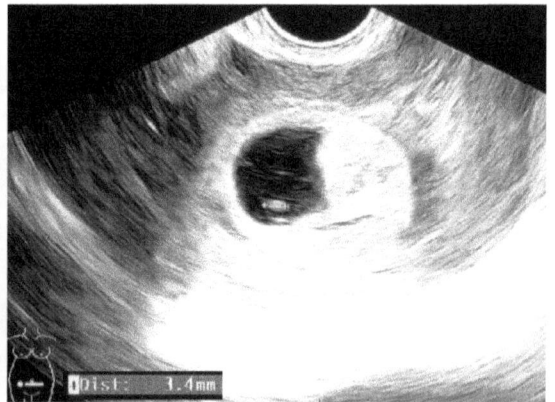

67h

Ultrasound Services in an Early Pregnancy and Acute Gynaecological Unit. Book 2

232

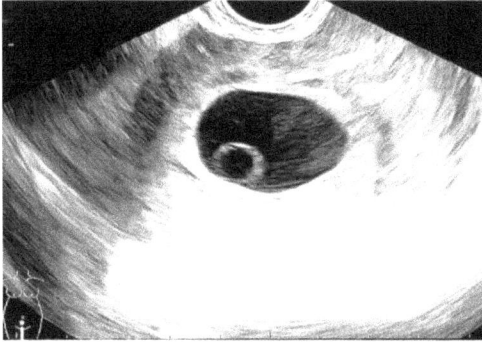

67i

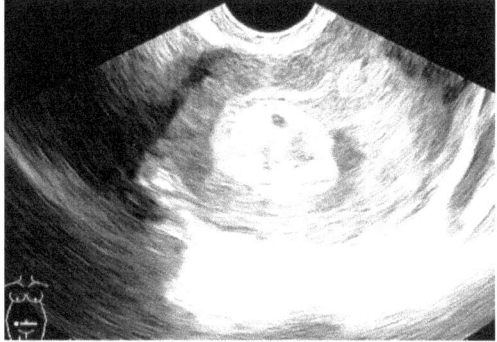

67j

a.   What could have been done to improve the quality of the images?
b.   Are there any worry some things on the images?
c.   Please write the scan report based on the images above.
d.   Should the Sonographer bring this woman back and why or why not?

68

This woman was referred with a history of pain. ?left ovarian cyst. The left ovary was not seen separately. The right ovary not shown here had a corpus luteum in it.

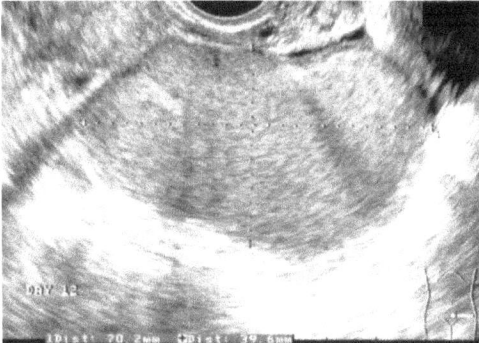

68a

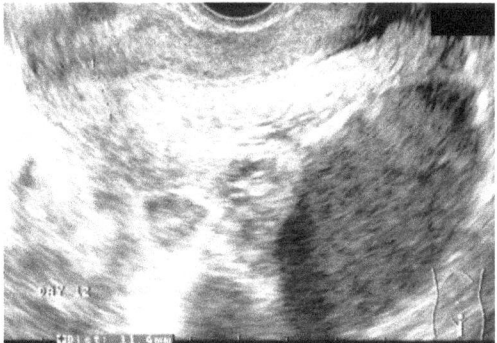

68b

Ultrasound Services in an Early Pregnancy and Acute Gynaecological Unit. Book 2

233

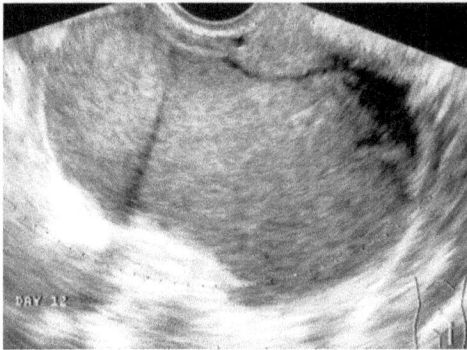

68c

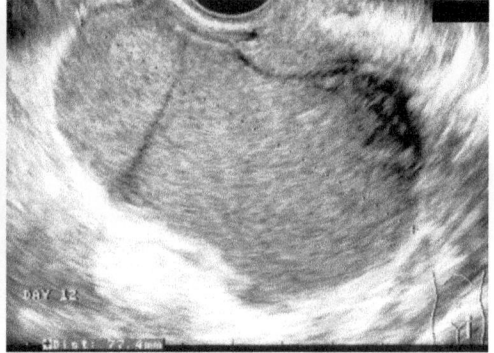

68d

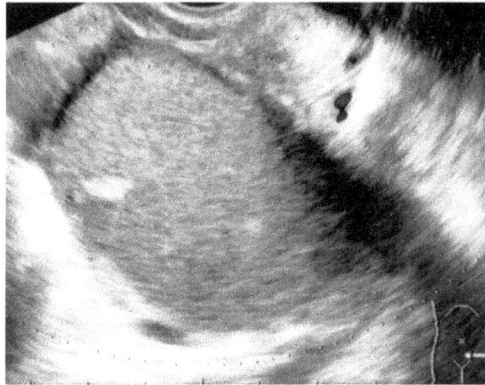

68e

a. Is there any ultrasound identifiable reason for this woman's pain.
b. Write an ultrasound report
c. Which condition may this woman be prone to.

69

This woman was referred with a history of pain in pregnancy. Single fetus with FHR and movements was seen but not shown here. Fetal measurements were equal to dates. Below are the images of the area of her pain.

Ultrasound Services in an Early Pregnancy and Acute Gynaecological Unit. Book 2

234

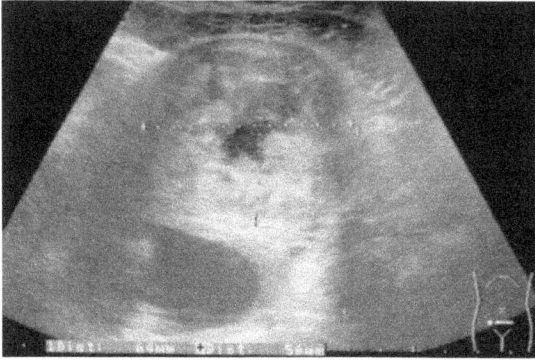
69a

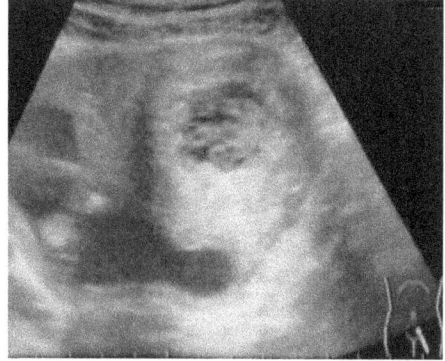
69b

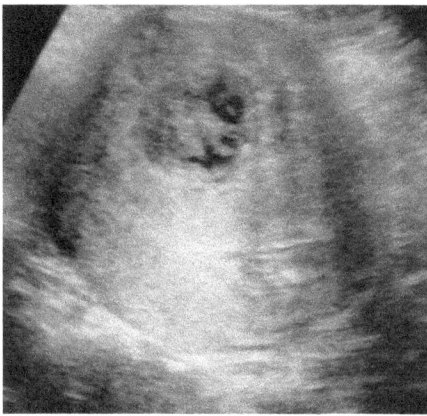
69c

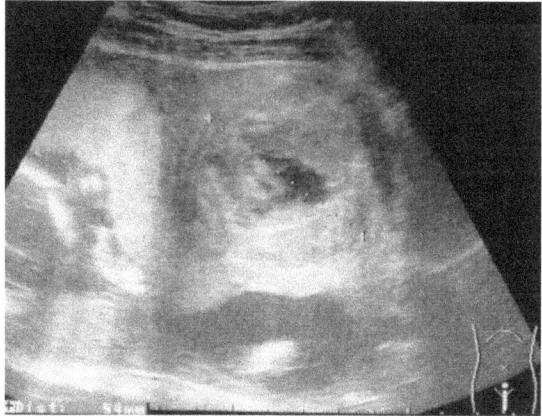
69d

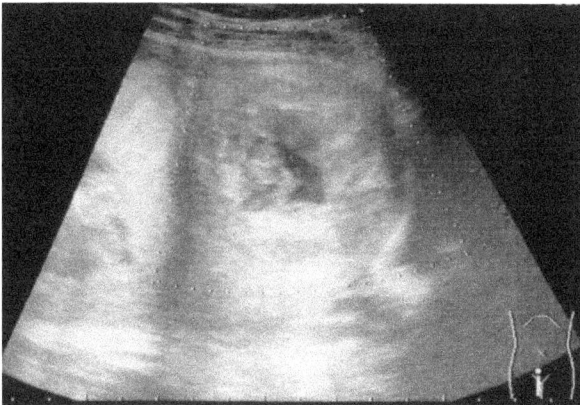
69e

a. Describe the ultrasound findings

b. What is the diagnosis?

Ultrasound Services in an Early Pregnancy and Acute Gynaecological Unit. Book 2

235

70

This woman was referred with a history of RIF pain. She was tender in the area of these findings.

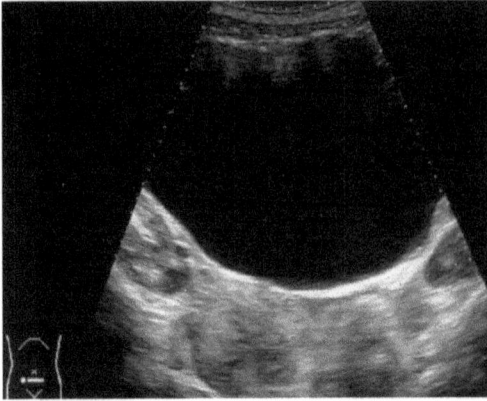

70a

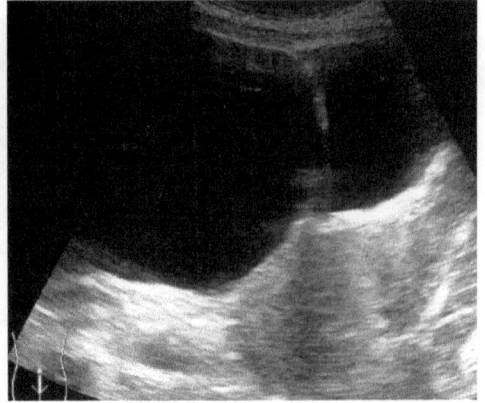

70b

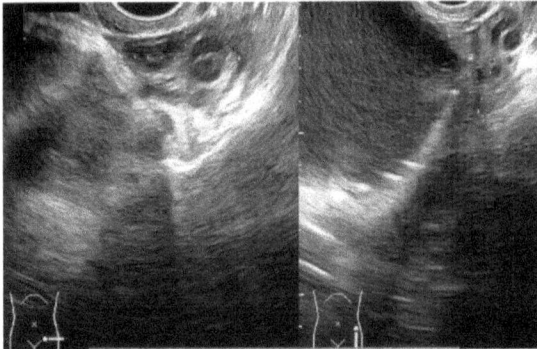

70c ++ 35 x 21 x 29mm

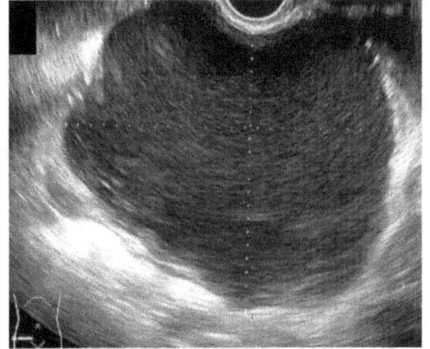

70d ++ 110 x 88mm

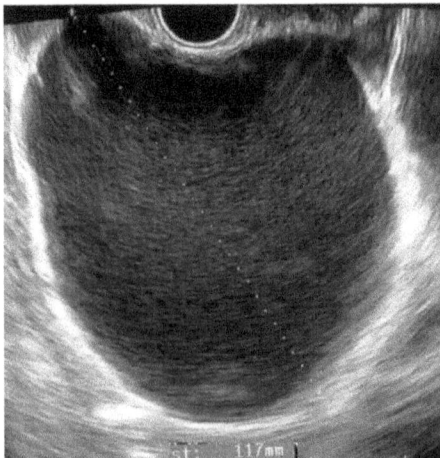

70.e

Ultrasound Services in an Early Pregnancy and Acute Gynaecological Unit. Book 2

236

a. Is there any ultrasound identifiable cause for her pain?

b. Write the ultrasound report.

c. In what ways can ultrasound assist in the management of this woman's pain?

71
This woman was referred with a history of RIF pain. On Zoladex for 3months.

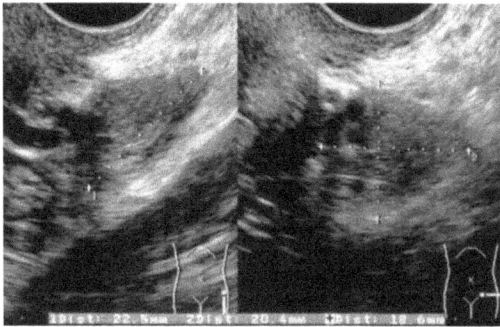
71.a

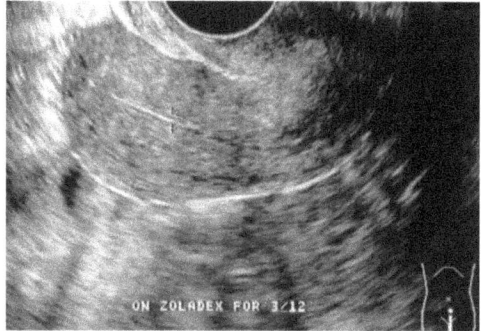
71.b

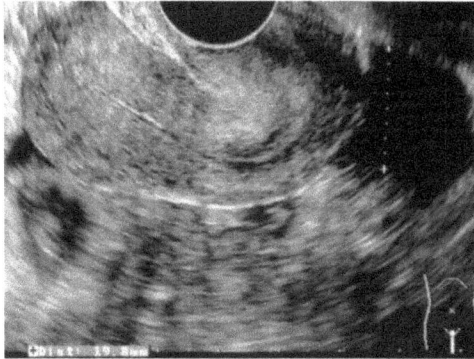
71.c

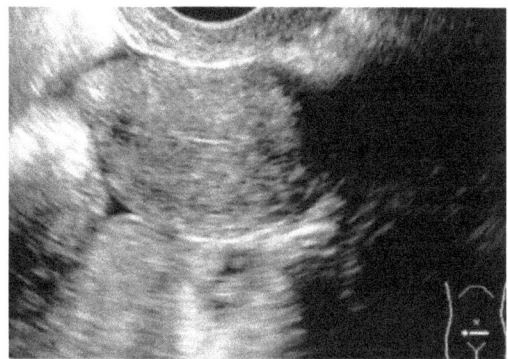
71.d

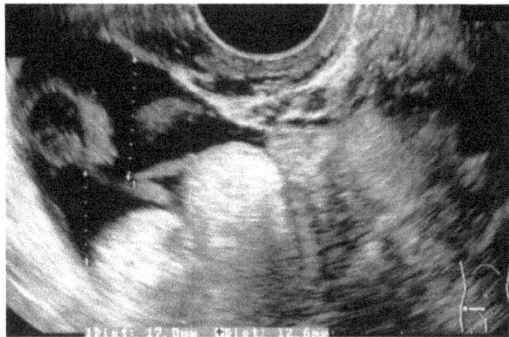
71.e

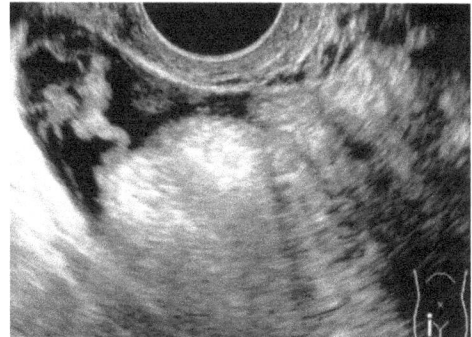
71f

Ultrasound Services in an Early Pregnancy and Acute Gynaecological Unit. Book 2

237

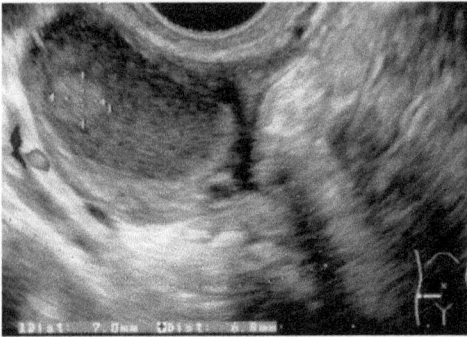
71.g

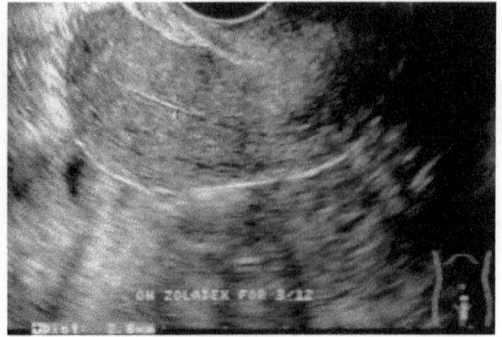
71.h

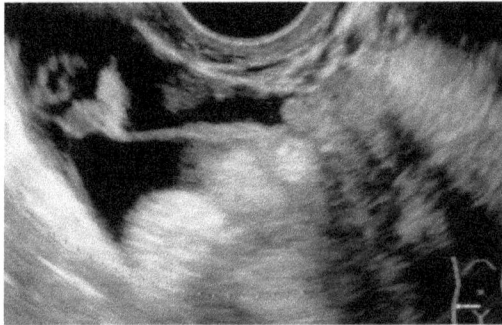
71.i

a. What or which question should the Sonographer ask and why?

b. What is Zoladex and what is it used for in women?

c. Is there any ultrasound identifiable challenge that the Sonographer might have encountered performing this scan?

d. Write the ultrasound report.

Ultrasound Services in an Early Pregnancy and Acute Gynaecological Unit. Book 2

238

72

This woman was referred with a history of PCO, LIF pain. GA according to the patient should be 10/40. FHB not shown was seen.

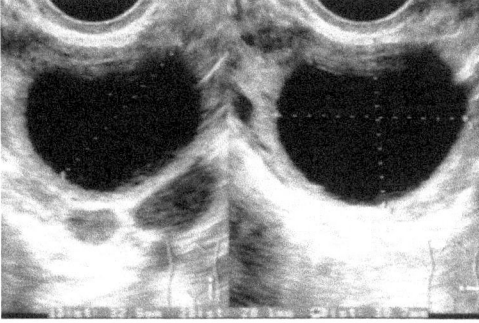

a

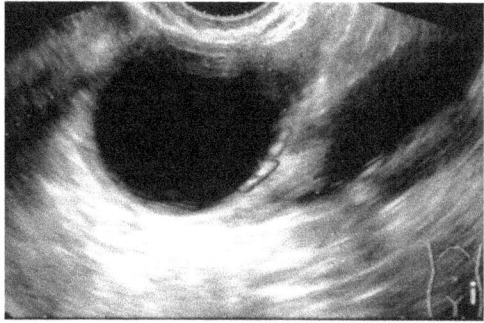

b

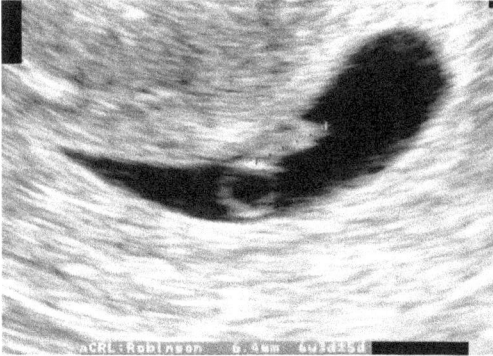

c

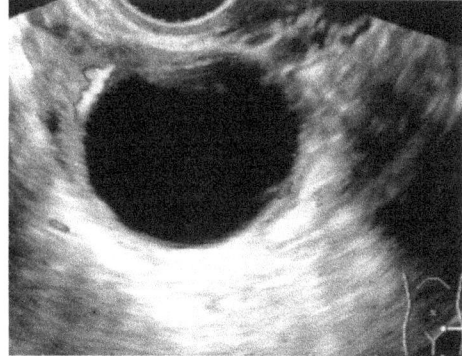

d

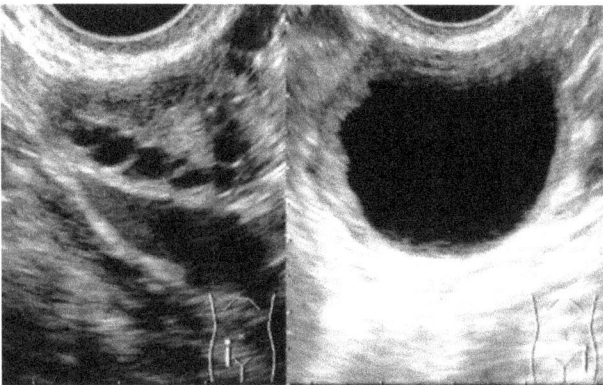

e

a.   Does this woman have PCO?

b.   Should the Sonographer go by the woman's GA calculation? Why or why not?

c.   Write the ultrasound report.

Ultrasound Services in an Early Pregnancy and Acute Gynaecological Unit. Book 2

239

73

This woman was referred for a dating scan at 12+5/30.

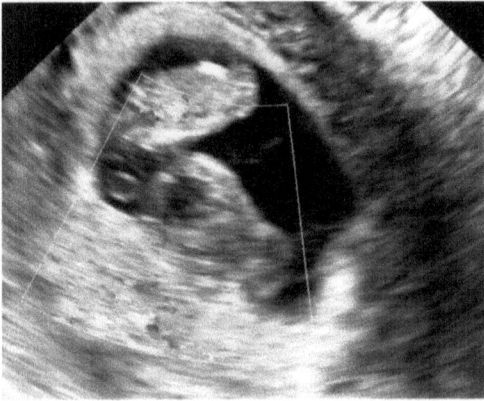

a

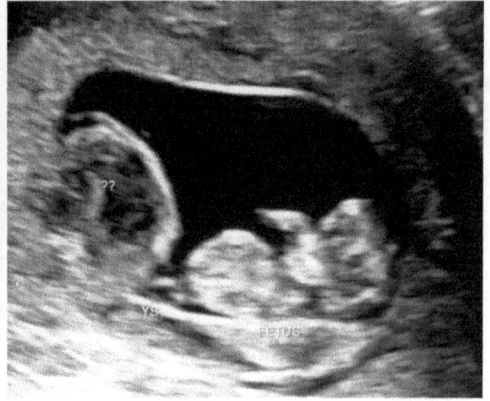

b

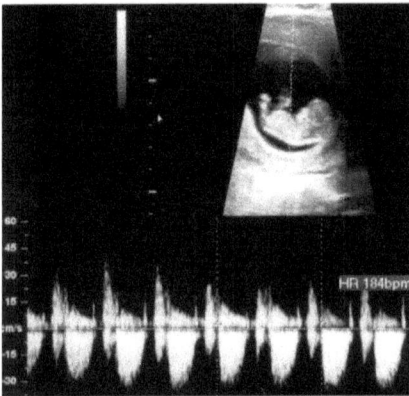

c

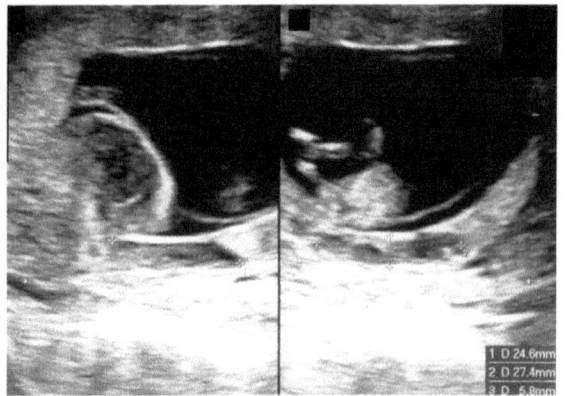

d

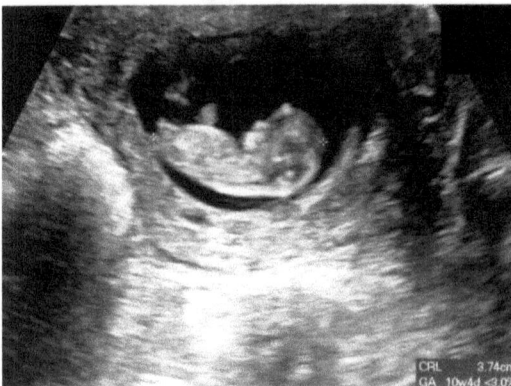

e

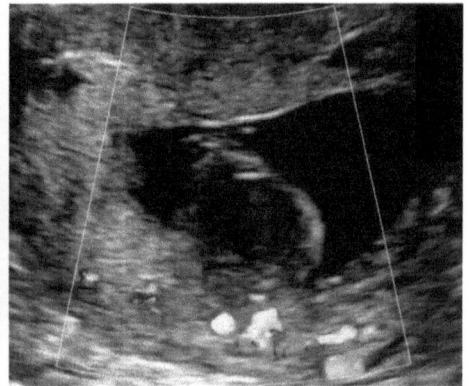

f

Ultrasound Services in an Early Pregnancy and Acute Gynaecological Unit. Book 2

240

a. Is there any worry some ultrasound identifiable feature?

b. Write an ultrasound report.

c. Will this woman need another scan before the routine anomaly scan? Why or why not?

74

This woman was referred with a history of post c/s 1/52 but no pvb. Both ovaries were not visualized.

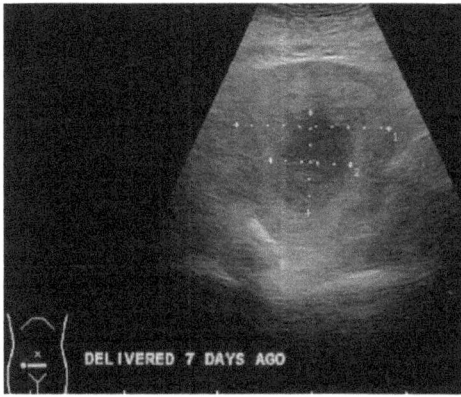

74.a

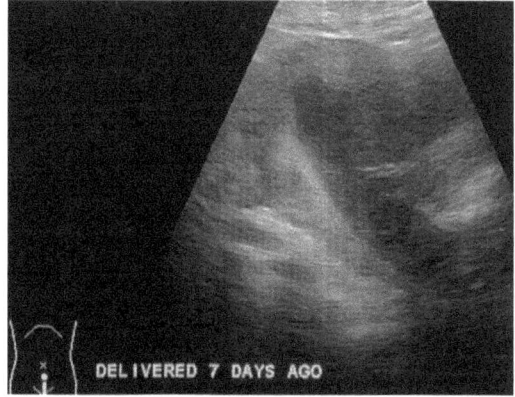

74.b

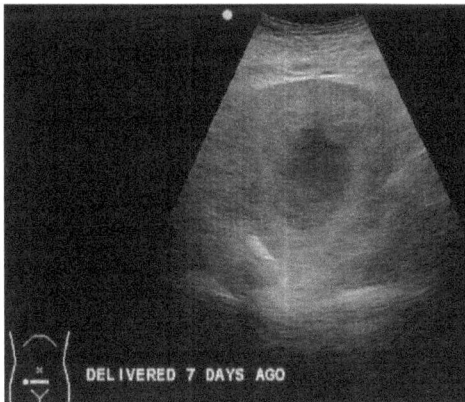

74.c

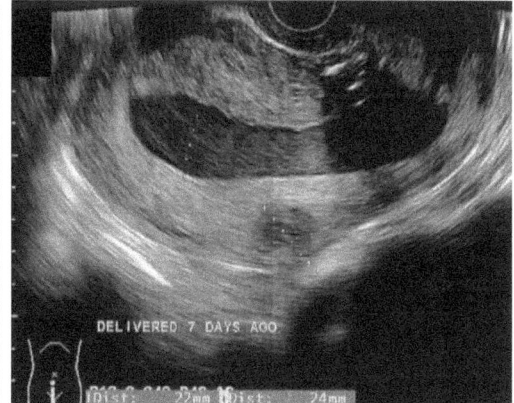

74.d

Ultrasound Services in an Early Pregnancy and Acute Gynaecological Unit. Book 2

241

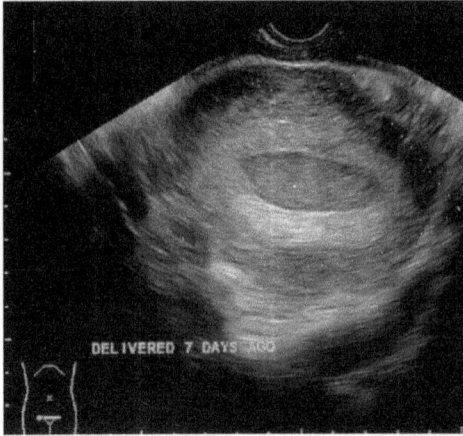

74.e

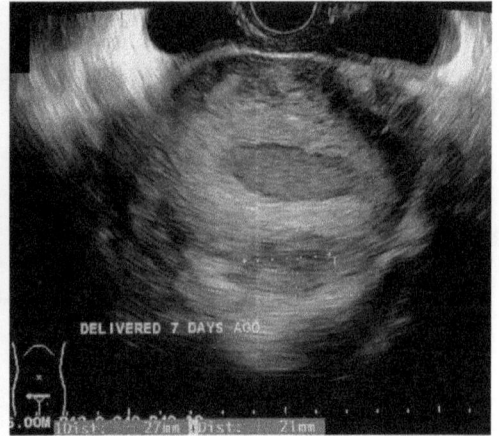

74.f

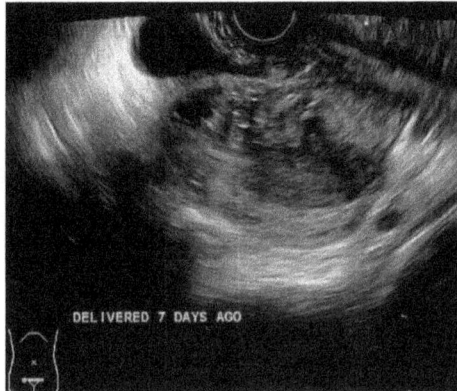

74.g

a. How was this woman scanned?

b. Write an ultrasound report.

c. Will this woman require another scan?

Ultrasound Services in an Early Pregnancy and Acute Gynaecological Unit. Book 2

242

75

This woman was referred with a history of pelvic pain in pregnancy.

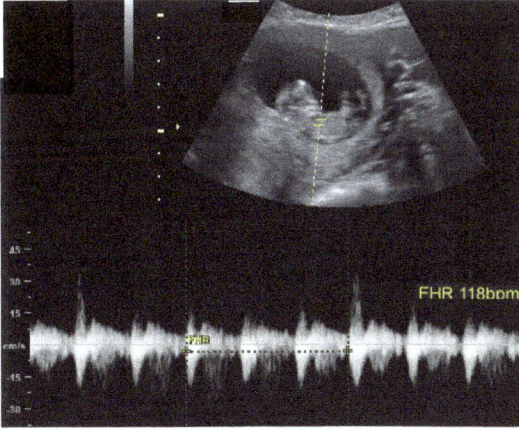

75.a

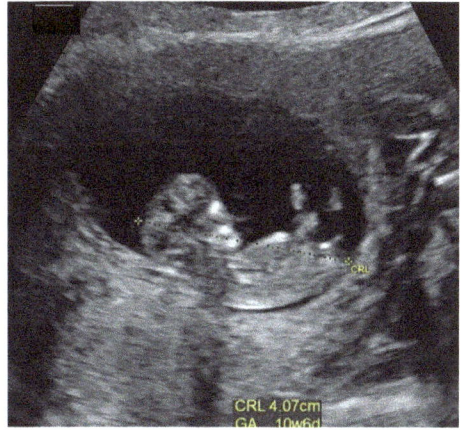

75.b

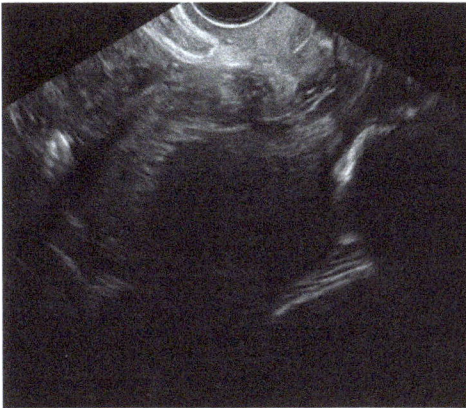

75.c

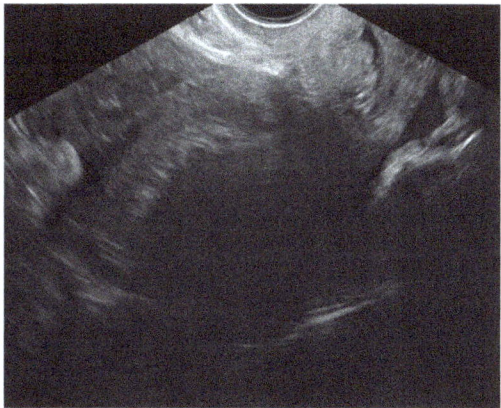

75.d

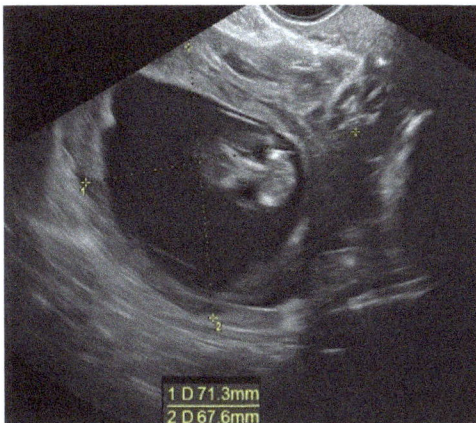

75.e

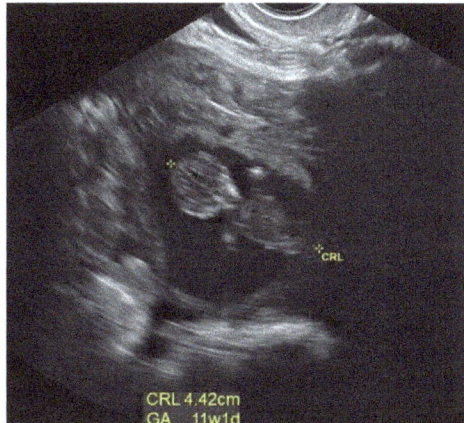

75.f

Ultrasound Services in an Early Pregnancy and Acute Gynaecological Unit. Book 2

243

a. How was this woman scanned?
b. Describe the ultrasound findings
c. What is your diagnosis and how have you arrived at your diagnosis?
d. Is there any ultrasound reason for the woman's pain?

76

This woman was referred post CT scan on day 8 of her cycle. No peristalsis or flow on Dopplers was noted in the structures shown in the following images.

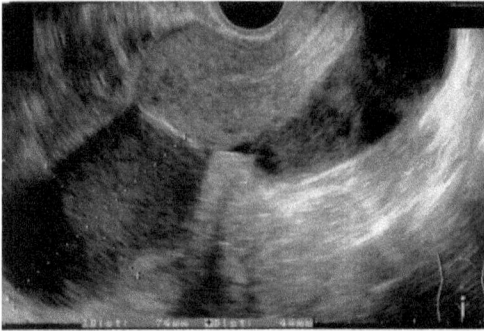

76.a

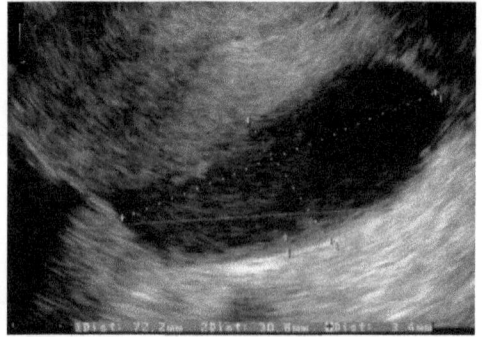

76.b

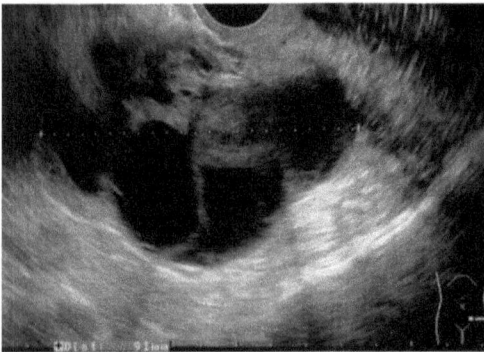

76.c

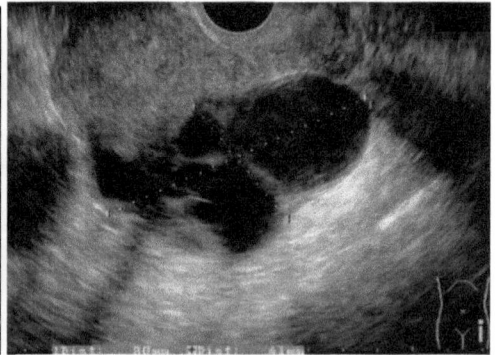

76.d

Ultrasound Services in an Early Pregnancy and Acute Gynaecological Unit. Book 2

244

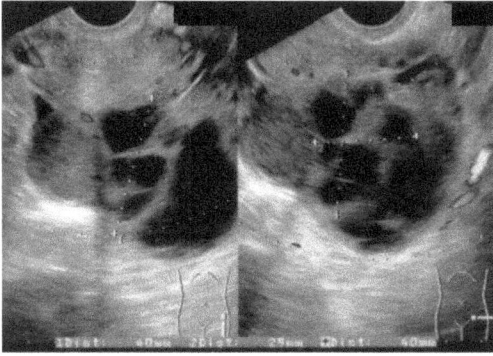

76.e

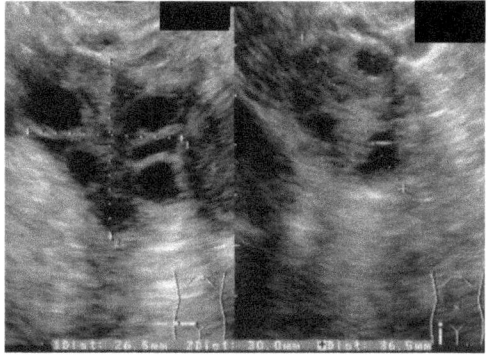

76.f

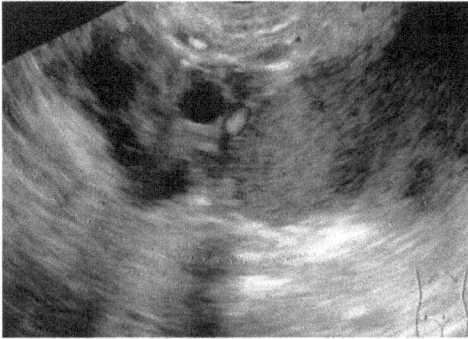

76.g

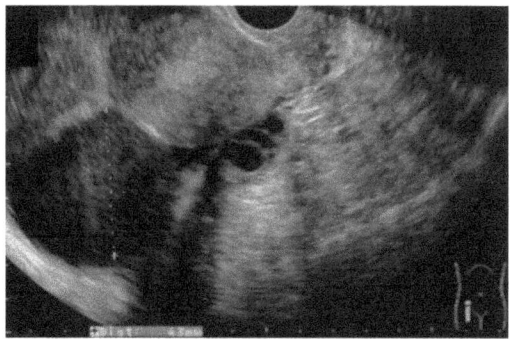

76.h

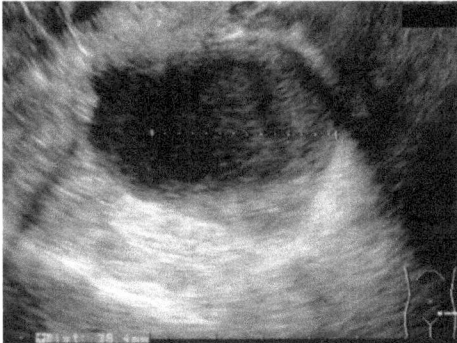

76.I

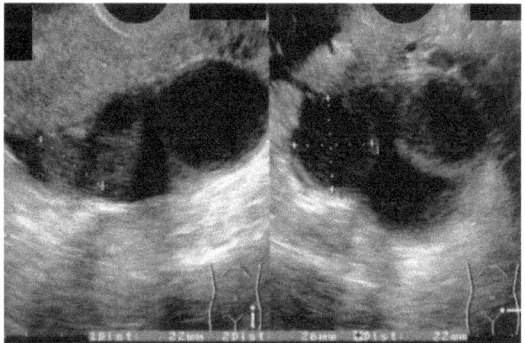

76.j

Ultrasound Services in an Early Pregnancy and Acute Gynaecological Unit. Book 2

245

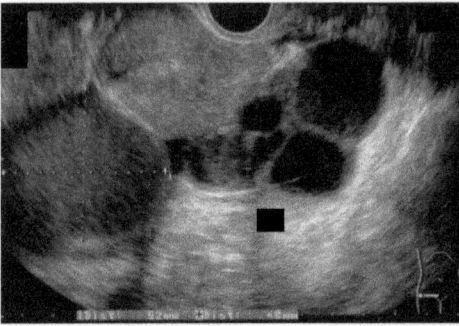

76.k

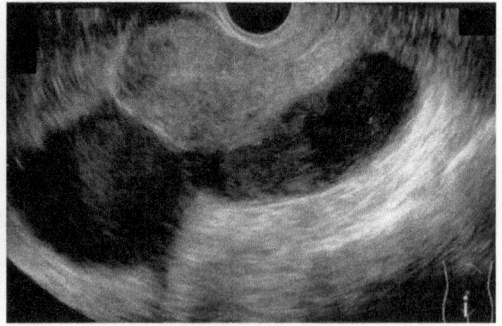

76.l

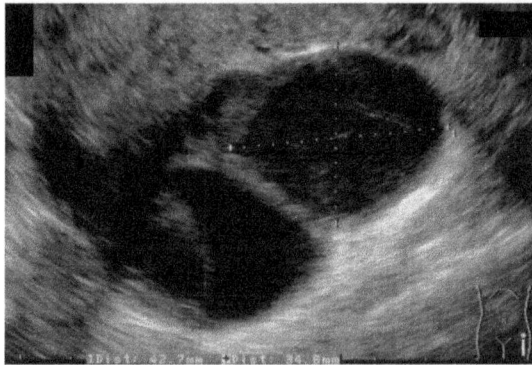

76.m

a. Describe the ultrasound appearances

b. How may ultrasound be used in the management of this woman?

77

This woman was referred with a history of light bleeding and pelvic cramps. GA by date = 6/40.

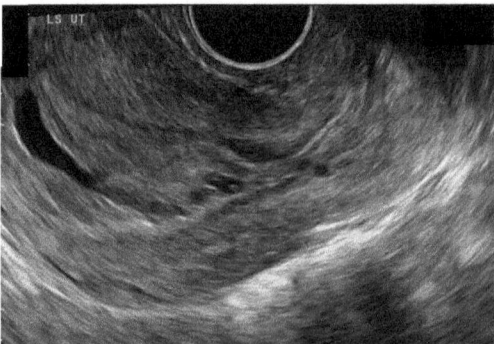

77a

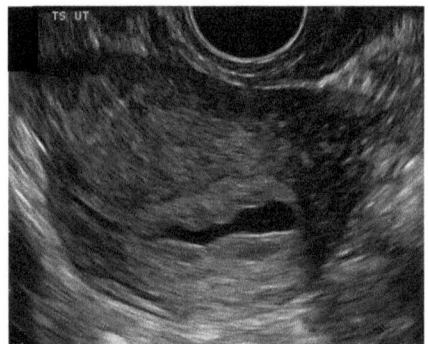

77b

Ultrasound Services in an Early Pregnancy and Acute Gynaecological Unit. Book 2

246

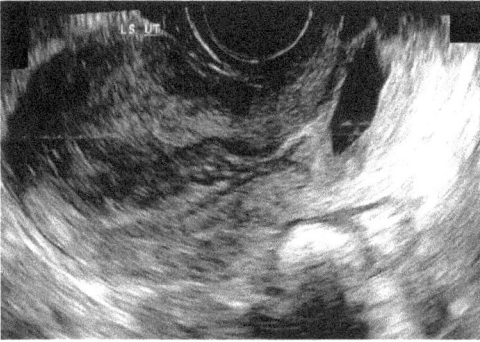

77c

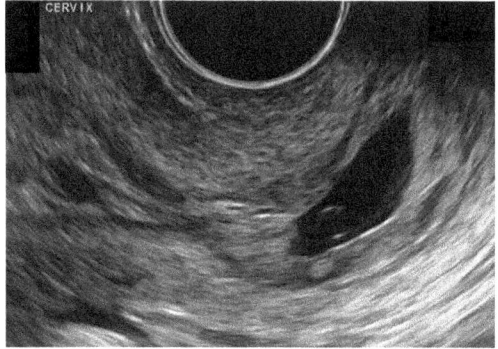

77d

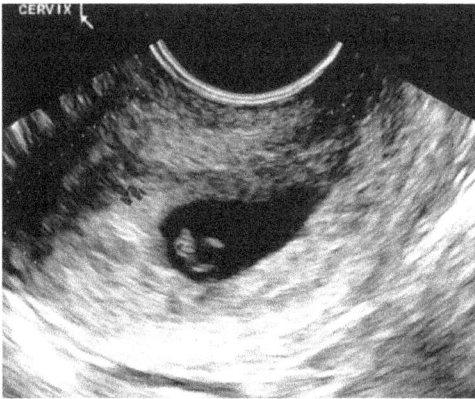

77e

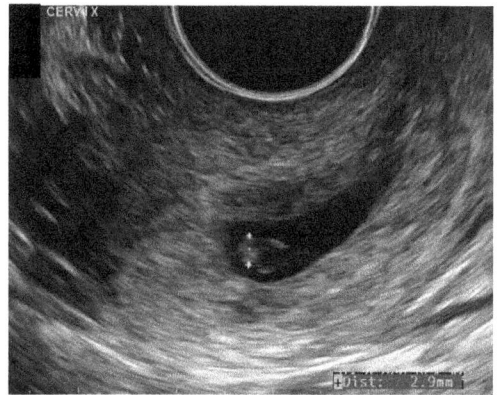

77f

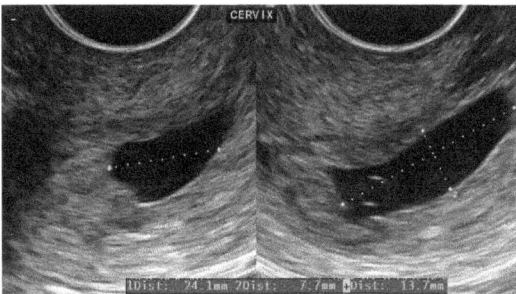

77.g

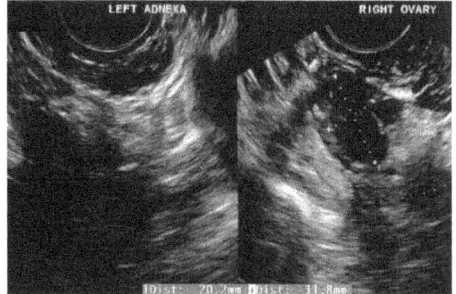

77.h

a. Describe the ultrasound findings
b. What is the ultrasound diagnosis?

Ultrasound Services in an Early Pregnancy and Acute Gynaecological Unit. Book 2

247

78

This woman was referred with a history of pelvic pain. FHB x 2 not shown here were noted. Natural conception. CRL's = date. No free fluid was seen in the POD or pelvis.

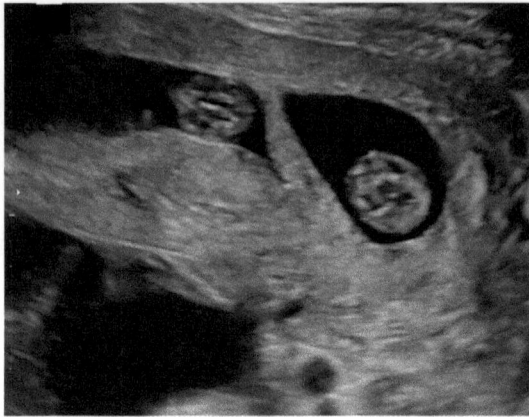

78a

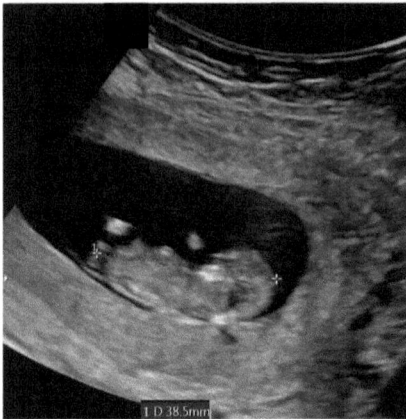

78b

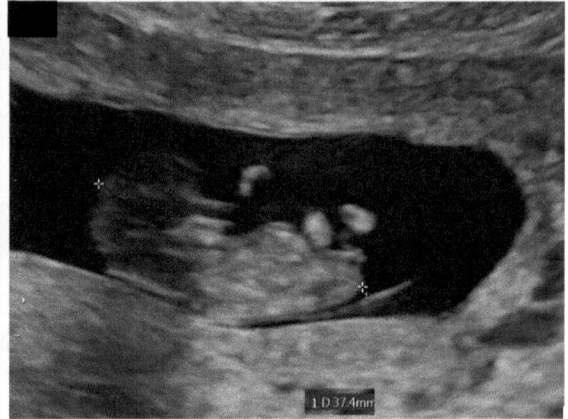

78c

Ultrasound Services in an Early Pregnancy and Acute Gynaecological Unit. Book 2

248

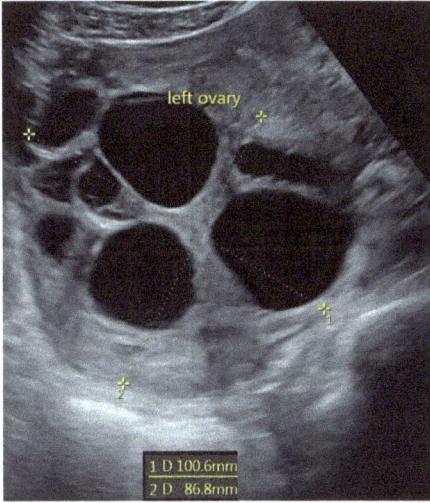

78d

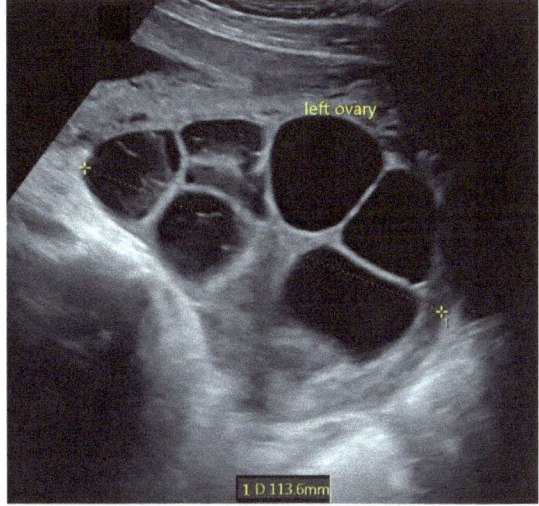

78e

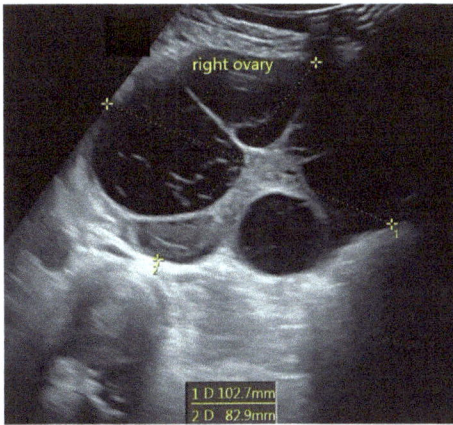

78f

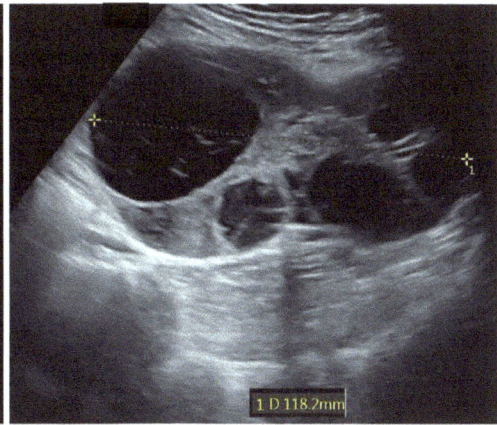

78g
right ovary

a. Does the sonographer need to check the upper abdomen in this case?
b. Why or why not?
c. Describe the ultrasound findings
d. What is the diagnosis or impression?
e. Is there any ultrasound identified cause of the pelvic pain in this woman?
f. What is the role of ultrasound in the management of this pregnancy?

Ultrasound Services in an Early Pregnancy and Acute Gynaecological Unit. Book 2

249

79

This patient in her late teens was referred with a history of acute and severe pelvic and abdominal pain. Negative pregnancy test result. Day 11. Ultrasound examination was limited by the patients' discomfort.

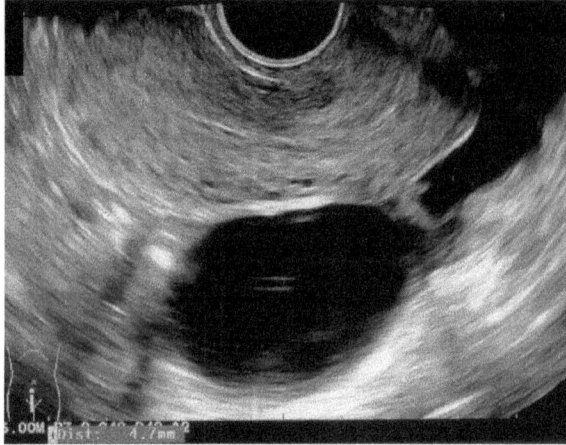

79.a

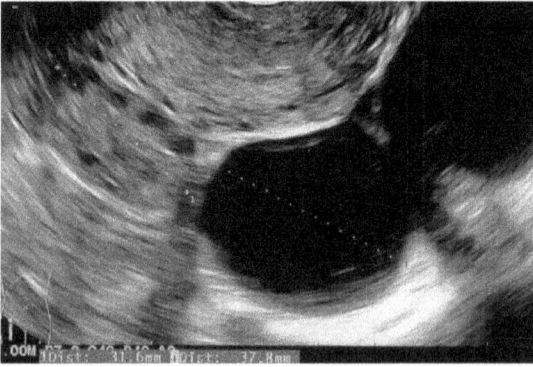

79.b

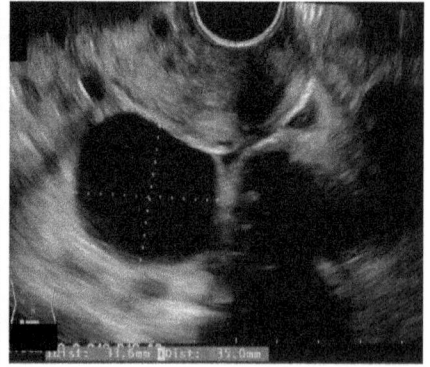

79.c

Ultrasound Services in an Early Pregnancy and Acute Gynaecological Unit. Book 2

250

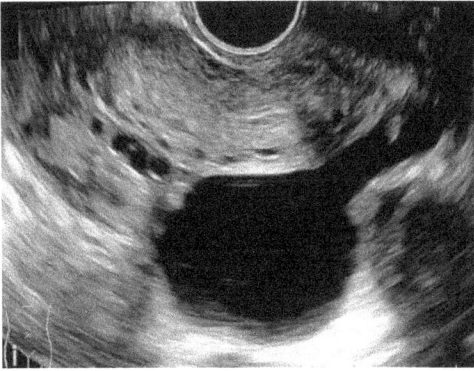

79.d

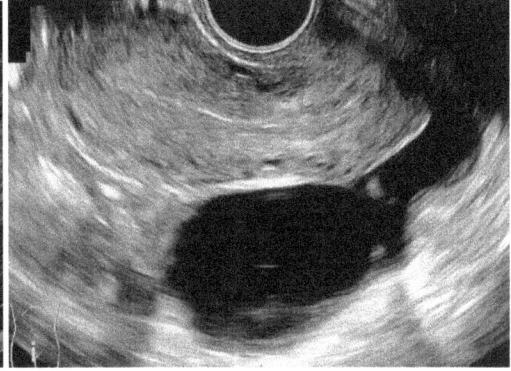

79.e

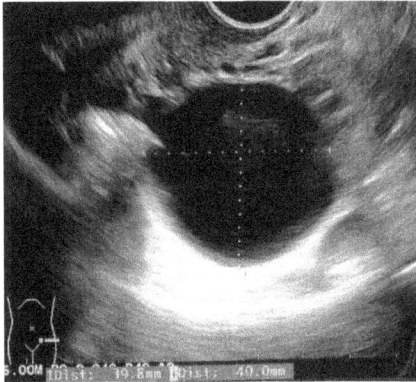

79.f

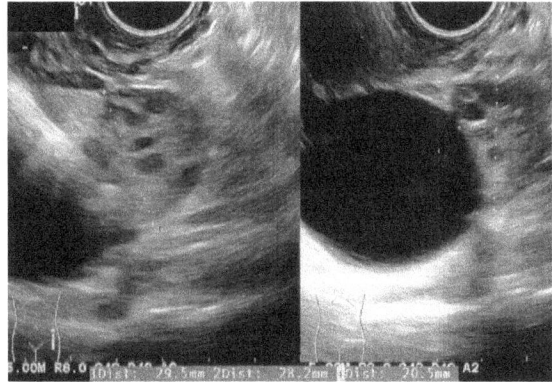

79.g

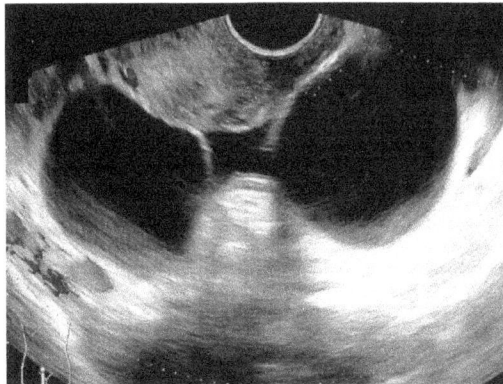

79h

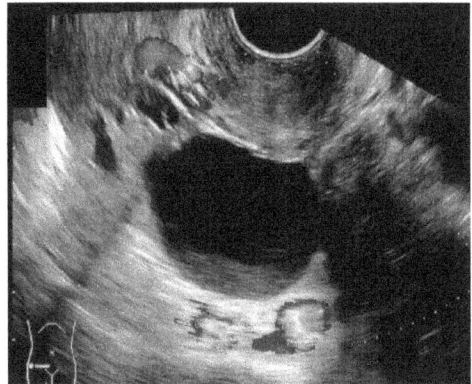

79.i

a. Describe the ultrasound appearances.

b. Will this woman need further imaging?

c. In what ways could ultrasound be used in the management of this woman?

Ultrasound Services in an Early Pregnancy and Acute Gynaecological Unit. Book 2

251

80

This woman was referred at 11+4/40 with a history of bleeding in pregnancy.

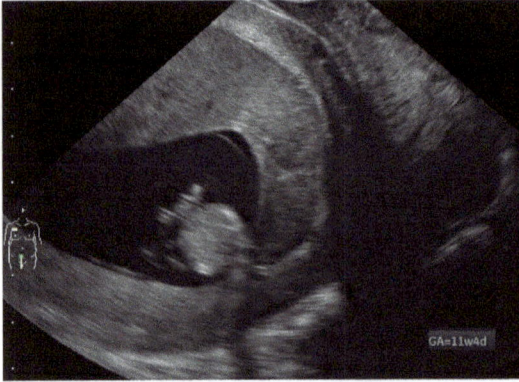

80a

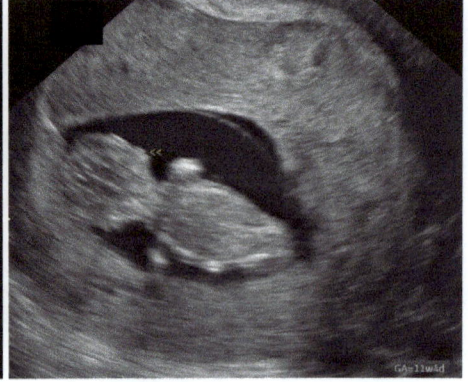

80b

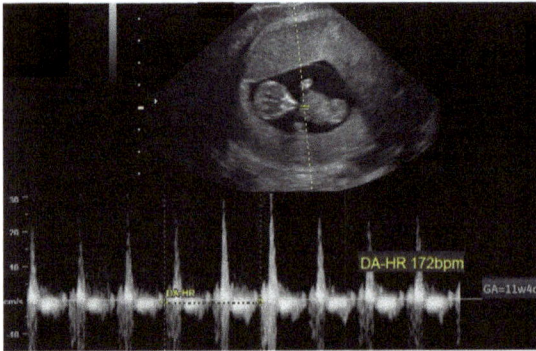

80c

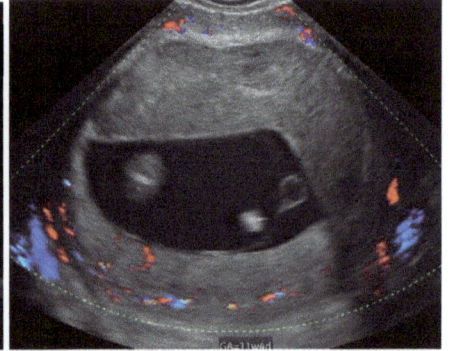

80d

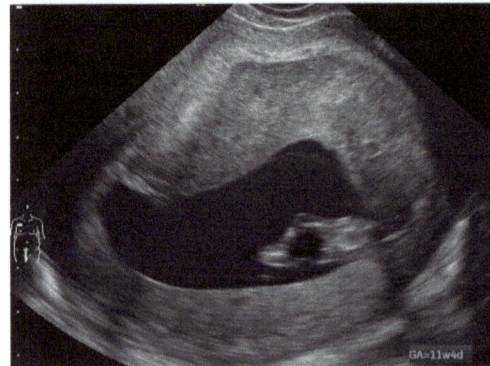

80e

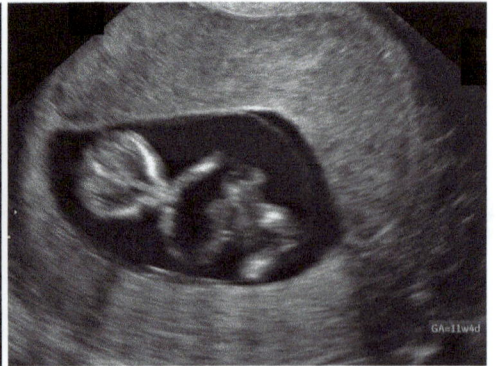

80f

Ultrasound Services in an Early Pregnancy and Acute Gynaecological Unit. Book 2

252

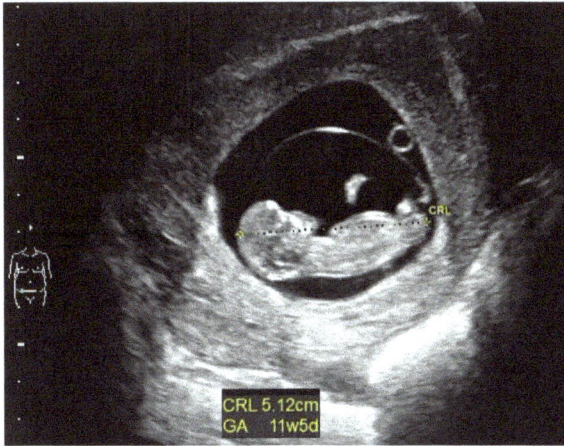

80g

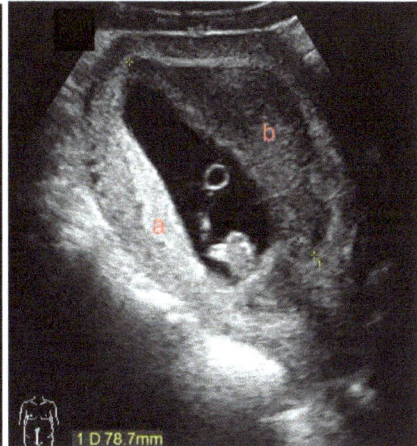

80h

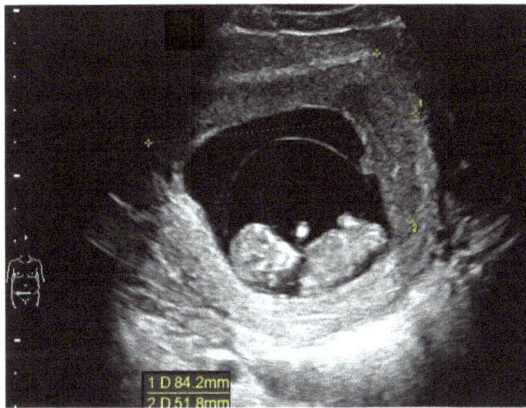

80i

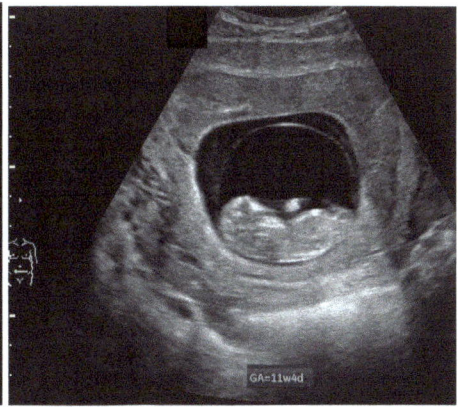

80j

a. Identify a –b in 80h?
b. How was this woman scanned?
c. Write the ultrasound report
d. What is the clinical implication of this finding?

Ultrasound Services in an Early Pregnancy and Acute Gynaecological Unit. Book 2

253

81
This patient was referred because of pvb in early pregnancy.

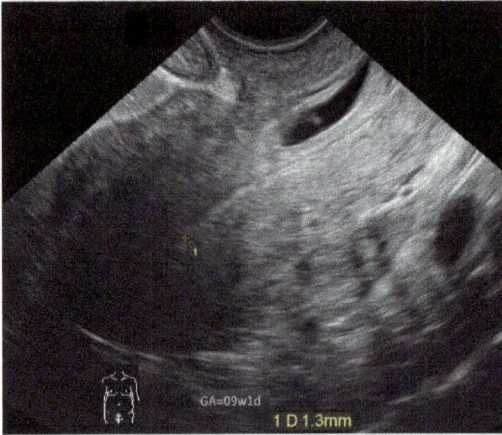

7.81a

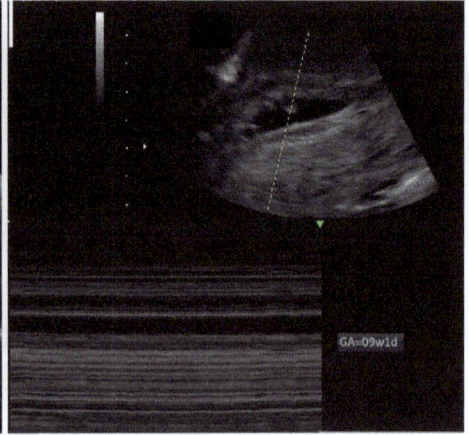

7.81b

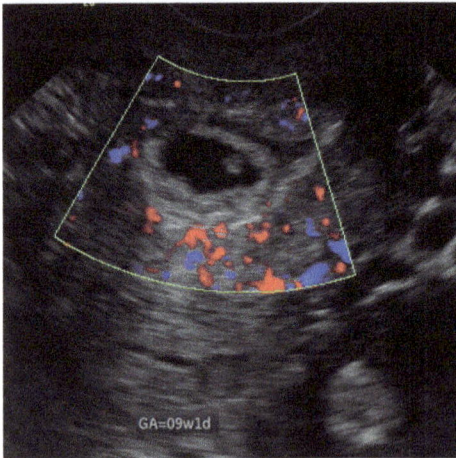

7.81c

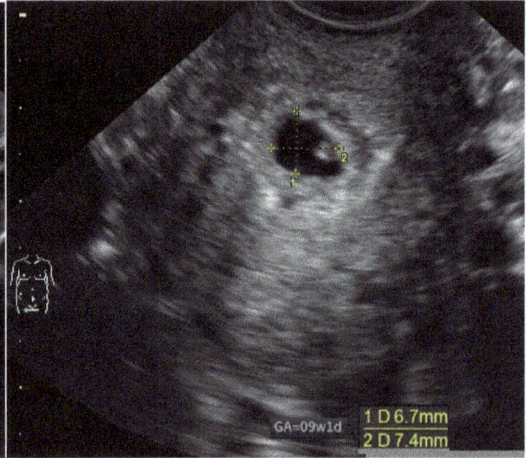

7.81d

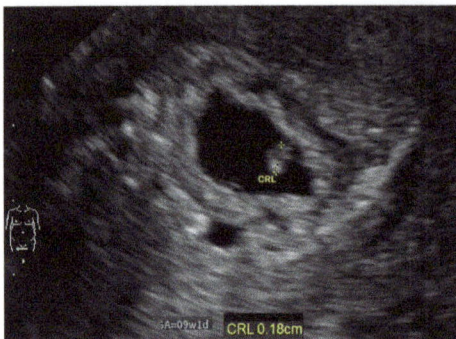

7.81e

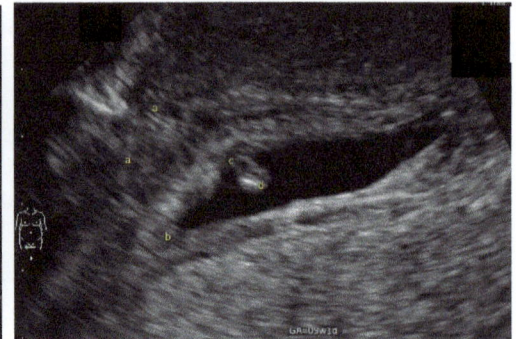

7.81f

Ultrasound Services in an Early Pregnancy and Acute Gynaecological Unit. Book 2

254

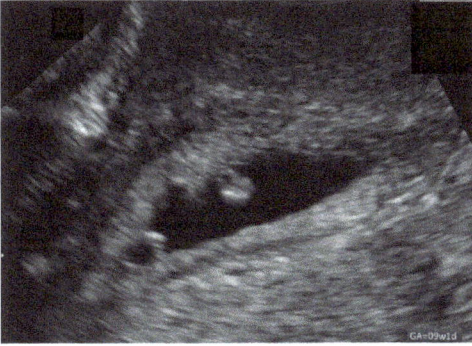

7.81g

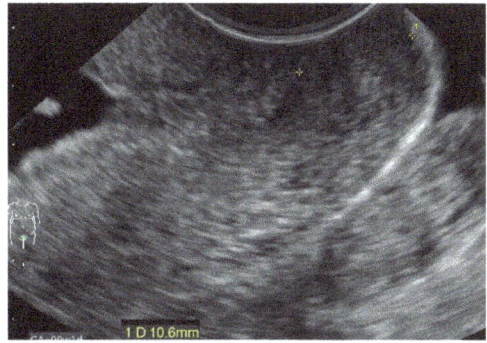

7.81h

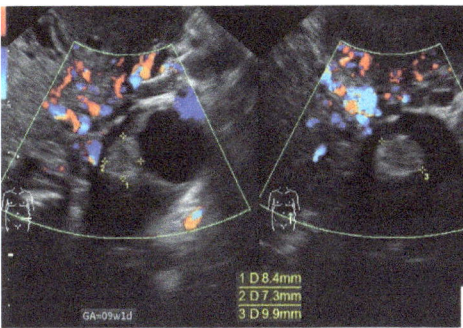

7.81i

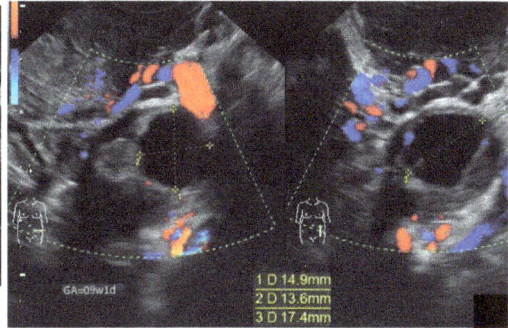

7.81j

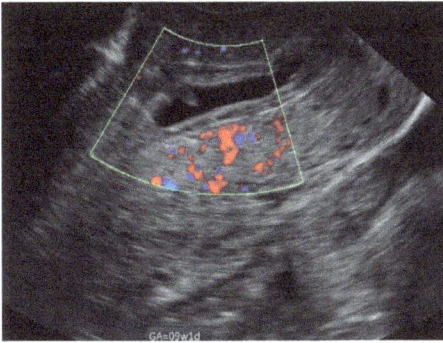

7.81k

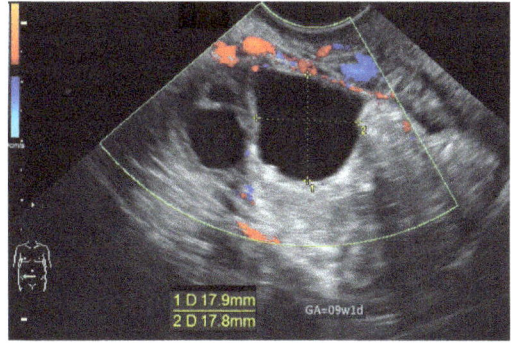

7.81l

Ultrasound Services in an Early Pregnancy and Acute Gynaecological Unit. Book 2

255

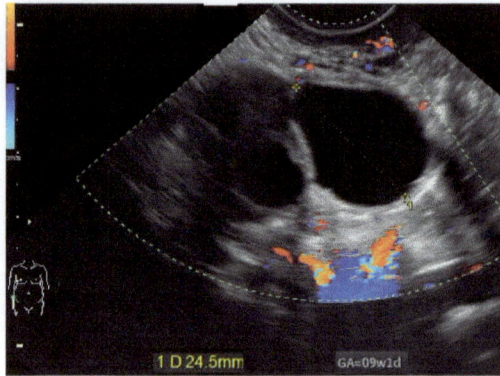

7.81m

a. Describe the ultrasound findings
b. What is the ultrasound diagnosis?

82

This patient in her thirties was referred because of pv bleeding and maternal anxiety. Previous subchorionic hematoma. Denies any trauma but tender in the pelvis. Measurements = date. Closed cervix seen but not shown here.

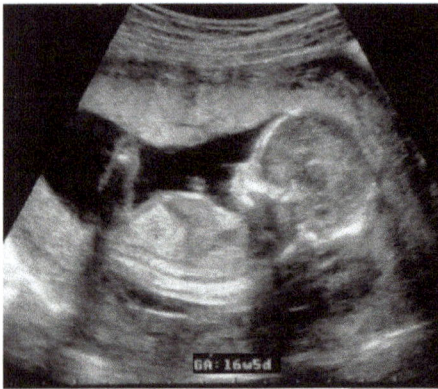

7.82a

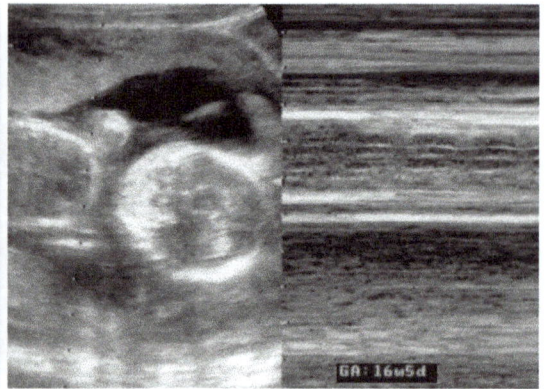

7.82b

Ultrasound Services in an Early Pregnancy and Acute Gynaecological Unit. Book 2

256

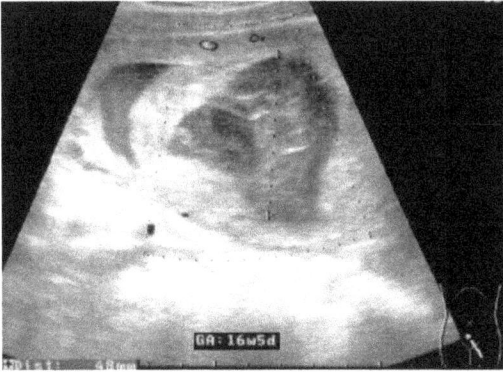

7.82c

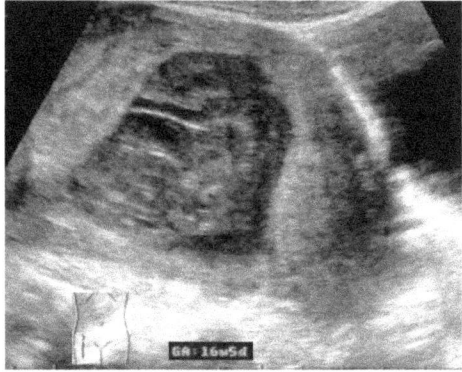

7.82d

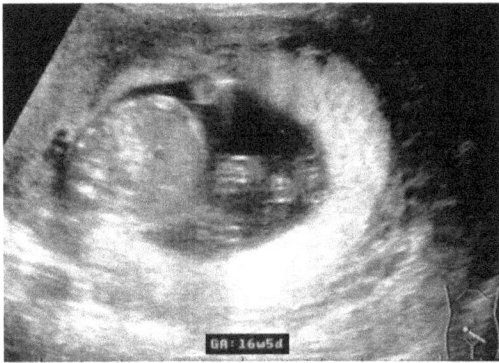

7.82e

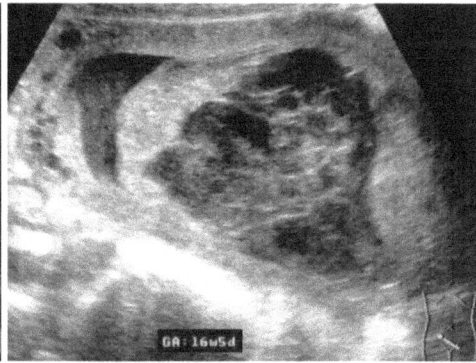

7.82f

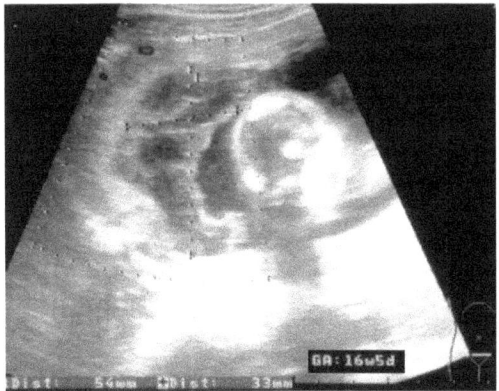

7.82g

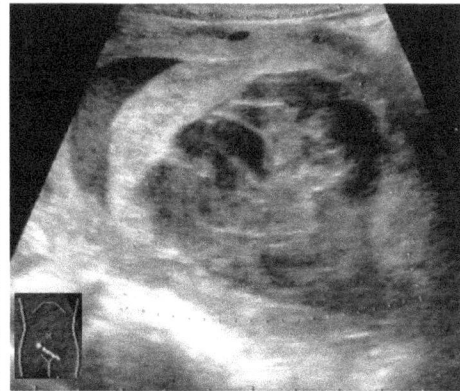

7.82h

Ultrasound Services in an Early Pregnancy and Acute Gynaecological Unit. Book 2

257

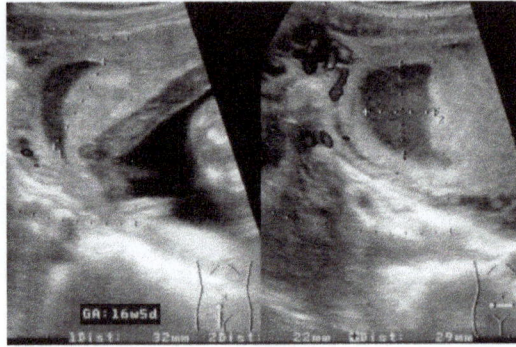

7.82i

a. Describe the ultrasound findings
b. How could this finding affect the pregnancy?
c. What is the role of ultrasound on this occasion?

83

This woman was referred for a dating scan with a clinical history of unknown LMP. Both ovaries were not identified at this scan.

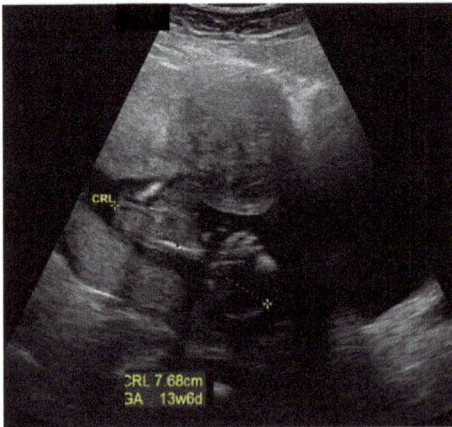

7.83a

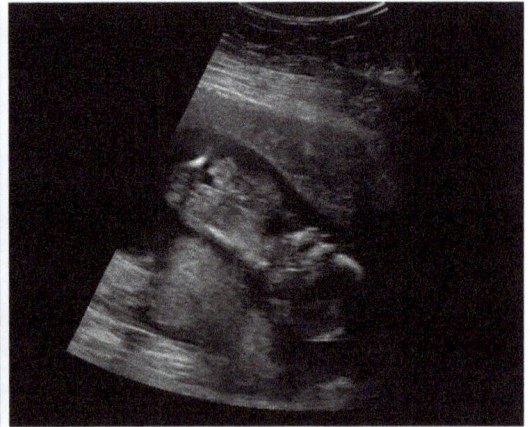

7.83b

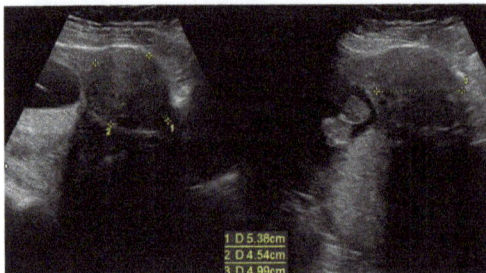

7.83c

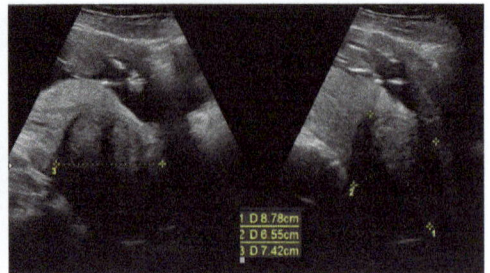

7.83d

Ultrasound Services in an Early Pregnancy and Acute Gynaecological Unit. Book 2

258

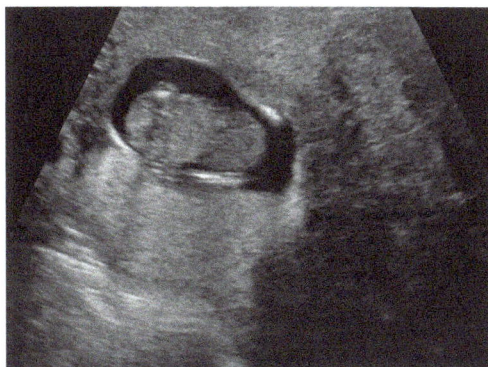

7.83e
TS abdo.

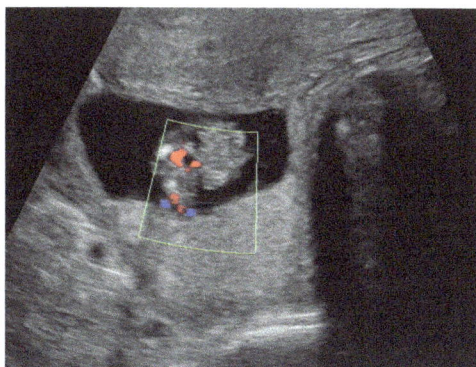

7.83f

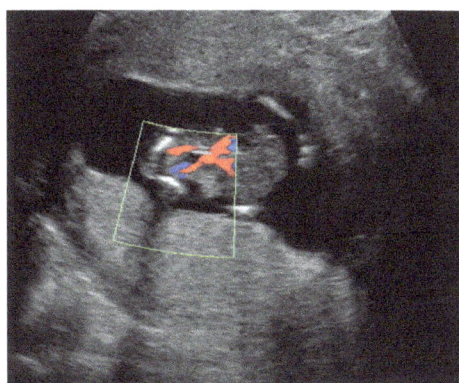

7.83g

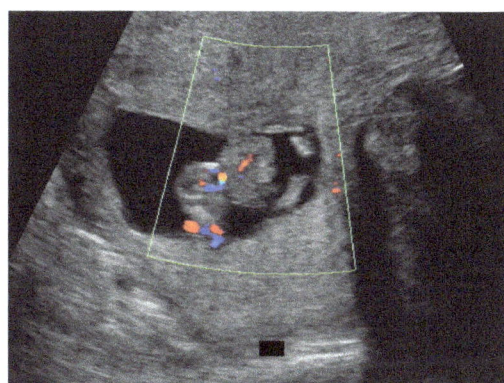

7.83h TS Pelvis

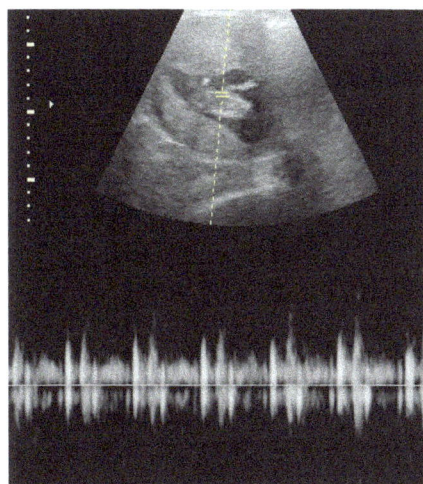

7.83i

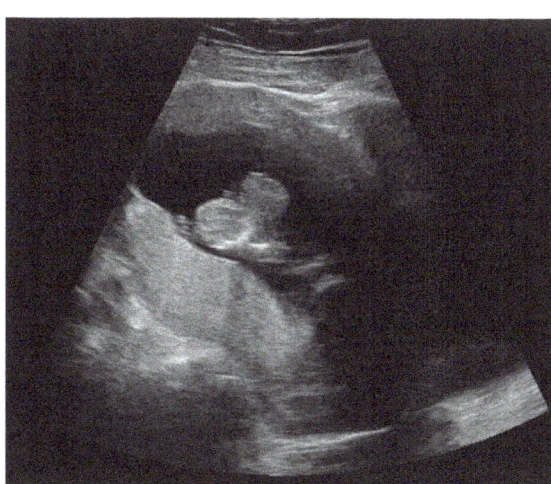

7.83j

Ultrasound Services in an Early Pregnancy and Acute Gynaecological Unit. Book 2

259

a. Is there any reason that could make the examination challenging for the Sonographer?
b. Write an ultrasound report of the examination.
c. What is the diagnosis and differentials?
d. How will the findings affect this pregnancy management?

84

This woman in her late thirties was referred because of continous pv bleed and maternal anxiety.

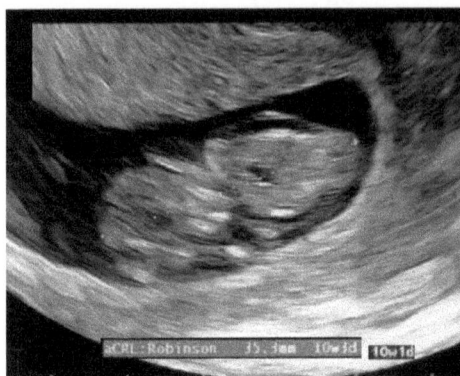
7.84a

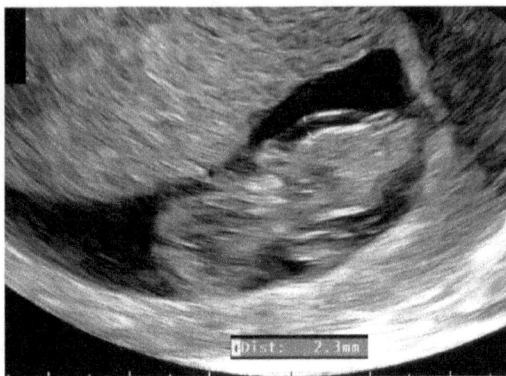
7.84b

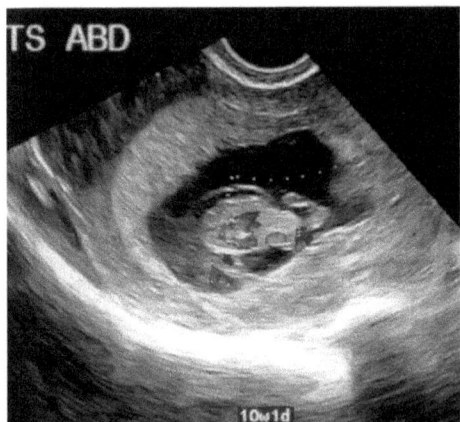
7.84c

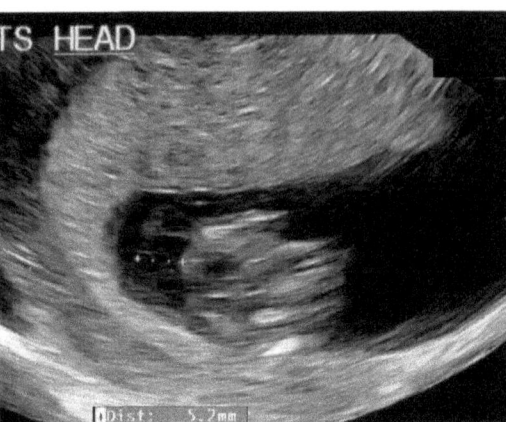
7.84d

Ultrasound Services in an Early Pregnancy and Acute Gynaecological Unit. Book 2

260

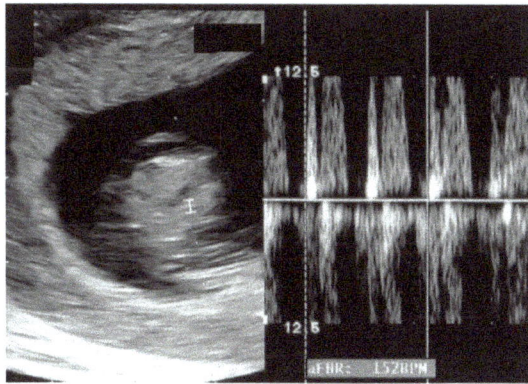

7.84e

a. Is there any worry some feature in this fetus?
b. Write the ultrasound report
c. How may ultrasound be used in the management of this pregnancy?

85

This woman was referred with a clinical history of post medical TOP. ?RPOC. Below are the ultrasound findings in the uterus. Both ovaries were not identified.

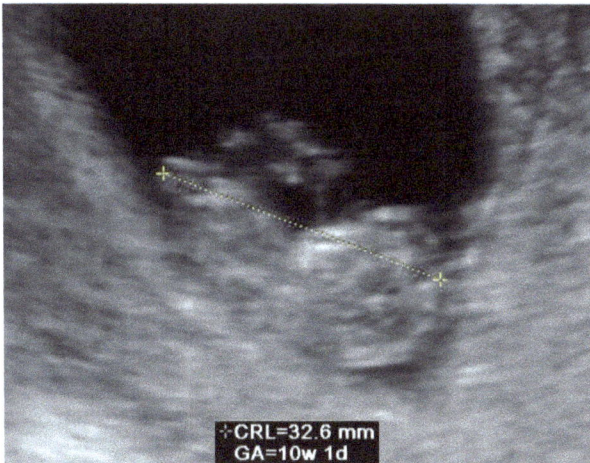

7.85a

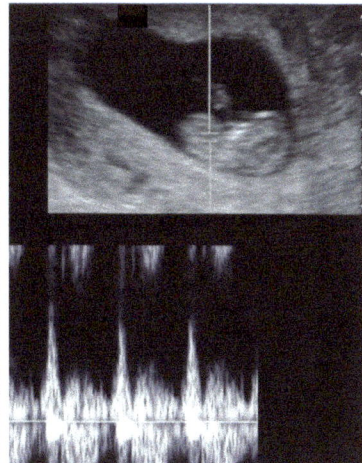

7.85b

Ultrasound Services in an Early Pregnancy and Acute Gynaecological Unit. Book 2

261

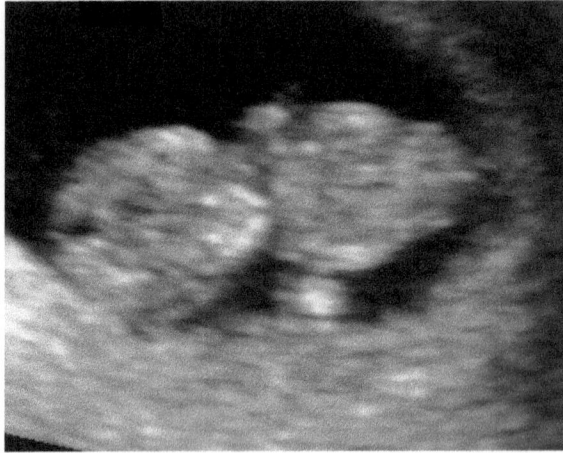

7.85c

a. Is there any evidence of RPOC?
b. Write the ultrasound report.

86

This woman was referred for a dating scan.

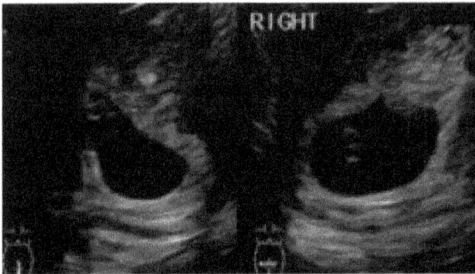

7.86a

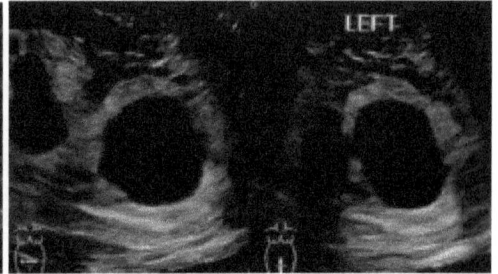

7.86b

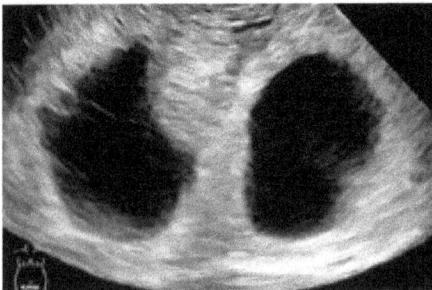

7.86c

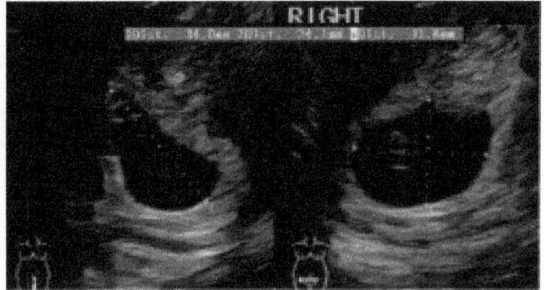

7.86d

Ultrasound Services in an Early Pregnancy and Acute Gynaecological Unit. Book 2

262

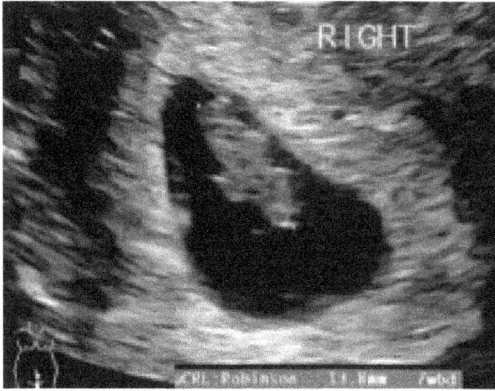

7.86e

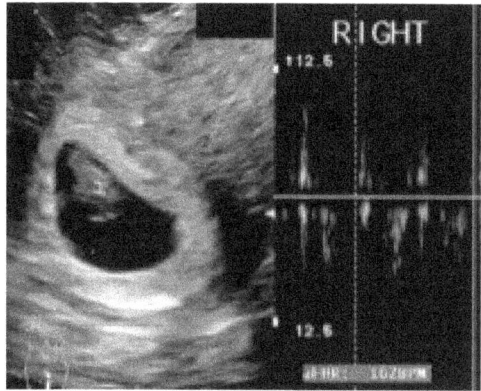

7.86f

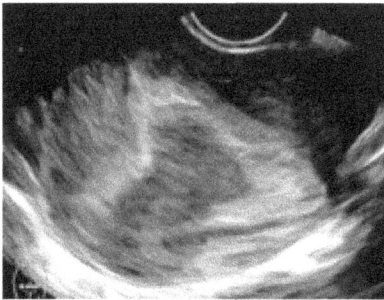

7.86g

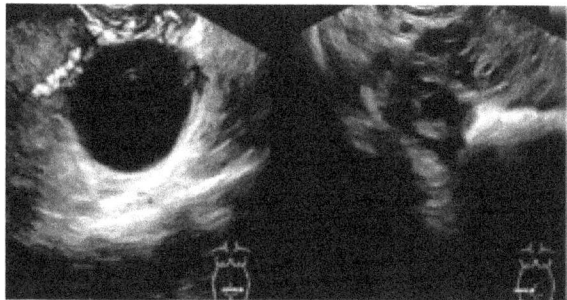

7.86h

Posterior io the gestational sacs

a. Is there any significant finding in 7.86c?
b. Which type of pregnancy is this and what confirms it?
c. Write the ultrasound report.
d. In what ways could ultrasound be useful in the management of this pregnancy?

Ultrasound Services in an Early Pregnancy and Acute Gynaecological Unit. Book 2

263

7.87

The images below were obtained during a dating scan.

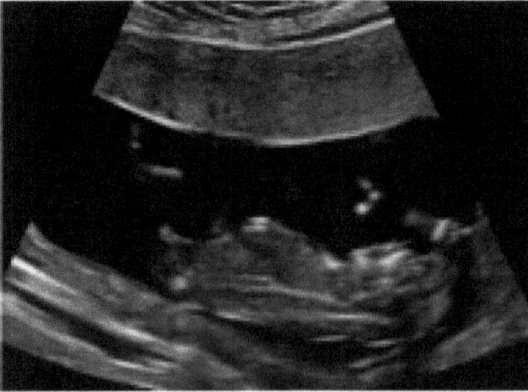

7.87a

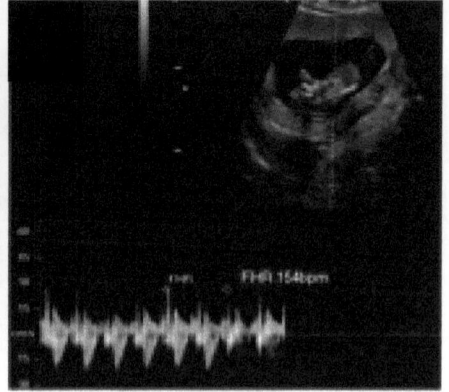

7.87b

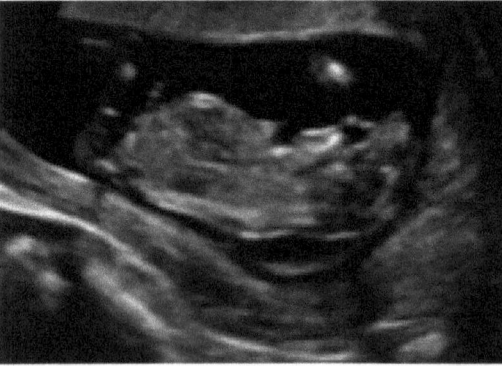

7.87c

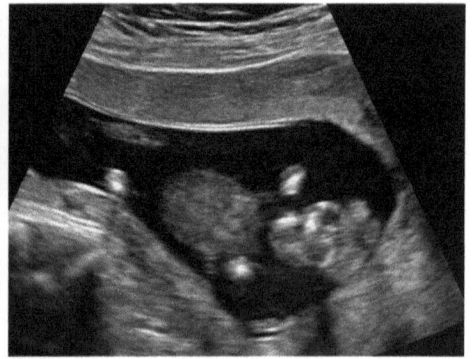

7.87d

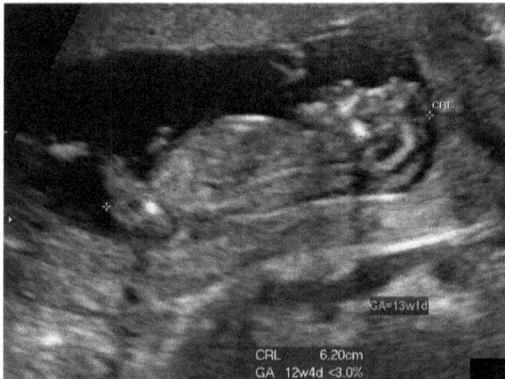

7.87e

a. What challenges may the Sonographer encounter and why?

Ultrasound Services in an Early Pregnancy and Acute Gynaecological Unit. Book 2

264

b. Describe the ultrasound appearance in 7.87d

c. Describe the ultrasound findings.

d. What is the ultrasound diagnosis?

e. What is the significance of this finding?

f. Why is this abnormality sometimes missed?

7.88

This woman was referred with a history of 3/7pv bleeding and hyperemesis. GA by LMP = 15+4/40. The right ovary was not identified at the time of the scan.

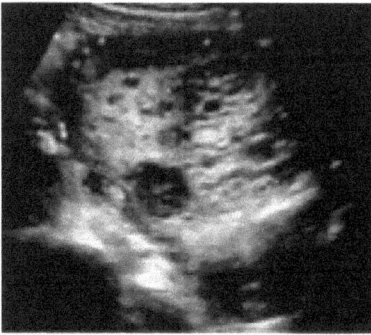 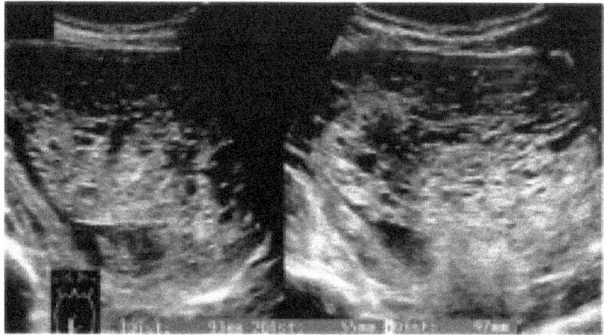

| 7.88a | 7.88b |

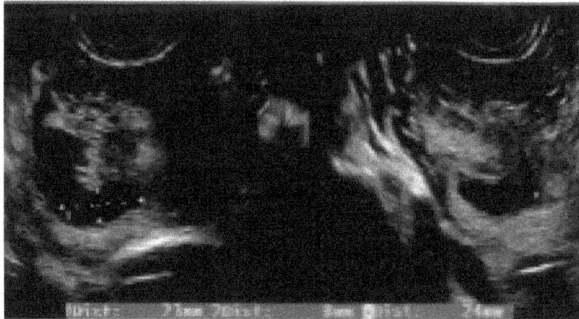

7.88c

a. Describe the ultrasound findings.

b. What is the ultrasound diagnosis?

c. How is this ultrasound appearance different from that of a missed miscarriage?

Ultrasound Services in an Early Pregnancy and Acute Gynaecological Unit. Book 2

265

7.89

This woman was referred with a history of hyperemesis and now pv bleeding. GA as previously calculated at this examination was 8/40. Left ovary was not visualised on the scan.

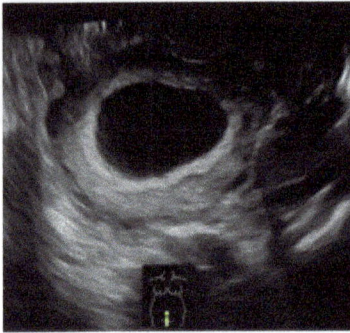

7.89a

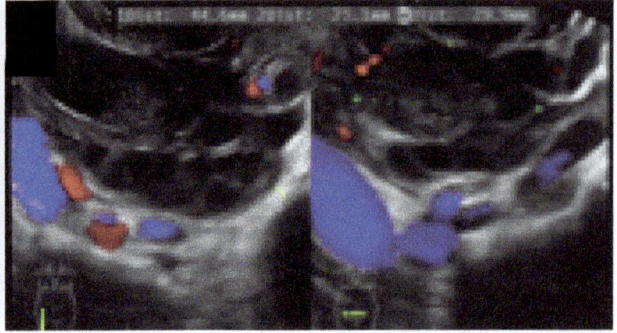

7.89b

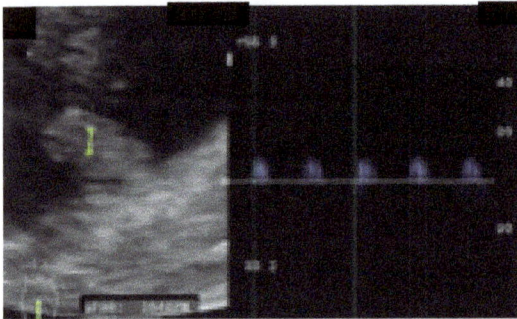

7.89c

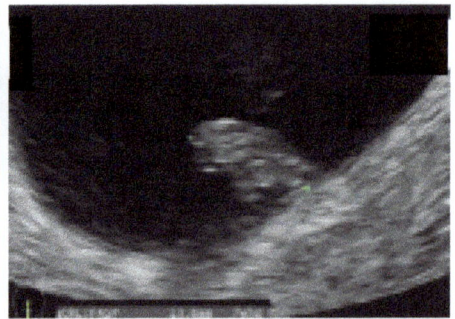

7.89d

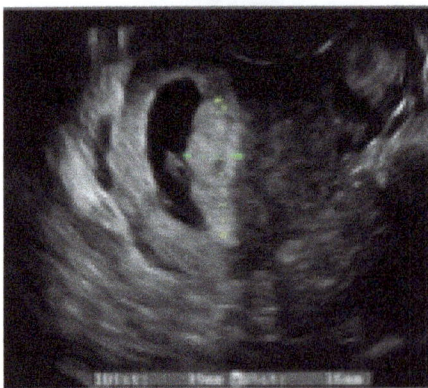

7.89e

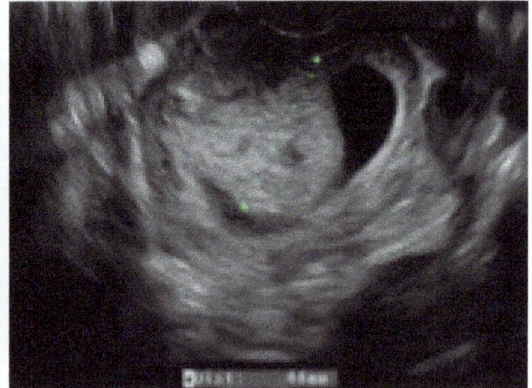

7.89f

a. Is there anything that should be of concern to the Sonographer?

b. Describe the ultrasound appearances.

c. What is the diagnosis?

Ultrasound Services in an Early Pregnancy and Acute Gynaecological Unit. Book 2

266

7.90

Post IVF treatment. 2 fresh ET. Painful and distended abdomen. GA by IVF treatment = 4/40.

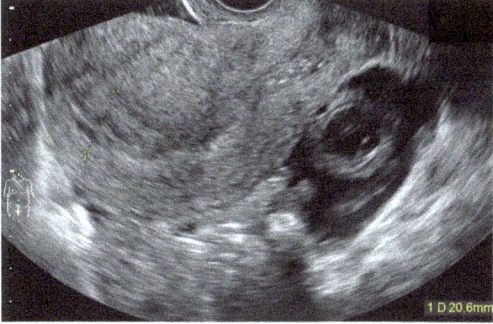

7.90a

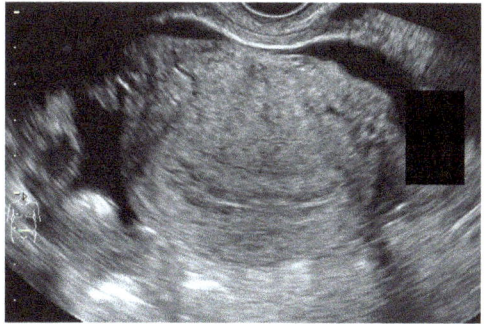

7.90b

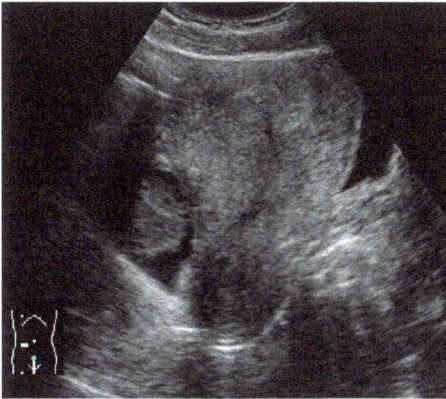

7.90c

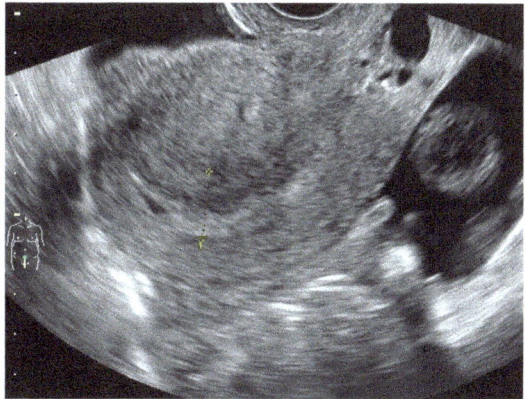

7.90d

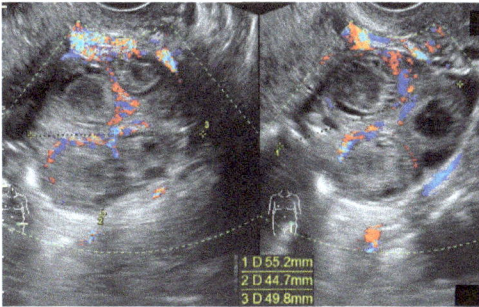

7.90e

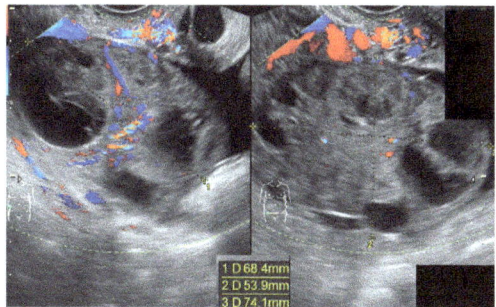

7.90f

Ultrasound Services in an Early Pregnancy and Acute Gynaecological Unit. Book 2

267

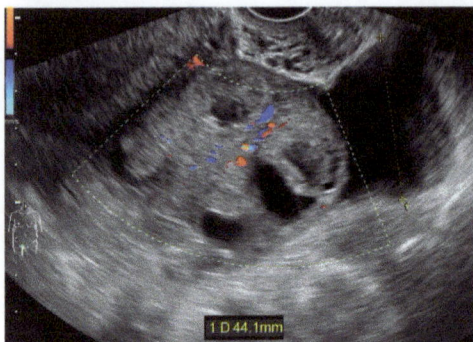

7.90g

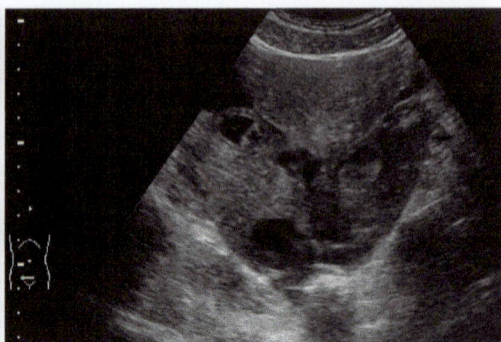

7.90h

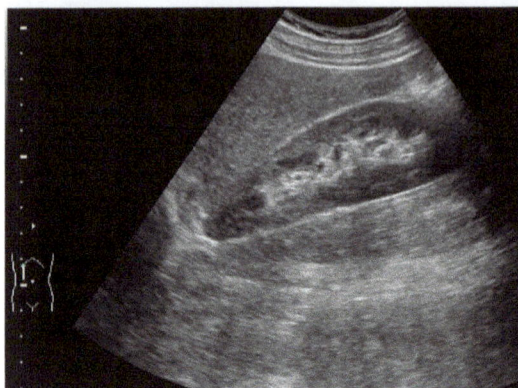

7.90i

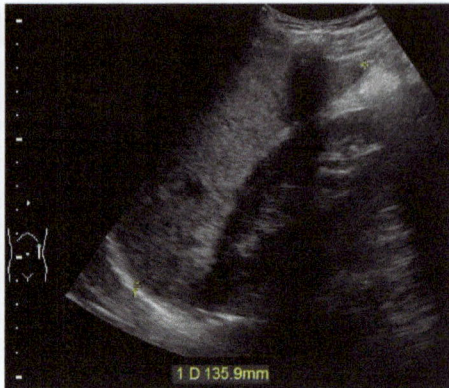

7.90j

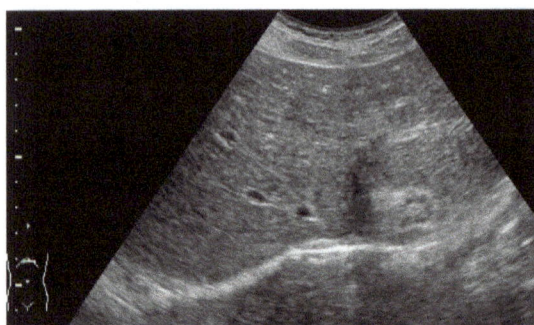

7.90k

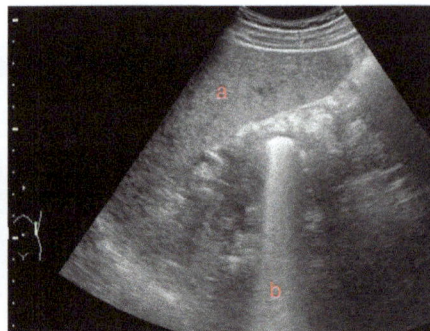

7.90l

a. Identify a –b in 7.90l
b. Which medical conditions is the woman prone to?
c. Why was the upper abdomen scanned?
d. Describe the ultrasound findings?
e. How can ultrasound be used in the management of this pregnancy?

Ultrasound Services in an Early Pregnancy and Acute Gynaecological Unit. Book 2

268

91

This woman referred at 6+3/40 with a history of abdominal cramps, pvb and positive pregnancy test result. Past medical history of right ectopic pregnancy 2 years ago and ovarian cyst surgery. Below are the ultrasound findings. CRL not shown here were 1.5mm and 1.6mm.

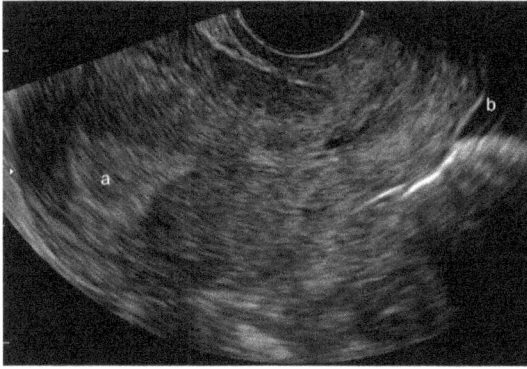

7.91a

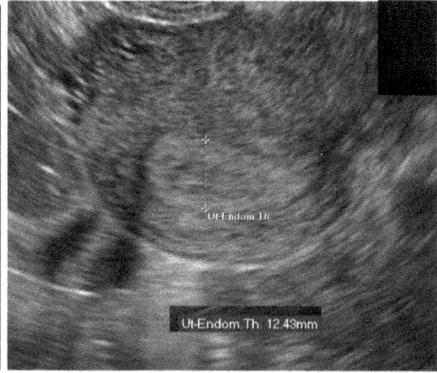

7.91b

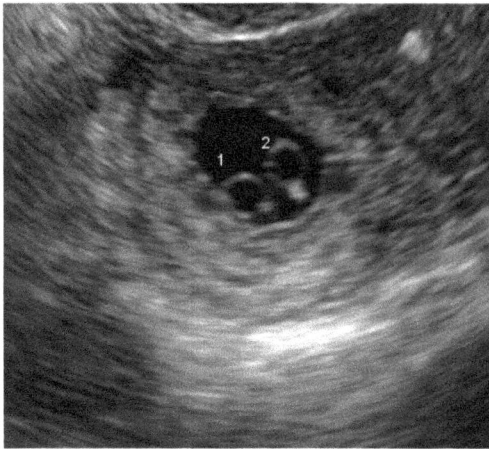

7.91c

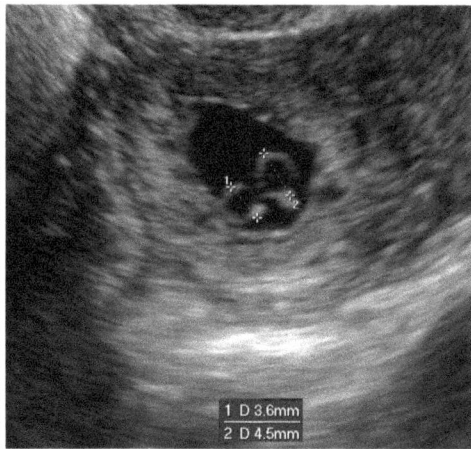

7.91d

Ultrasound Services in an Early Pregnancy and Acute Gynaecological Unit. Book 2

269

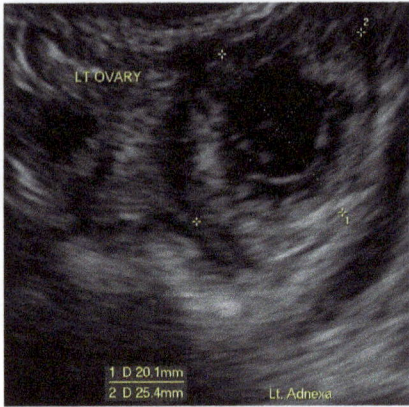

7.91e

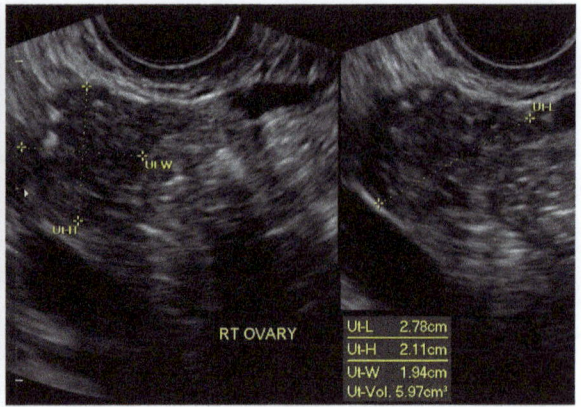

7.91f

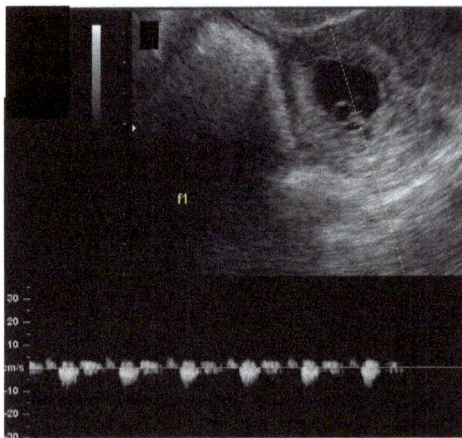

7.91g

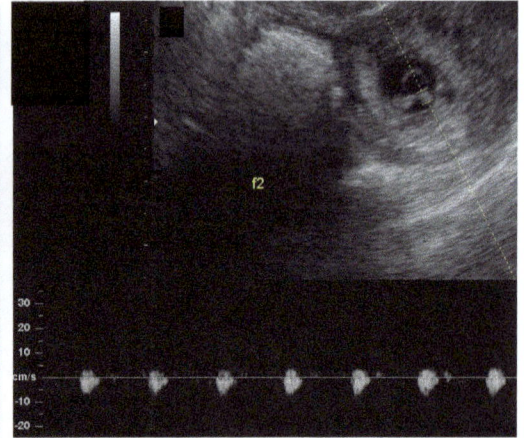

7.91h

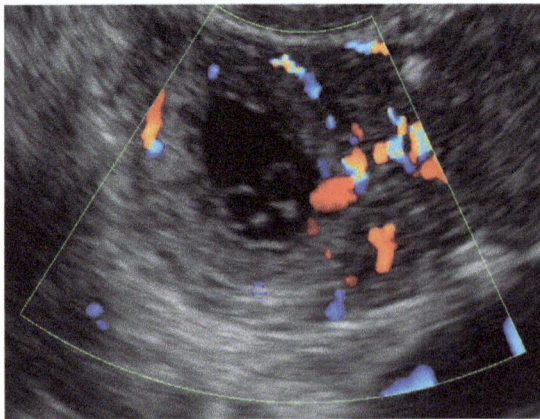

7.91 i

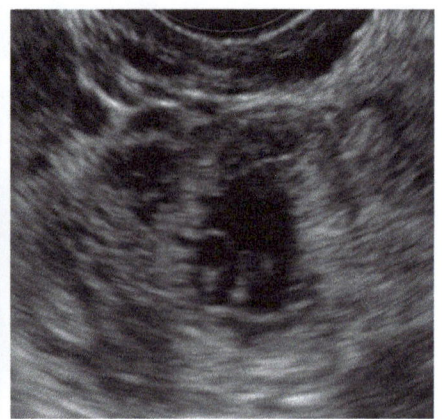

7.91j

Ultrasound Services in an Early Pregnancy and Acute Gynaecological Unit. Book 2

270

a. Identify a and b in 7.91.a

b. Describe the ultrasound findings

c. What is the diagnosis and how often does this occur?

92

This woman was referred because of anxiety at 9+3/40.

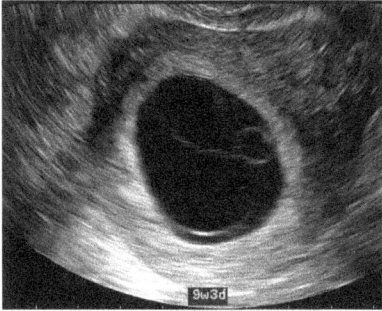

7.92a

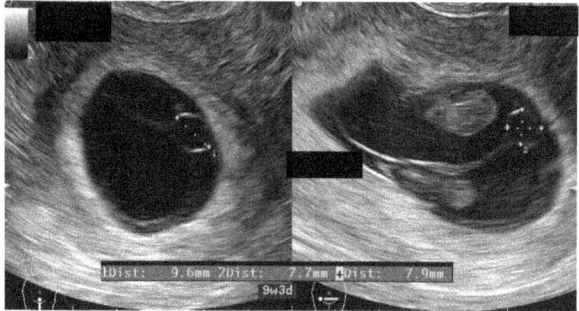

7.92b

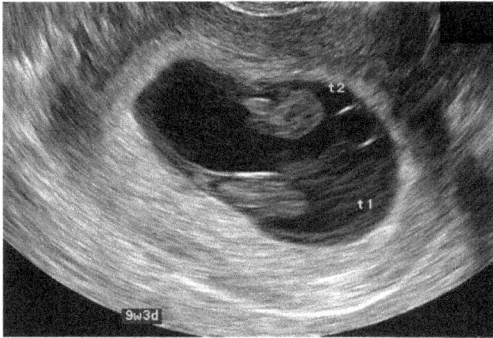

7.92c

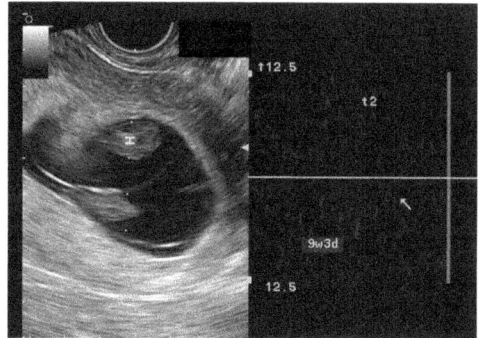

7.92d

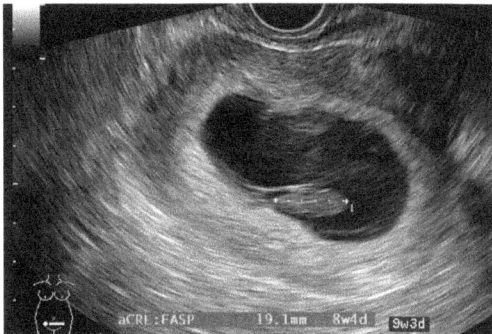

7.92e

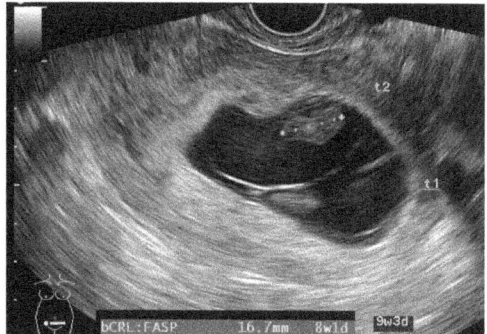

7.92f

Ultrasound Services in an Early Pregnancy and Acute Gynaecological Unit. Book 2

271

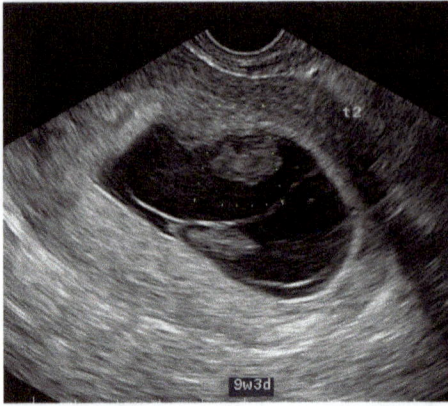

7.92g

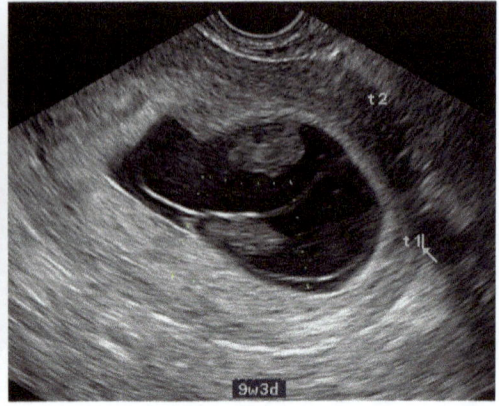

7.92h

a. Which type of pregnancy is this?

b. Describe the ultrasound findings

c. What is the ultrasound diagnosis?

93

This woman was referred with a history of falling from staircase 1/7 earlier.

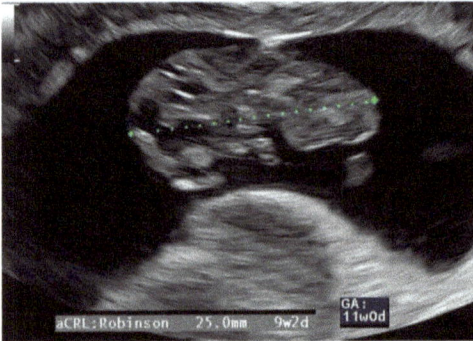

93.a

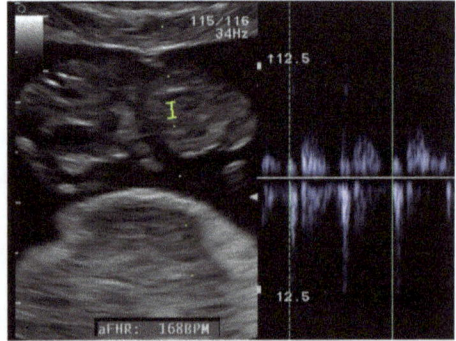

93.b

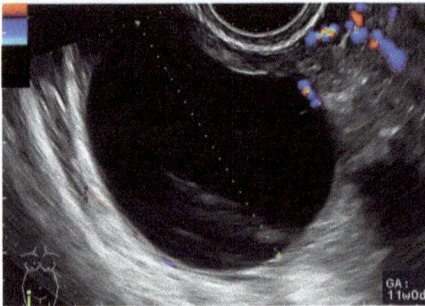

93.c

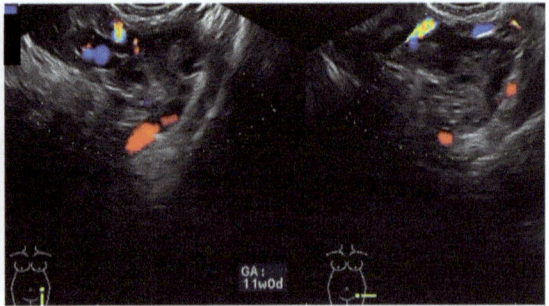

93.d ++ 50mm

Ultrasound Services in an Early Pregnancy and Acute Gynaecological Unit. Book 2

272

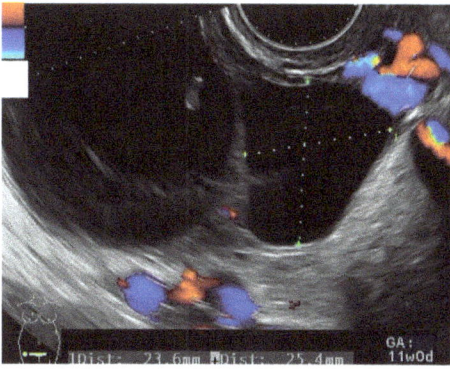

7.93e

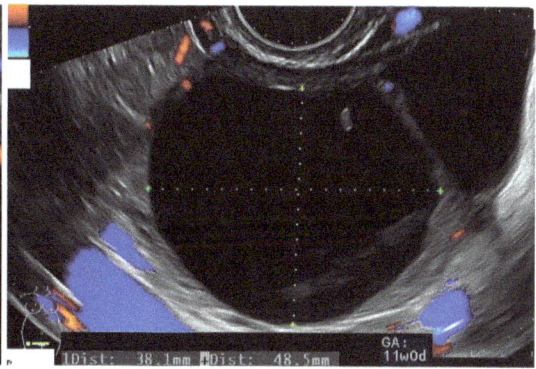

7.93f

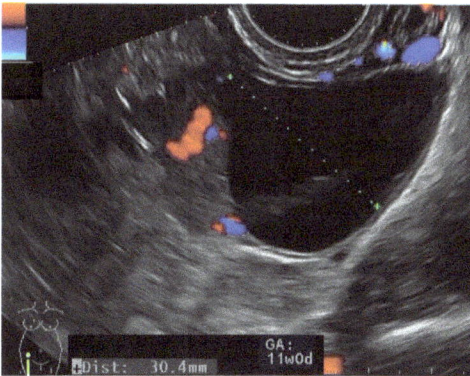

7.93g

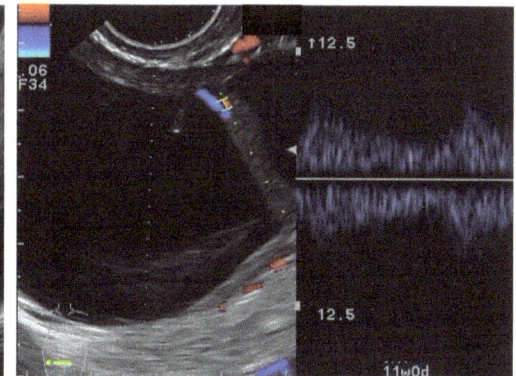

7.93h

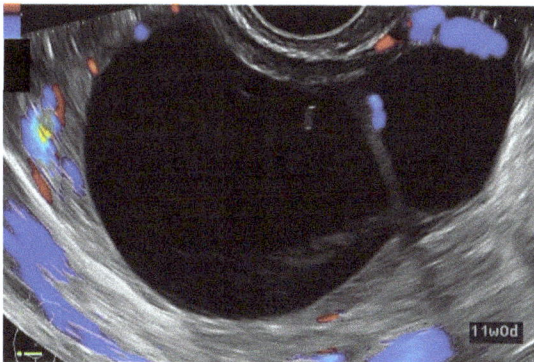

7.93i

a. What is the aim of the examination?
b. Describe the ultrasound findings.

Ultrasound Services in an Early Pregnancy and Acute Gynaecological Unit. Book 2

273

94

This woman was referred for a scan 6/7 post delivery with a clinical history of ?collection. Both ovaries were not identified.

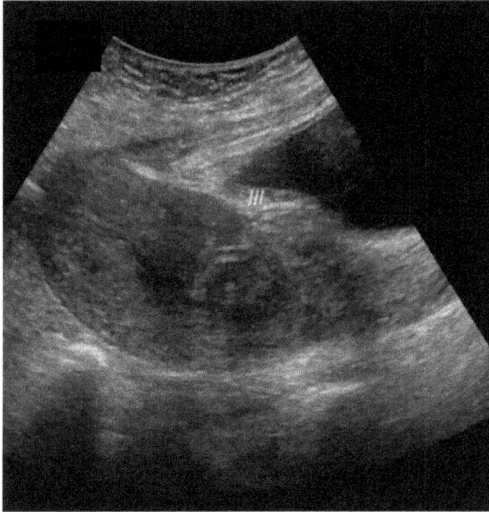

7.94.a

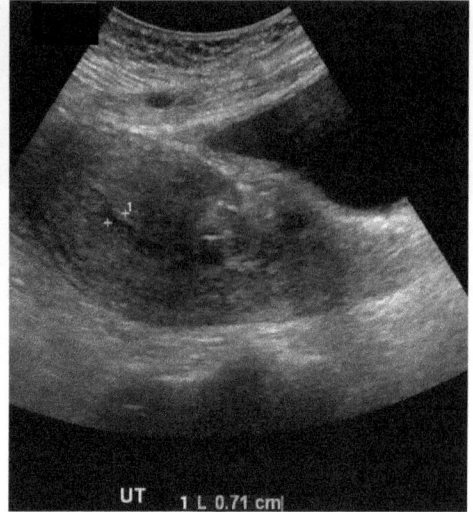

7.94.b

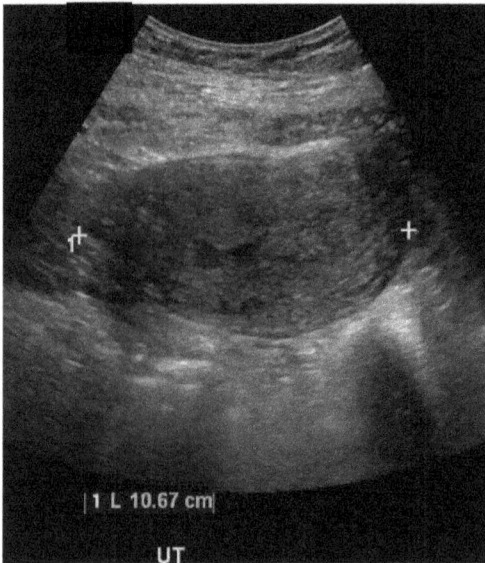

7.94.c

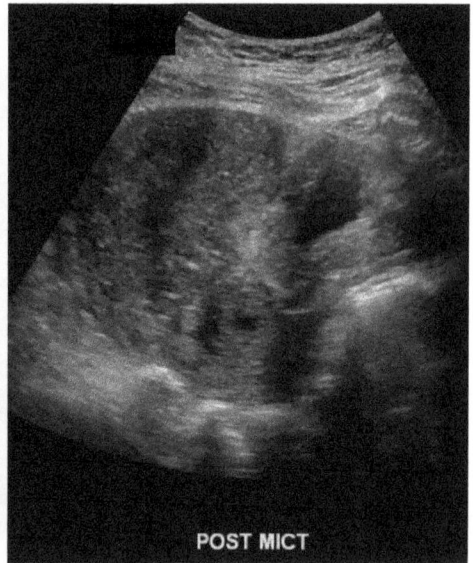

7.94.d

a. How did this woman deliver her baby and what supports your impression?

b. Write the ultrasound report

Ultrasound Services in an Early Pregnancy and Acute Gynaecological Unit. Book 2

274

95

This woman was referred with a clinical history of abdominal pain and pv bleeding for 3/7. 2 frozen embryos transferred. GA by IVF treatment =6/40. Previous scan was inconclusive. Patient was tender in the LIF.

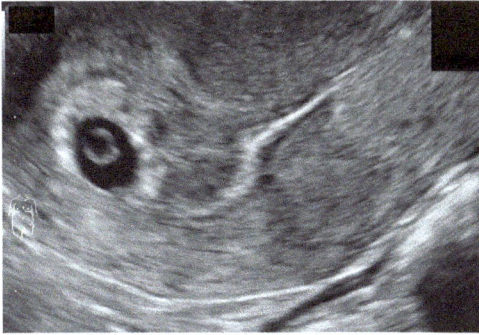

7.95a

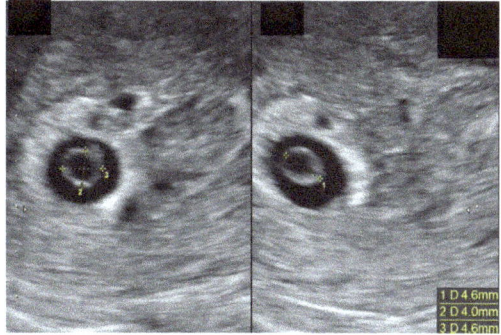

7.95b

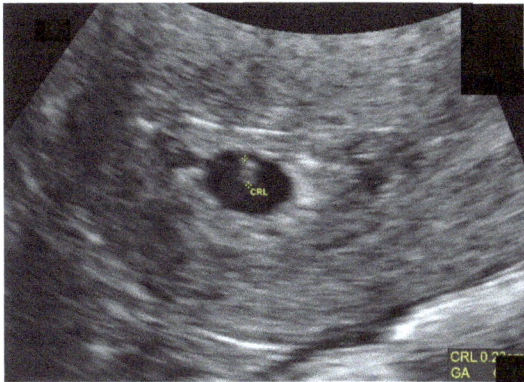

7.95c

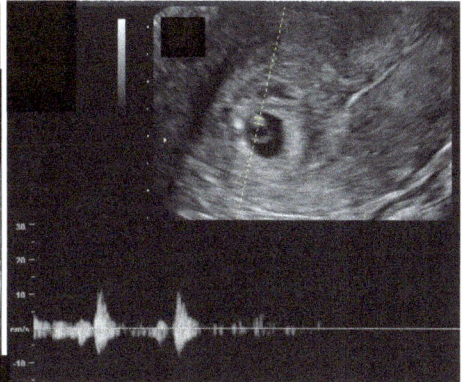

7.95d

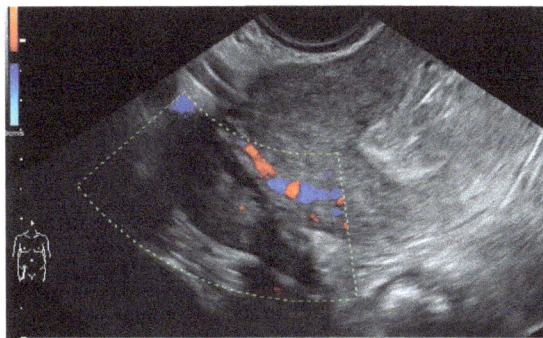

7.95e

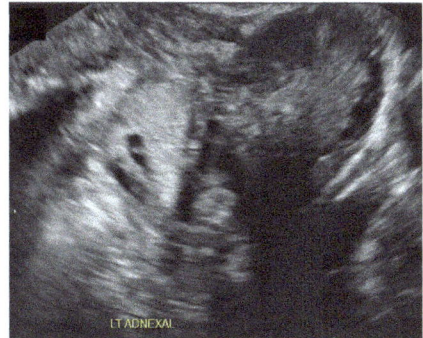

7.95f

Ultrasound Services in an Early Pregnancy and Acute Gynaecological Unit. Book 2

275

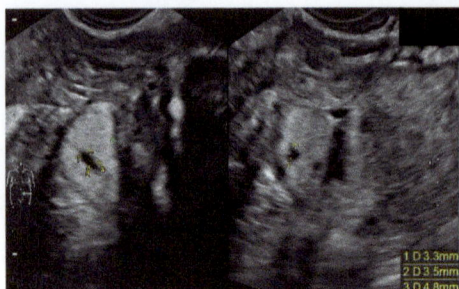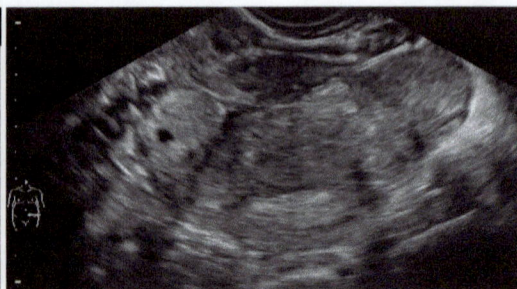

7.95g   **7.95h**

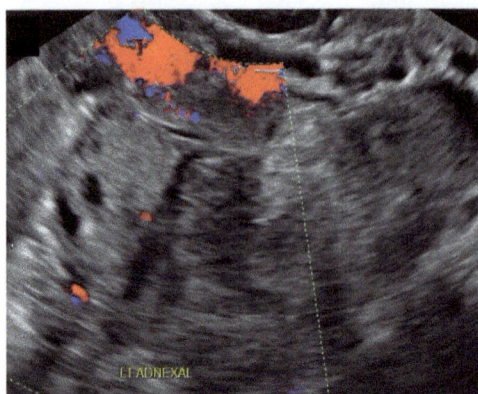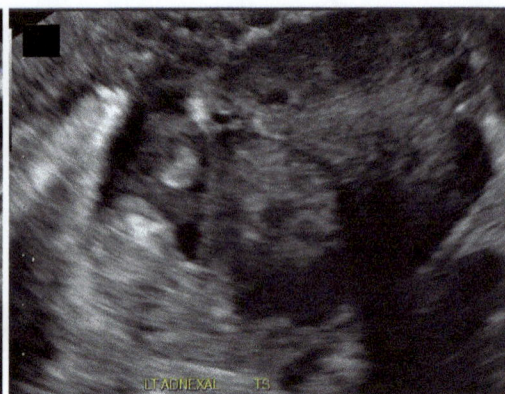

7.95i   **7.95j**
45 x 24 x 39mm

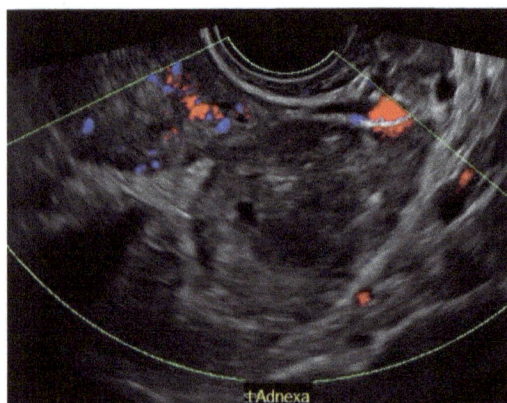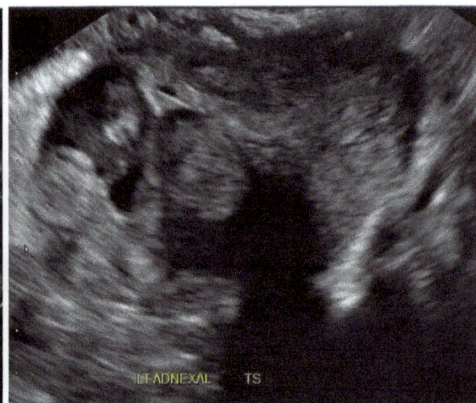

7. 95k   **7.95l**

a. Describe the ultrasound findings
b. What is the diagnosis?
c. How could ultrasound be used to manage this pregnancy?

Ultrasound Services in an Early Pregnancy and Acute Gynaecological Unit. Book 2

276

96

This woman was referred with a history of pelvic pain. LMP 2-3 weeks before.

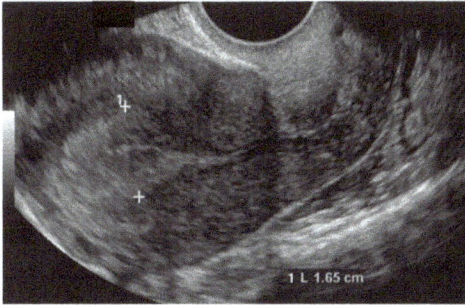

7.96a

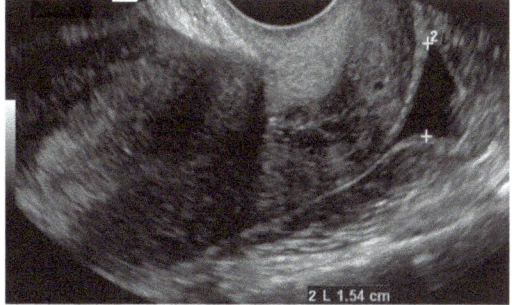

7.96b

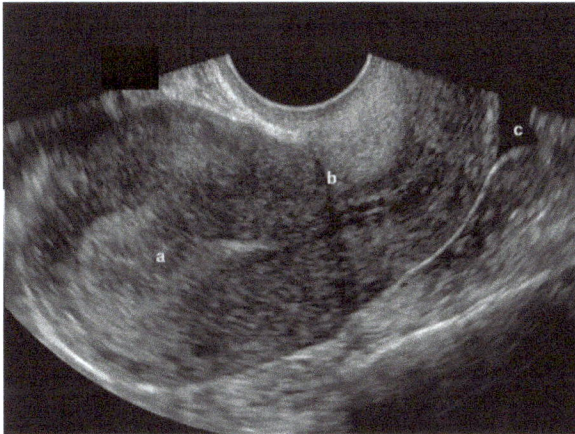

7.96c

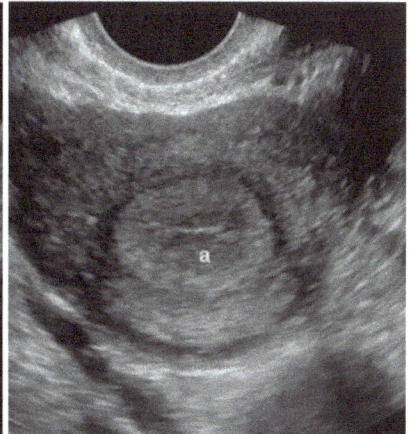

7.96d

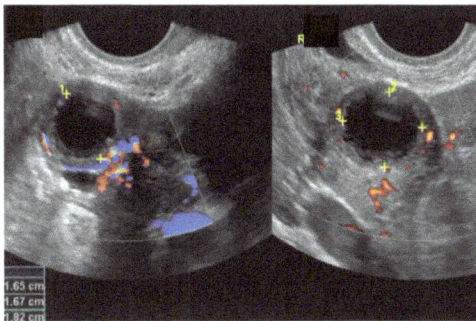

7.96e

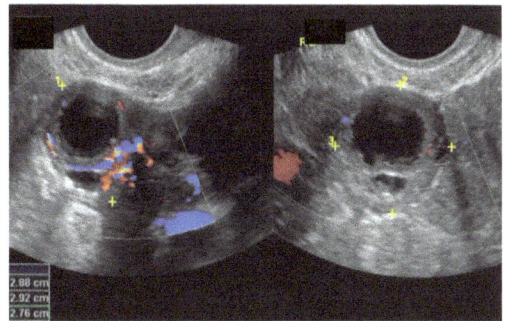

7.96f

Ultrasound Services in an Early Pregnancy and Acute Gynaecological Unit. Book 2

277

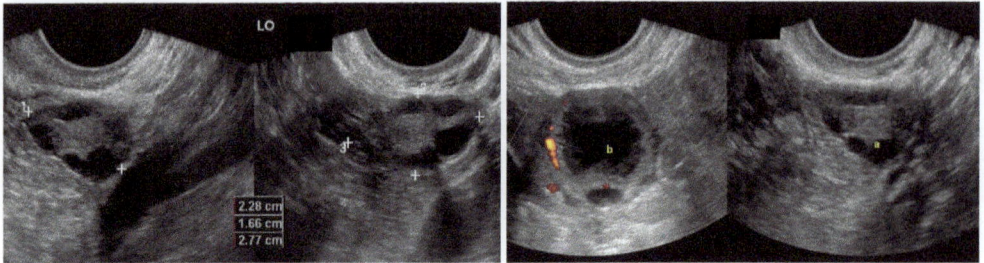

7.96g   **7.96h**

a. Identify sections 96c and d
b. Identify a-c in 96c-d and h
c   In which phase of the menstrual cycle is this woman?
d. Write the ultrasound report

97

This is a follow up examination. Clinical history of pv spotting in pregnancy. EHB not shown here was seen. Both ovaries were not identified.

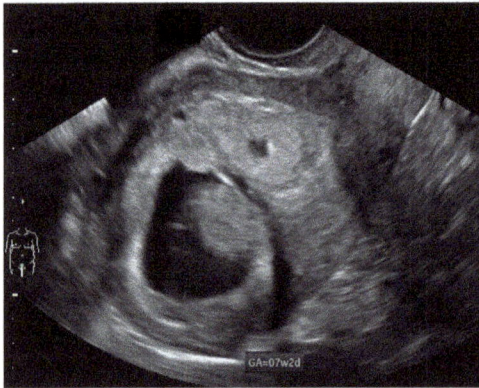

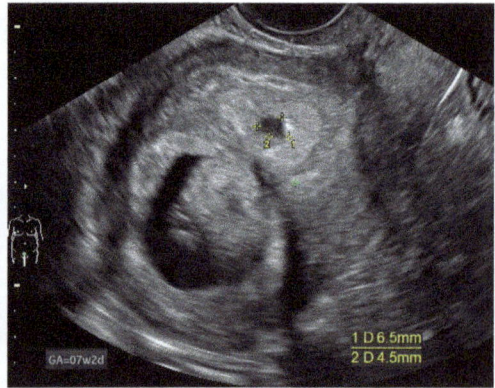

7.97a   **7.97b**

Ultrasound Services in an Early Pregnancy and Acute Gynaecological Unit. Book 2

278

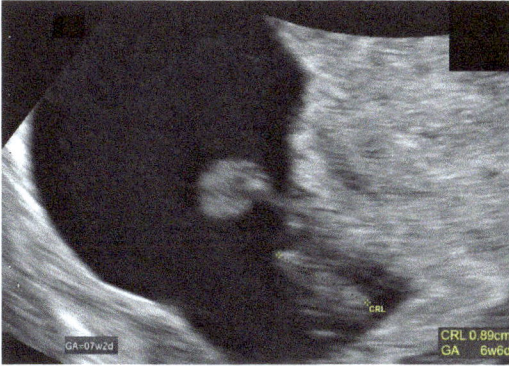

7.97c

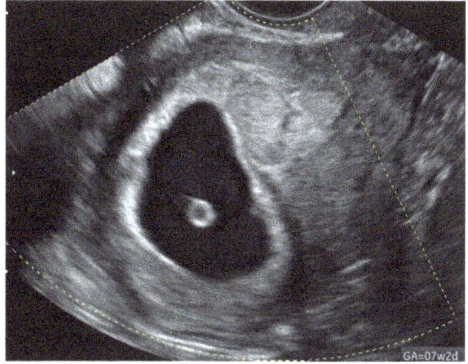

7.97d

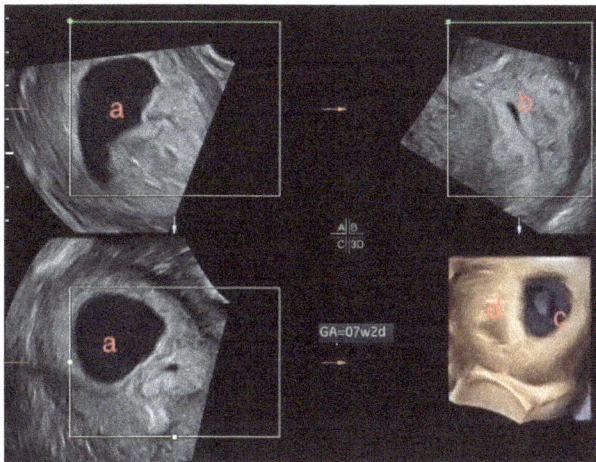

7.97e

a. Identify a-d in 97e.

b. Write the ultrasound report.

c. Can you identify the possible cause of this woman's bleeding?

Ultrasound Services in an Early Pregnancy and Acute Gynaecological Unit. Book 2

279

98

This woman was referred with a clinical history of pelvic pains. Below are the ultrasound findings on Day 21 of her cycle.

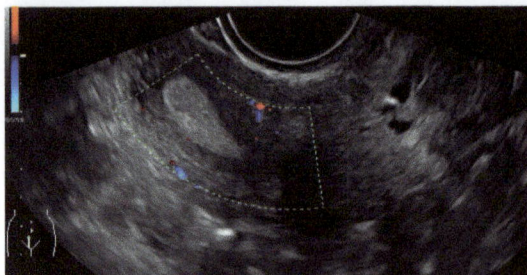

7.98a

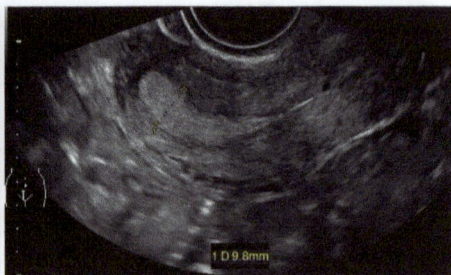

7.98b

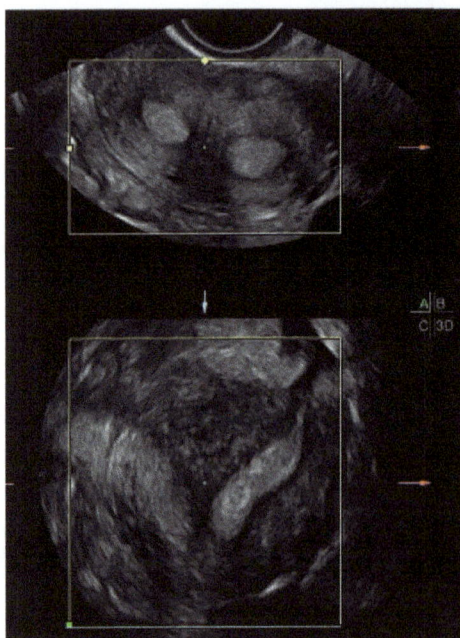

7.98c

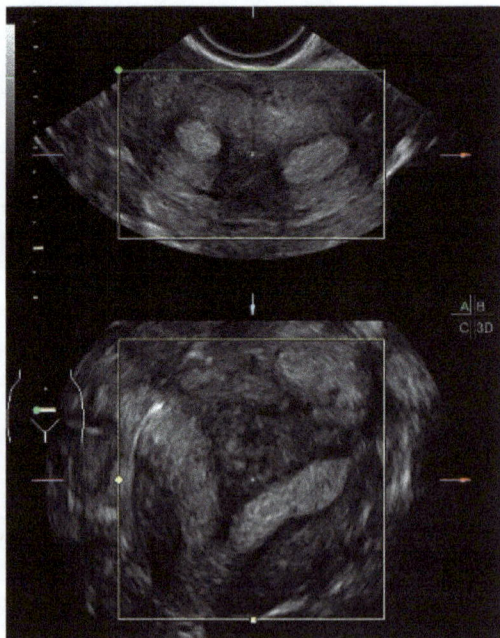

7.98d

Ultrasound Services in an Early Pregnancy and Acute Gynaecological Unit. Book 2

280

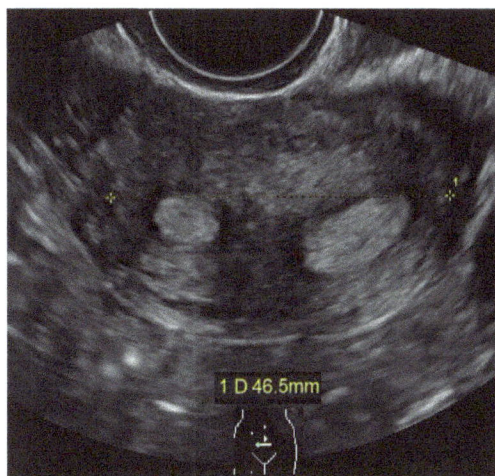

1 D 46.5mm

7.98f

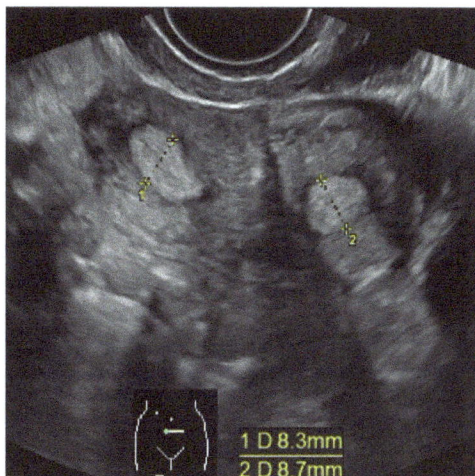

1 D 8.3mm
2 D 8.7mm

7.98f

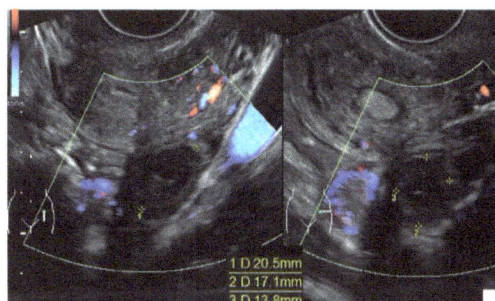

1 D 20.5mm
2 D 17.1mm
3 D 13.8mm

7.98g

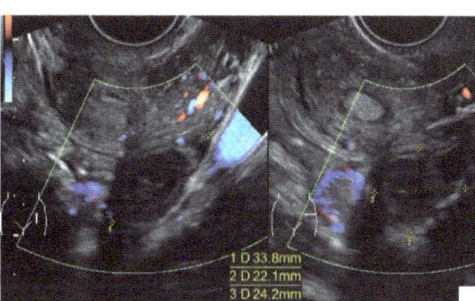

1 D 33.8mm
2 D 22.1mm
3 D 24.2mm

7.98h

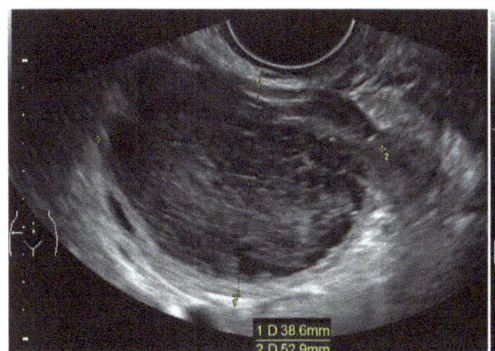

1 D 38.6mm
2 D 52.9mm

7.98i

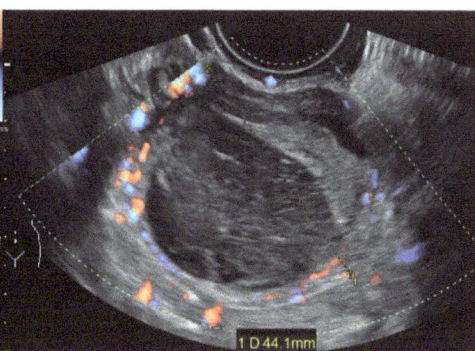

1 D 44.1mm

7.98j

Ultrasound Services in an Early Pregnancy and Acute Gynaecological Unit. Book 2

281

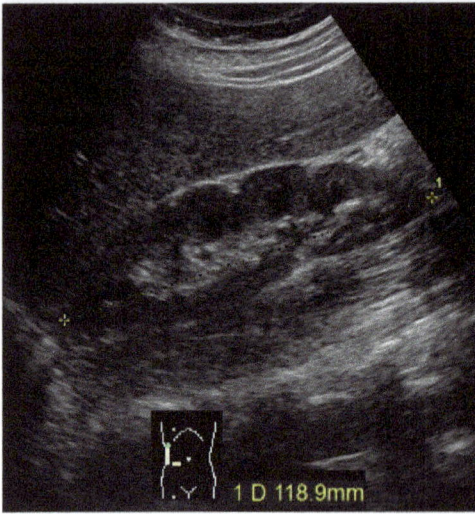

7.98k

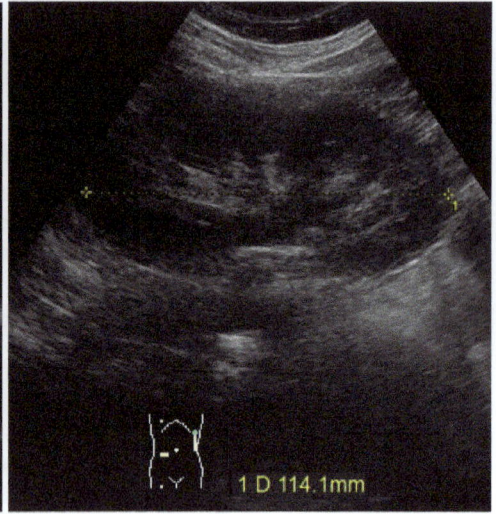

7.98l

a. Why did the Sonographer scan the patient's kidneys?
b. Write the ultrasound report
c. What is the differentials?

99

This woman was referred with a history of previous endometriosis. Below are some ultrasound and MRI images.

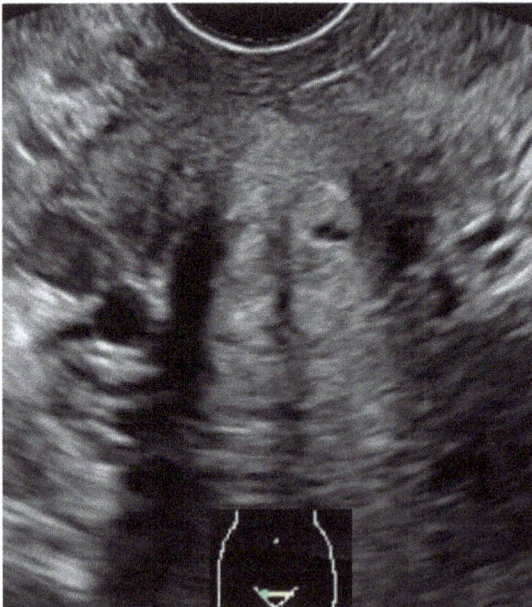

7.99a

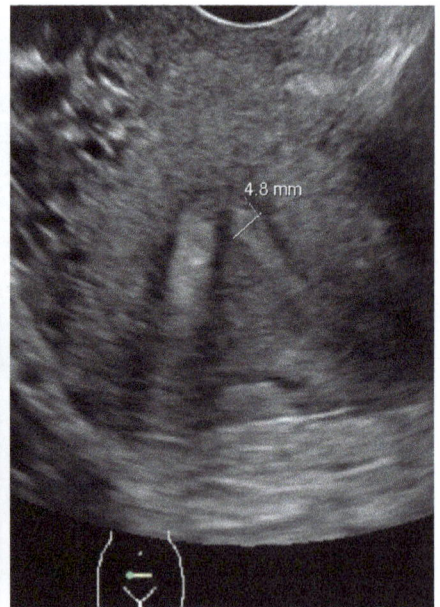

7.99b

Ultrasound Services in an Early Pregnancy and Acute Gynaecological Unit. Book 2

282

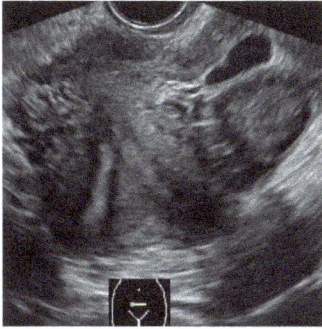
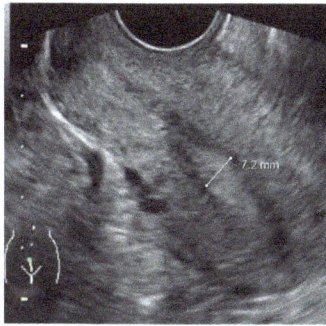
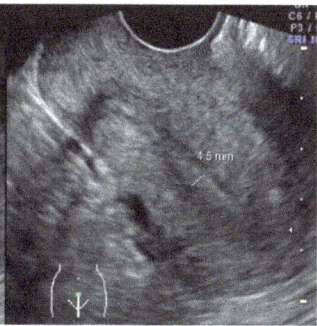

7.99c

7.99d

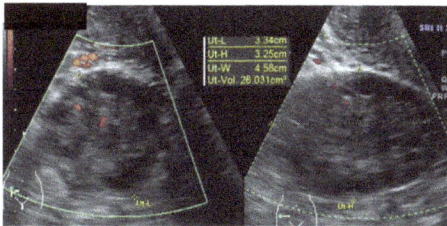
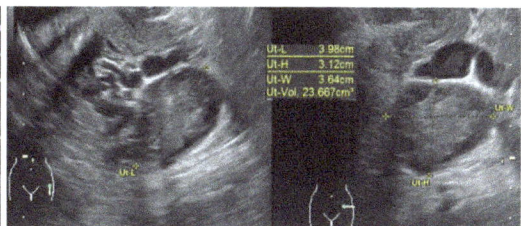

7.99e

7.99f

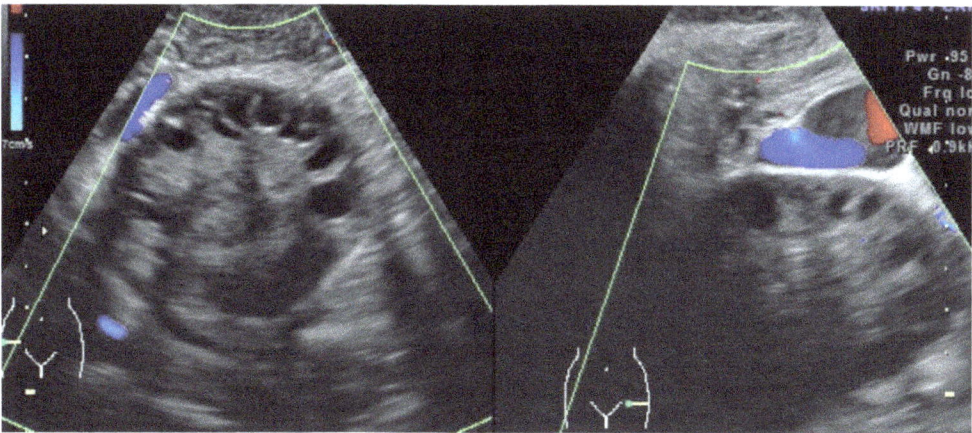

7.99g

Ultrasound Services in an Early Pregnancy and Acute Gynaecological Unit. Book 2

283

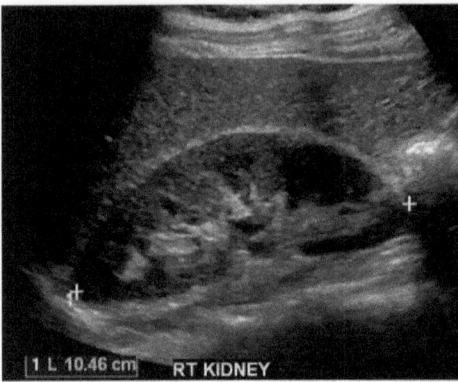

7.99h

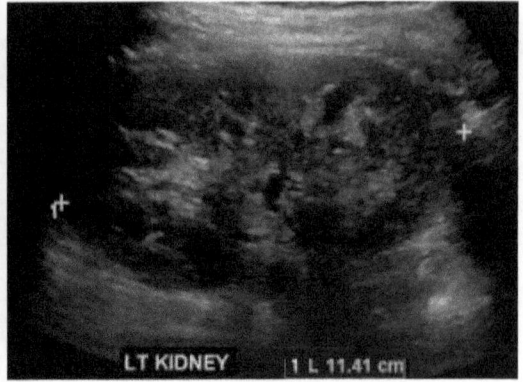

7.99i

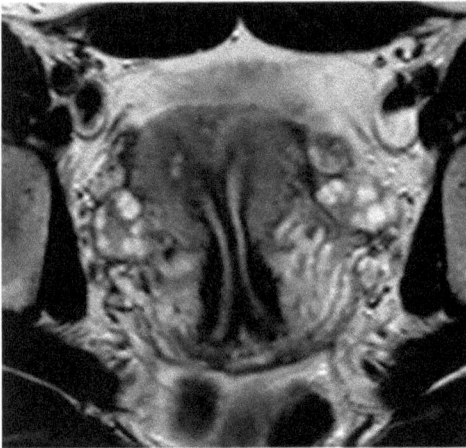

7.99j

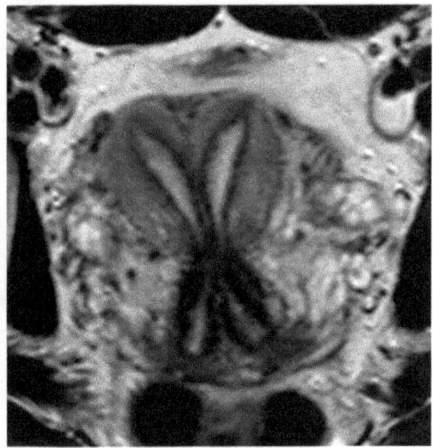

7.99k

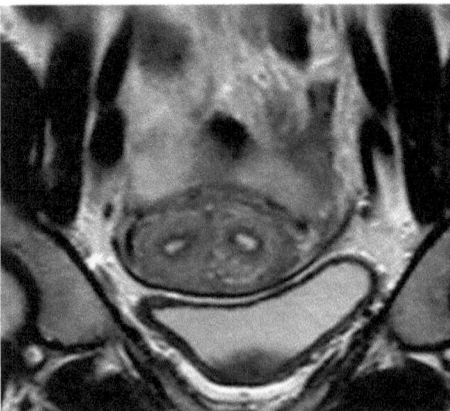

7.99l

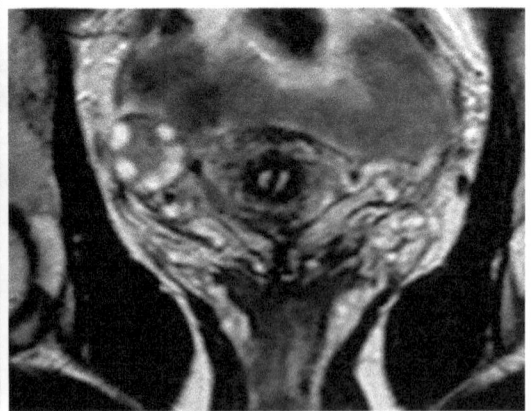

7.99m

a. Describe the ultrasound findings

b. What is the ultrasound diagnosis.

Ultrasound Services in an Early Pregnancy and Acute Gynaecological Unit. Book 2

284

100a.

Identify the following and indicate any clinical significance:

	IMAGE/S	What is it?	Clinical Significance
A	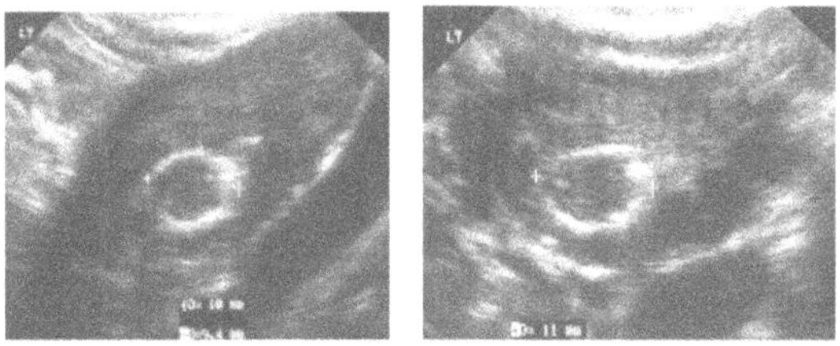		
B	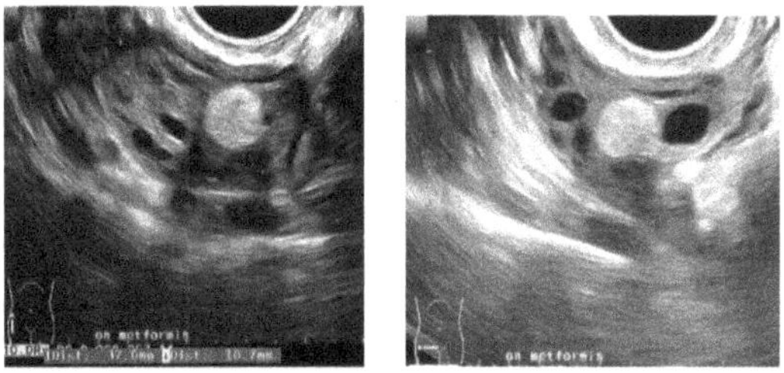		
C	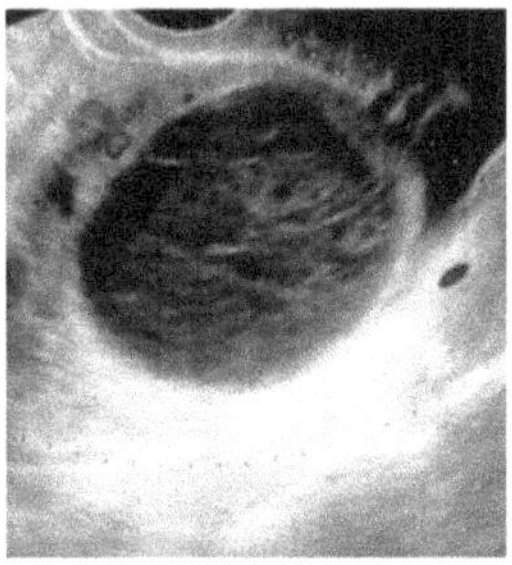		
D	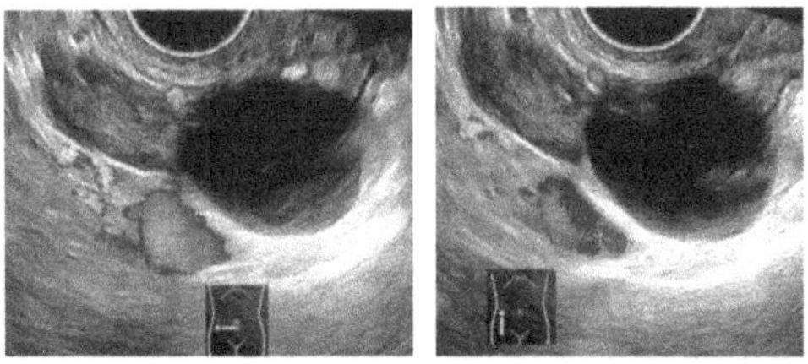		
E	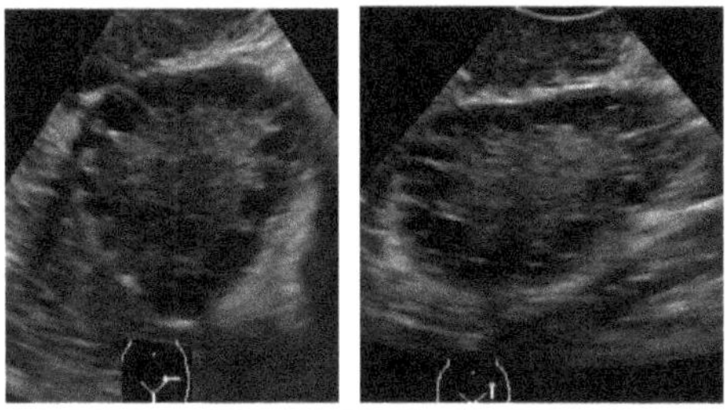		

Ultrasound Services in an Early Pregnancy and Acute Gynaecological Unit. Book 2

285

F			
G			
H			
I			
J			

Ultrasound Services in an Early Pregnancy and Acute Gynaecological Unit. Book 2

286

K			
L			
M			

100b.
Identify the following, where and the clinical significance if any:

	Image	What	Where	Clinical Significance
i				

Ultrasound Services in an Early Pregnancy and Acute Gynaecological Unit. Book 2

287

ii				
iii				
iv				

Ultrasound Services in an Early Pregnancy and Acute Gynaecological Unit. Book 2

288

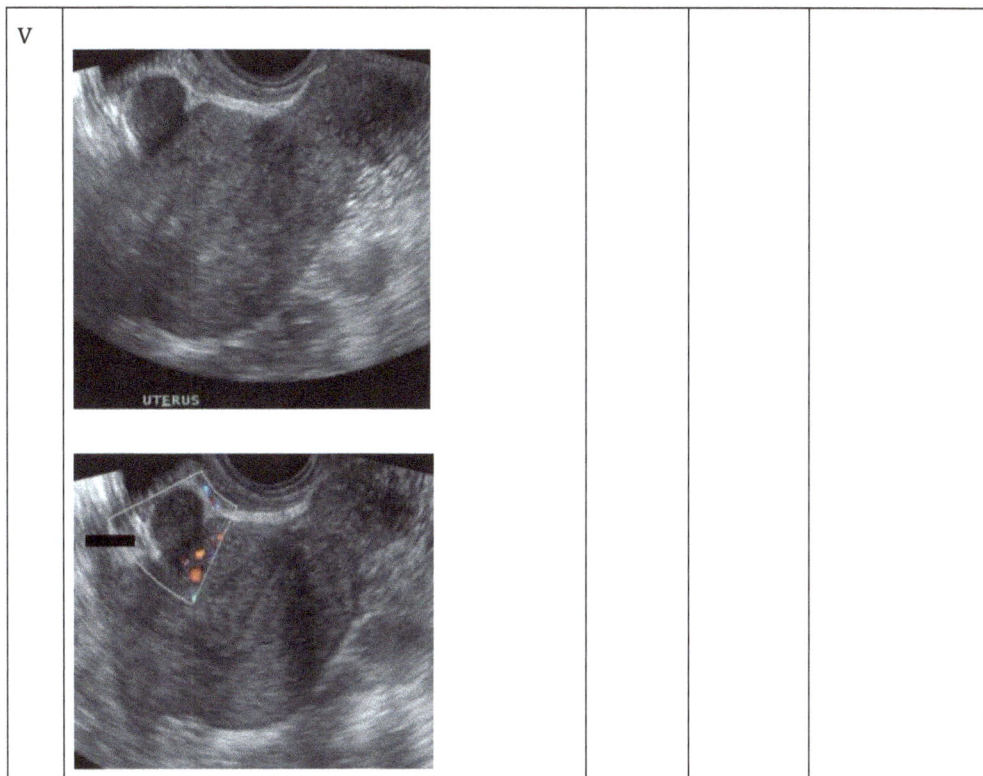

UTERUS

7.101

This lady was referred with a history of ?pvb,. FHB and movements were noted in F2.

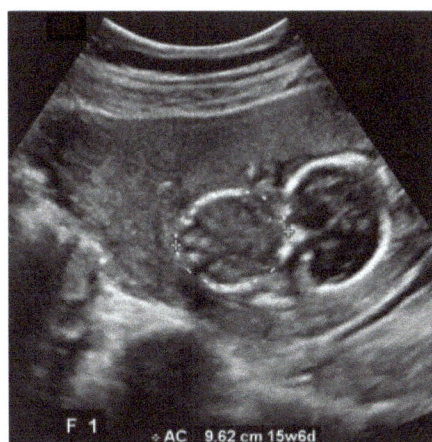

F 1   ⊹AC 9.62 cm 15w6d

7.101a

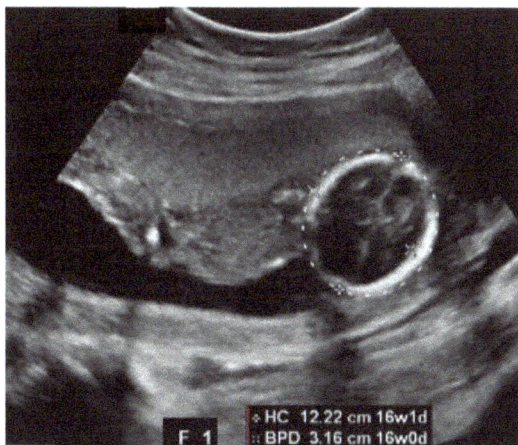

⊹HC 12.22 cm 16w1d
∷BPD 3.16 cm 16w0d

F 1

7.101b

Ultrasound Services in an Early Pregnancy and Acute Gynaecological Unit. Book 2

289

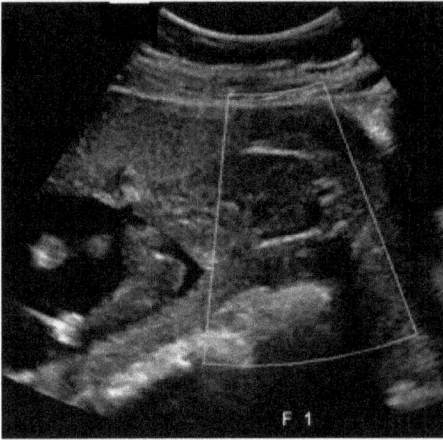

7.101c

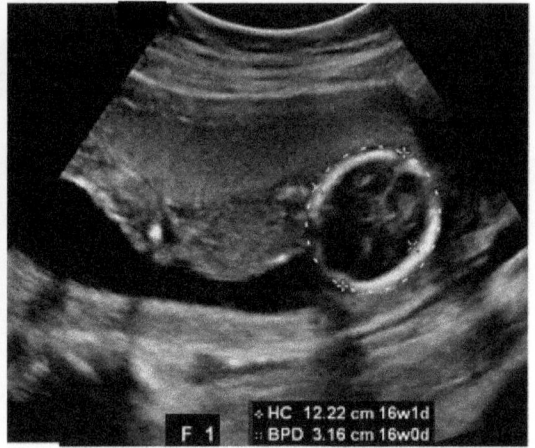

HC 12.22 cm 16w1d
BPD 3.16 cm 16w0d
F 1

7.101d

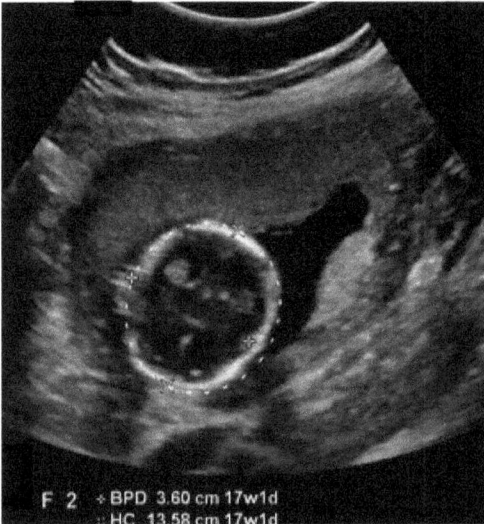

F 2   BPD 3.60 cm 17w1d
HC 13.58 cm 17w1d

7.101e

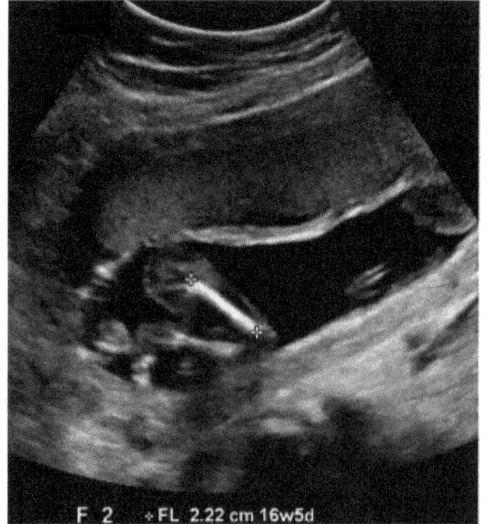

F 2   FL 2.22 cm 16w5d

7.101f

Ultrasound Services in an Early Pregnancy and Acute Gynaecological Unit. Book 2

290

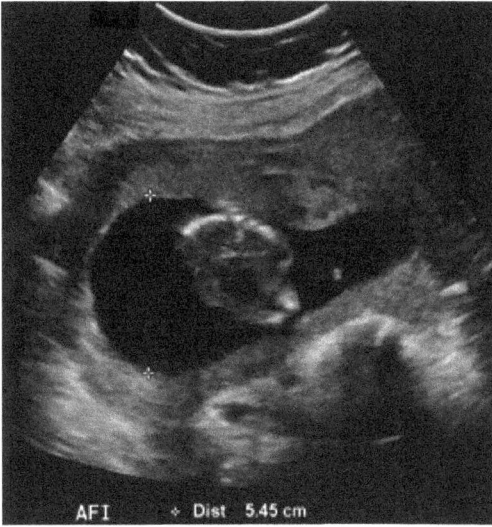

7.101g

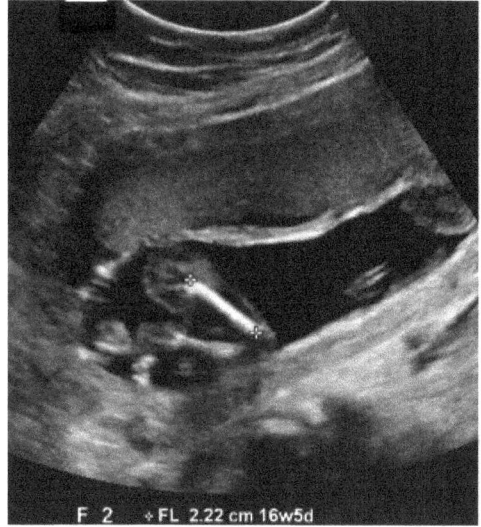

7.101h

a. What type of pregnancy has been shown?

b. Are there any challenges for the sonographer?

c. Describe the ultrasound appearances

d. What is your diagnosis?

e. How can ultrasound be used in the management of the pregnancy?

Ultrasound Services in an Early Pregnancy and Acute Gynaecological Unit. Book 2

291

Chapter 8

Answers to the 101 Case presentations and Quiz

In this chapter, answers will be provided to the questions in chapter 7. Any known additional information will be included. To avoid confusion, the images in this chapter will have similar labeling as in chapter 7.

ANSWERS

1a

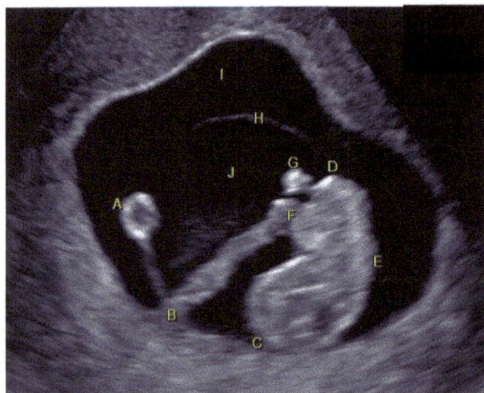

7.1a

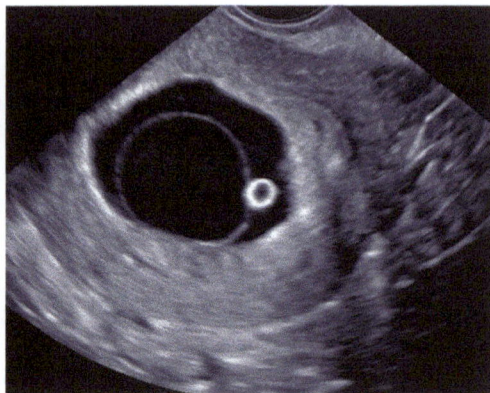

7.1b

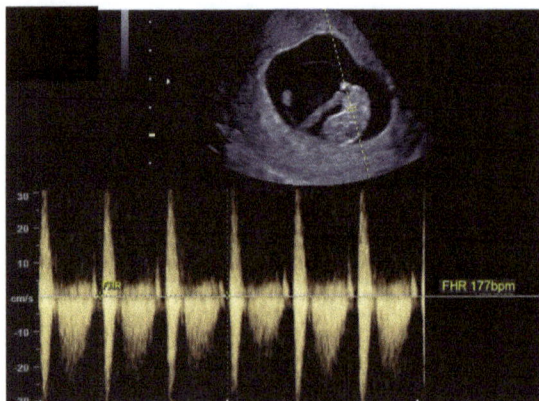

7.1c

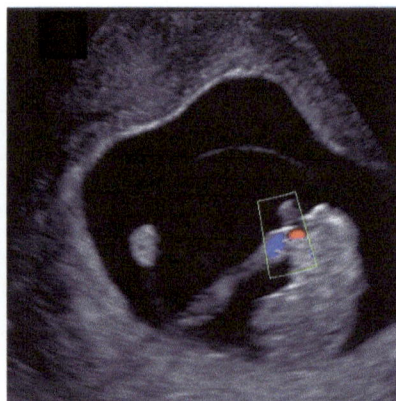

7.1d

Ultrasound Services in an Early Pregnancy and Acute Gynaecological Unit. Book 2

292

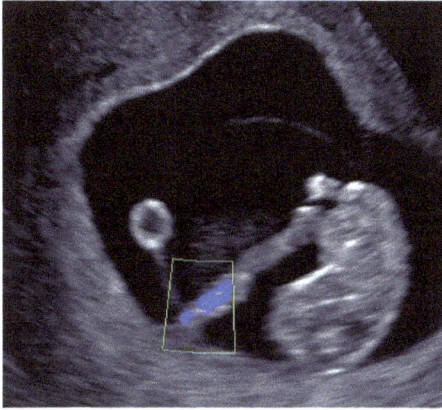

7.1e

7.1a

A. yolk sac

B. cord insertion to placenta .

C. head or crown

D. rump or bum

E. embryo back

F. cord insertion to the embryo's abdomen.

G. lower limb bud

H. amniotic membrane or amnion

I. chorionic cavity

J. amniotic cavity

1b

The embryo is between 8 –9+/40. This is because the limb buds are just beginning to be seen and the yolk sac is seen outside the amniotic membrane as from 8+/40. FHB has been claimed to be at it's maximum 177bpm at 9/40.
This embryo was 8+6/40 by CRL.

1c

The yolk sac (smaller, more hyper echoic and directly outside the amniotic membrane) and the amniotic membrane (thinner but bigger circle in the gestational sac)

1d

Colour Doppler box in 7.1d is at the cord insertion into the embyronic abdomen and in 7.1e the Colour Doppler box is the cord insertion to the placenta.

Ultrasound Services in an Early Pregnancy and Acute Gynaecological Unit. Book 2

293

7.2a

TS showing lower limbs at 12+4/40. Can you identify a-d ?

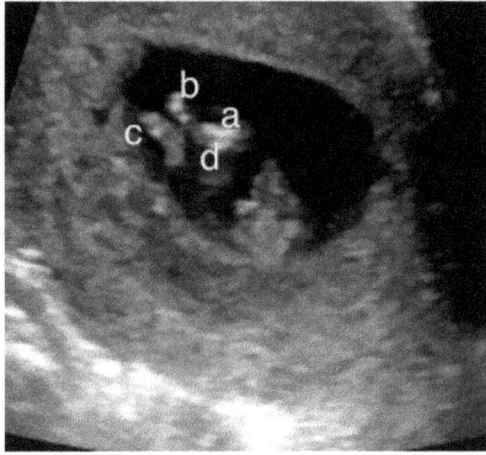

7.2a

a –right tibia, b-right foot, c-left foot, d- right fibula.

7.2b

TS at the level of the fetal thorax showing both hands and face at 12+4/40.

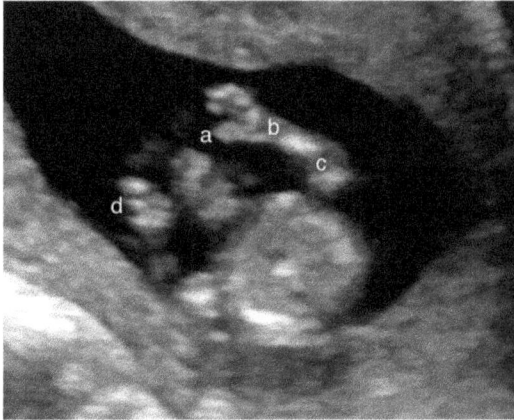

a- left thumb
b- left wrist
c- left elbow
d- right hand

Ultrasound Services in an Early Pregnancy and Acute Gynaecological Unit. Book 2

294

7.2c

12/40. Identify a-g.

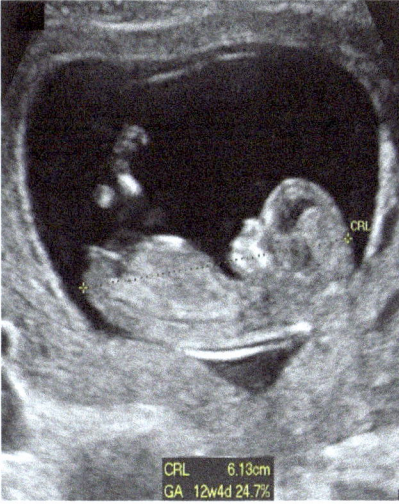 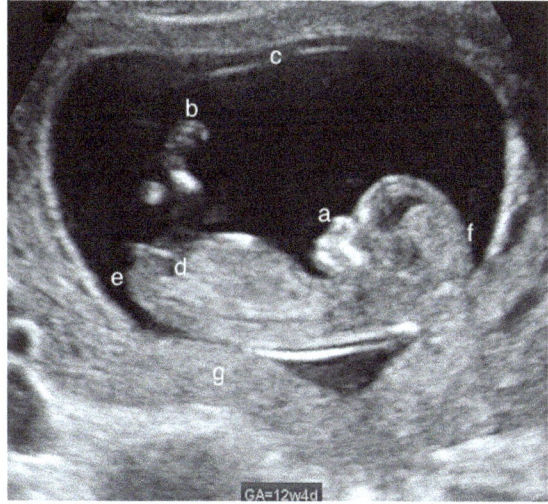

7.2c	7.2cc

Saggital view of the fetus

a-tip of the nose, b- foot, c-amniotic membrane or amnion, d-urinary bladder,
e-fetal rum or bum or bottom, f-crown or head, g-posterior placenta

7.2d

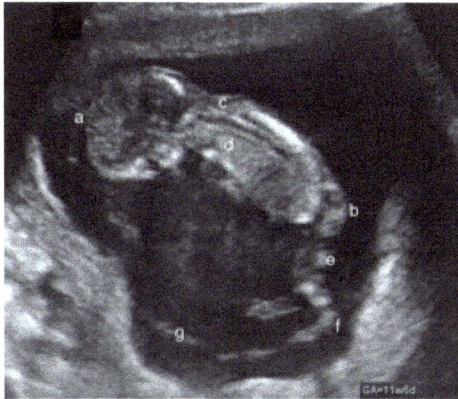

7.2d

(oblique sagittal view)

a-head or crown, b-bottom or bum orrump, c- spine, d-ribs, e-femur, f-heel,
g-amniotic membrane or amnion

Ultrasound Services in an Early Pregnancy and Acute Gynaecological Unit. Book 2

295

7.2e

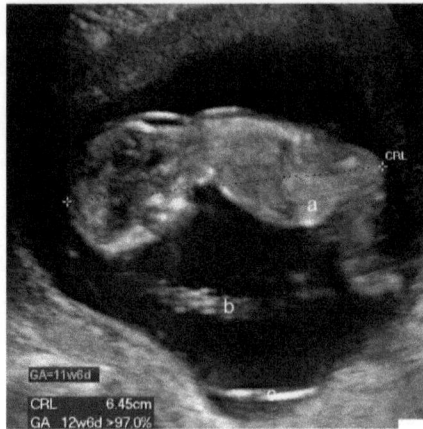

7.2e
Sagittal view

a-small intestine, b-cord, c-amnion or amniotic membrane

7.2f

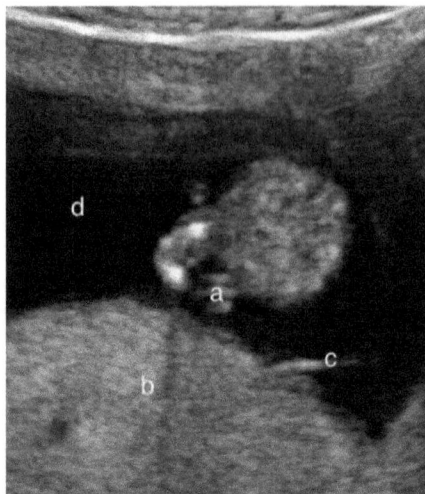

7.2f
TS view of the abdomen at the level of the cord insertion

a-cord insertion into the embryonic abdomen, b-posterior placenta, c, amniotic membrane or amnion, d-amniotic fluid.

Ultrasound Services in an Early Pregnancy and Acute Gynaecological Unit. Book 2

296

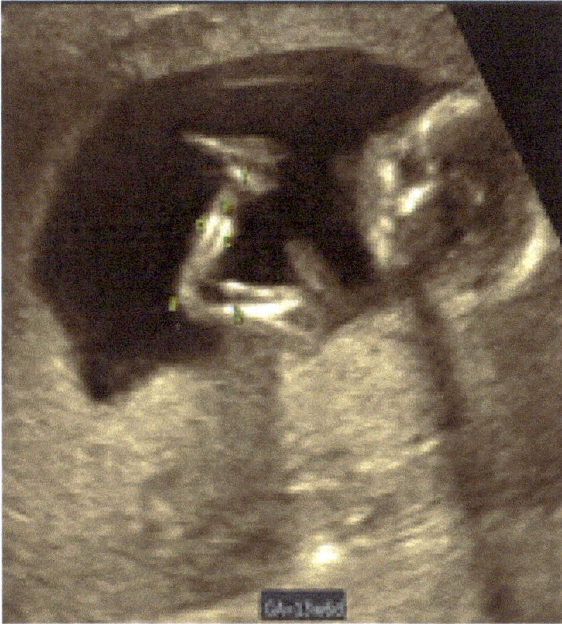

7.2g
a-elbow, b- humerus, c-ulna, d-radius

7.2h

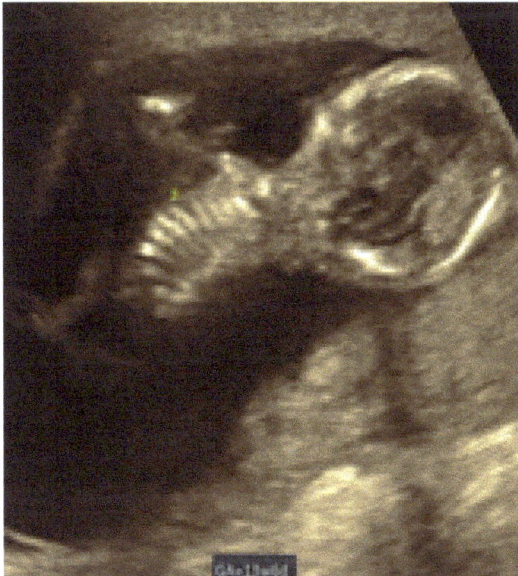

7.2h
a-ribs

Ultrasound Services in an Early Pregnancy and Acute Gynaecological Unit. Book 2

297

7.2i

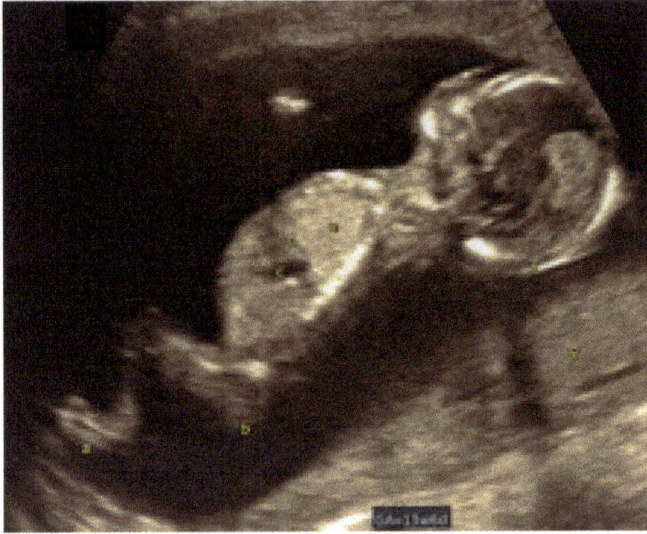

7.2i
sagittal view of the fetus
a-foot, b-bottomor bum or rump, c-stomach, d-diaphragm, e-left lung, f-cranium, g-placenta

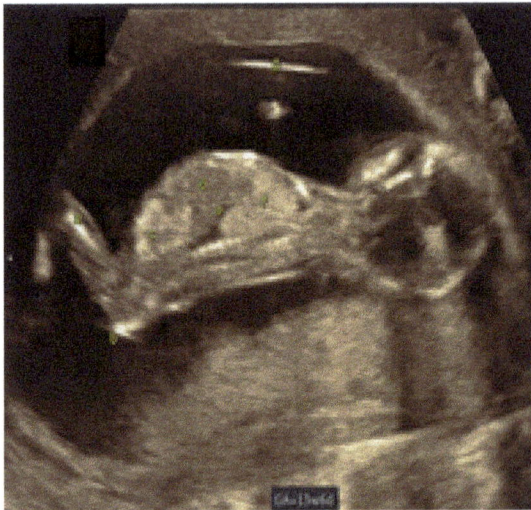

7.2j
a-Femur, b-bottom or bum or rump, c-small intestine, d-liver, e-diaphragm, f-right lung, g -amniotic membrane

Ultrasound Services in an Early Pregnancy and Acute Gynaecological Unit. Book 2

298

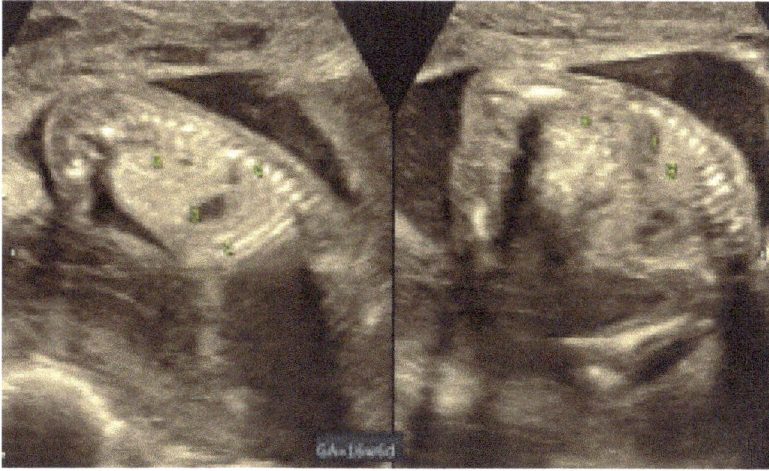

7.2k

a-Left kidney, b- stomach, c-ribs, d-spine, e-right kidney, f-diaphragm, g-right lung

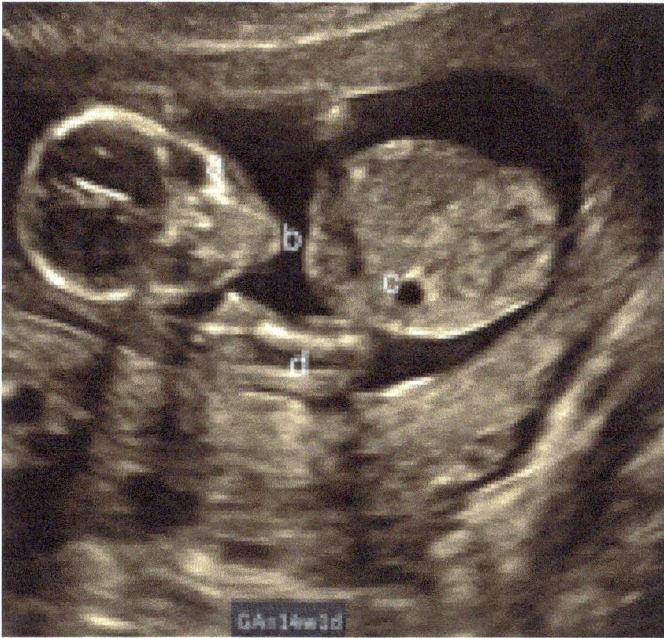

7.2l

a-orbit, b-chin, c-stomach, d- forearm

Ultrasound Services in an Early Pregnancy and Acute Gynaecological Unit. Book 2

299

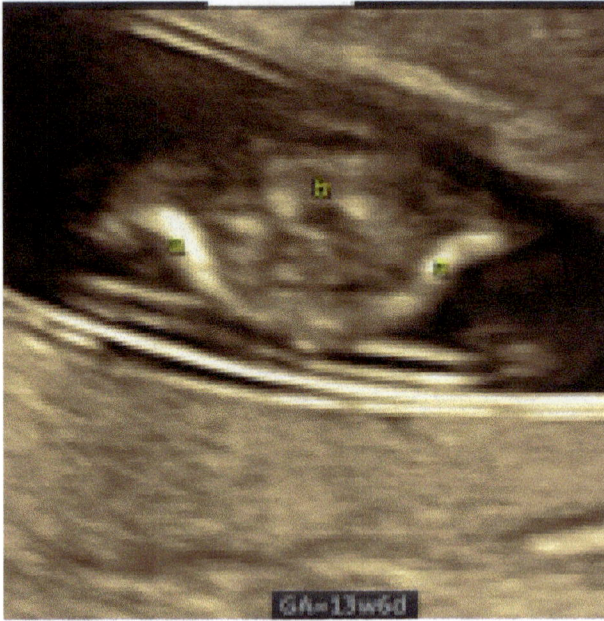

7.2m
TS of the level of the clavicles
a. clavicle, b- TS Spine

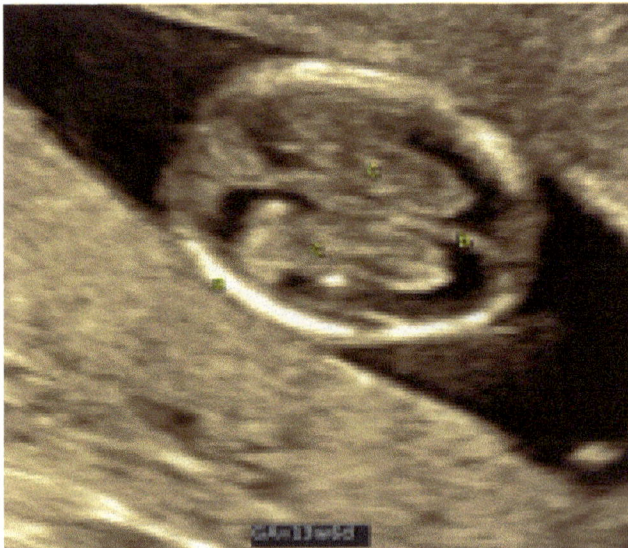

7.2n
view showing the choroid plexus

Ultrasound Services in an Early Pregnancy and Acute Gynaecological Unit. Book 2

300

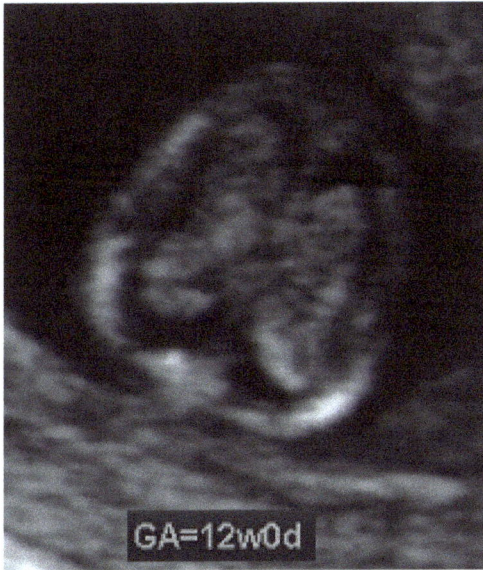

7.2o

a- ossified portion of the calvarium, b- falx cerebri, c-choroid plexus.
* the choroid plexus should have a butterfly shape at this stage in a normal
pregnancy as above.

7.3a

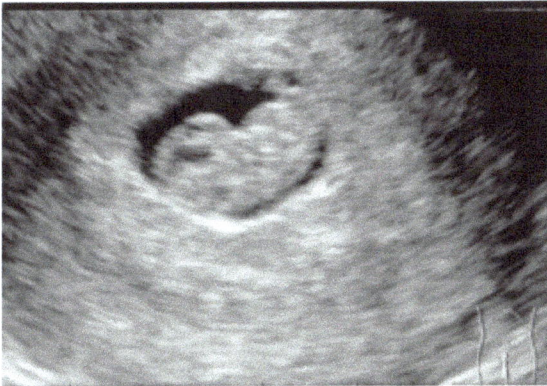

7.3a

There is reduced amniotic fluid making in impossible to distinguish YS or
amniotic membrane.

* compare this image with 7.1a. Both embryos are about the same GA.
*Follow up scan later showed a missed abortion or miscarriage.

Ultrasound Services in an Early Pregnancy and Acute Gynaecological Unit. Book 2

301

7.3b

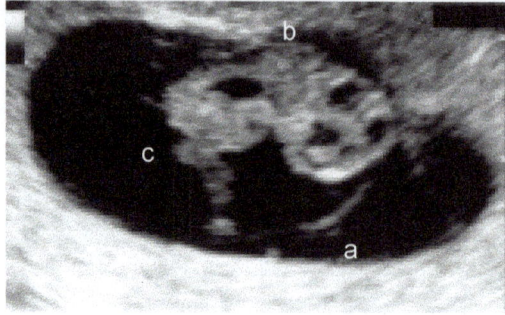

7.3b

There is an unusual cystic entity in the abdomen.

*Follow up scan 3 weeks later showed a missed abortion.

7.4a

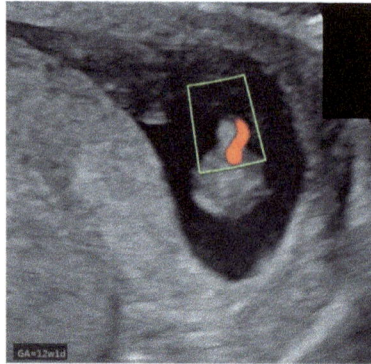

7.4a

TS of the abdomen at the level of the cord insertion (Colour Doppler box)

7.4b

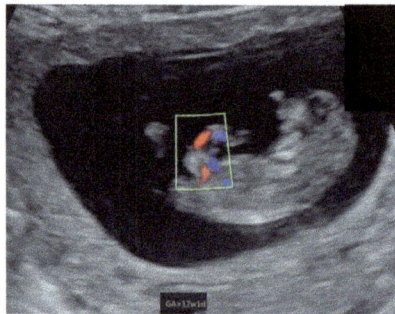

7.4b

Sagittal view of fetus showing the cord insertion (Colour Doppler box)

Ultrasound Services in an Early Pregnancy and Acute Gynaecological Unit. Book 2

302

7.4c

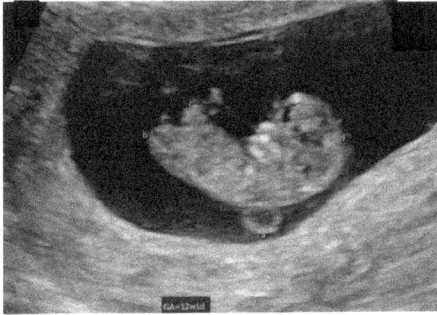

7.4c
Sagittal view of fetus
a- yolk sac, b- rump or bum or bottom, c- cord insertion, d- head or crown

7.4d

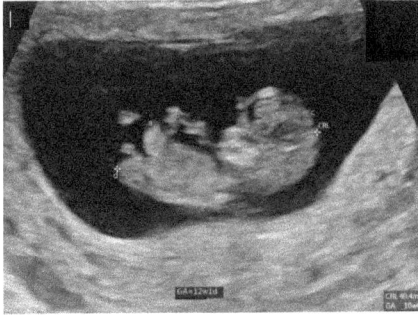

7.4d
Sagittal view of fetus
a- herniated gut, b- cord, c- crown or head, d- rump or bum or bottom, e- fetal back

7.4e

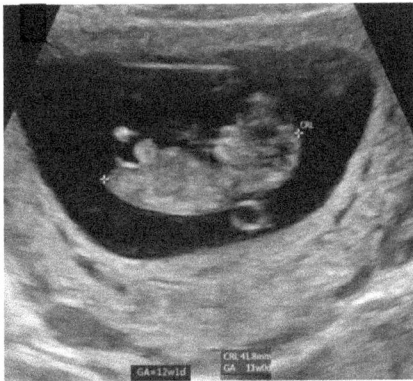

7.4e
Sagittal view of fetus.
CRL = 41.8mm = 11/40

Ultrasound Services in an Early Pregnancy and Acute Gynaecological Unit. Book 2

303

7.4f

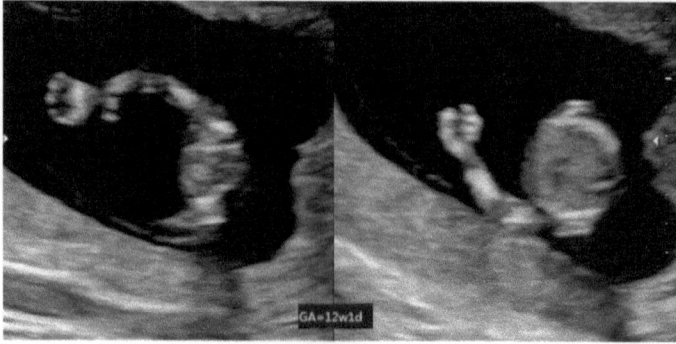

7.4f
Views of both upper limbs

7.4g

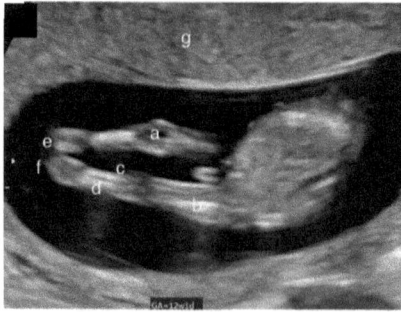

7.4g
view of both lower limbs
a- right knee joint, b- left femur, c- left tibia, d- left fibula, e- right foot
f – left foot, g- anterior placenta

7.4h

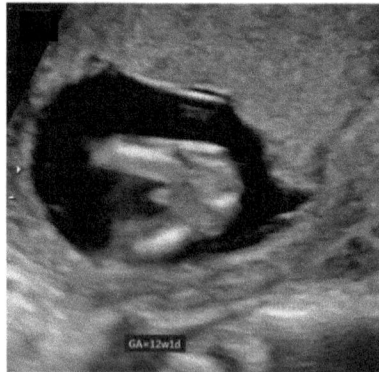

7.4h
view showing both femurs and the fetal gender

Ultrasound Services in an Early Pregnancy and Acute Gynaecological Unit. Book 2

304

7.4i

Fetus is 11/40 (7.4e).

7.4j

What - the Sonographer would need to redate the pregnancy using the CRL NOT the LMP date which initially worked out the fetal gestational age (GA) to be 12+1/40.

Why- So that:

a. The screening tests are not missed but booked appropriately (NT screening and anomaly scan)
b. IUGR is not missed later in the pregnancy
c. Normal growing fetus is not seen or treated as an IUGR fetus
d. The pregnancy can be delivered on time.

7.5a

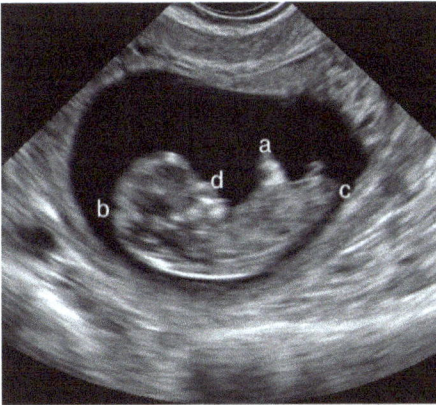 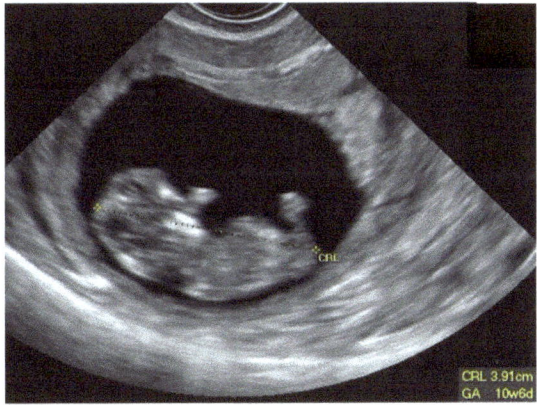

7.5a	**7.5b**

7.5a a- physiological gut herniation, b- crown or head, c- bottom or bum or rump d-tip of the nose

Ultrasound Services in an Early Pregnancy and Acute Gynaecological Unit. Book 2

305

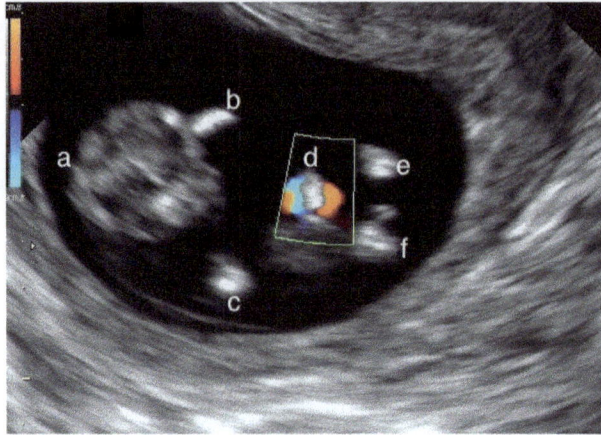

7.5c

7.5c
a-crown or head, b-left hand, c - right upper limb, d-herniated gut and cord
e-left leg, f- right leg

b. No there is nothing wrong with the fetal abdomen at this GA.

There is physiological herniation of the gut at the base of the umbilical cord in the abdomen. This finding is normal at this GA.

7.6

a. There is a 32 x 37 x 4mm predominantly hypoechoic area seen the anterior wall of the uterus. This is likely to represent a subchorionic hematoma or hemorrhage.

b. Date the pregnancy as the CRL > GA by LMP.

c. An intrauterine pregnancy, yolk sac, fetus seen (7.6.a-f) CRL = 54= 12+1/40 (7.6c). FHB and movements not shown were reported to have been seen. The placenta is posterior (7.6c-d).

   Impression: subchorionic hematoma, differentials being unfused amnion,

d. Subchorionic haemorrhage or haematomas have been linked to increased risk of miscarriage, still birth, placental abruption and preterm labor

* The subchorionic hemorrhage (subchorionic hematoma) collects between the uterine wall and the chorionic membrane and may leak through the cervical canal

Ultrasound Services in an Early Pregnancy and Acute Gynaecological Unit. Book 2

306

7.7

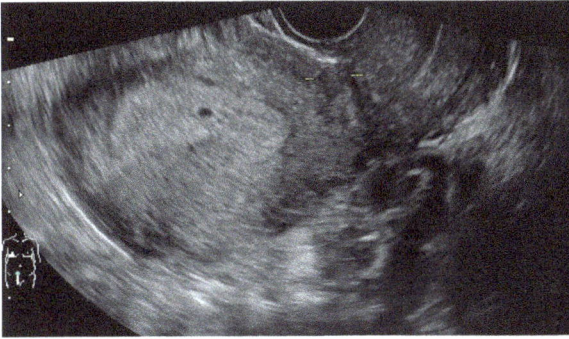
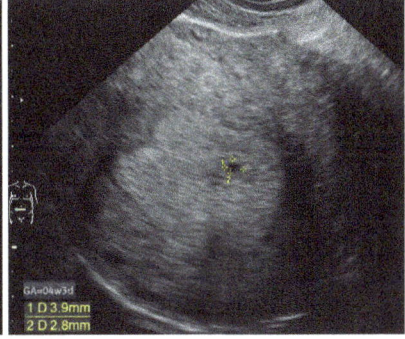

7.7a   **7.7b**

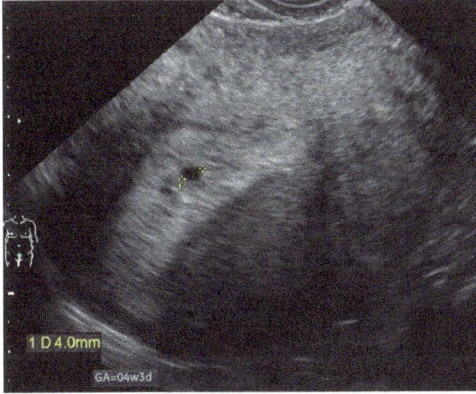
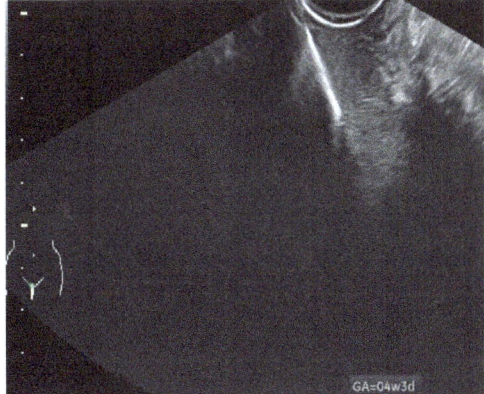

7.7c

a. Third pregnancy at least in view of the C/S scars in 7.7a

b. Copper T IUCD in 7.7d

c. The IUCD is in the cervical canal just above the os (7.7d)

d.   If the IUCD is incorrectly positioned or located as in this case or if the IUCD is in one of the horns of didelphys or bicornuate or septated uterus the patient can get pregnant in the other horn. It can also happen if the IUCD has been expelled without the patient knowing.

e. An anteverted uterus with a 4 x 4 x 3mm cystic entity in a thickened endometrium (7.7 a-c). This is probably an early intrauterine gestational sac. There is an IUCD in the cervical canal just above the os (7.7d). The right ovary is measuring 41 x 34 x 39mm - 28 mls (7.7e) and in it is a 18 x 16 x 21mm corpus

Ultrasound Services in an Early Pregnancy and Acute Gynaecological Unit. Book 2

307

luteum (7.7f). The left ovary is measuring 29 x 31 x 40mm - 18.8 mls (7.7g). ***Impression:*** Possible early intrauterine pregnancy. IUCD is incorrectly positioned in the cervical canal.

7.8

a. a. Left ovary in view of the cyst in it (7.8.d) Normal ultrasound appearance of the right ovary. (7.8.c)
b. The patient has had a previous left salpingectomy and this is a natural conception. The mechanism by which she got pregnant is most likely to be by *transperitoneal migration of the ovum*.
c. An IUP with an embryo with a CRL =13mm= 7+4/40. (7.8.b). EHB = 154bpm (7.8a). The right ovary appears sonographically normal (7.8.c) and there is a cyst in the left ovary (7.8.d) which is probably a corpus luteum.

Impression: An intrauterine pregnancy with EHB. Normal right ovary. Cyst in the left ovary.

- *Transperitoneal migration of the ovum*

There is the belief or suggestion that:

- Transperitoneal migration of ova resulting in intrauterine pregnancy is probably a common event yet rarely observed.
- The corpus luteum is visualized in the ovary opposite to the remaining tube in women who spontaneously conceived following unilateral salpingectomy as in the case above.

Ultrasound Services in an Early Pregnancy and Acute Gynaecological Unit. Book 2

308

7.9

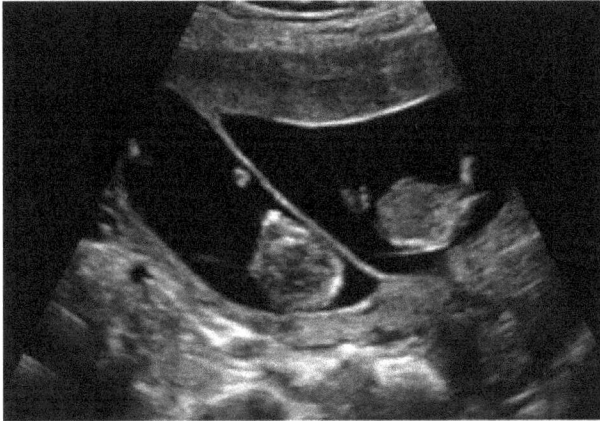

9.a

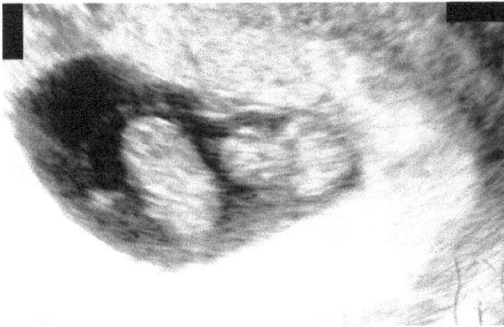

7.9b

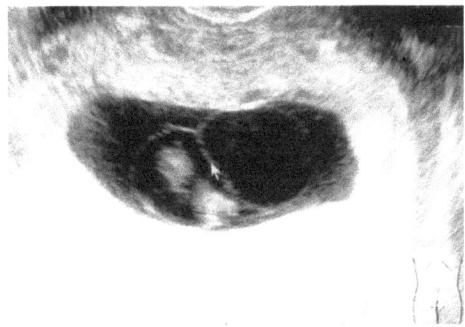

7.9c

a. Both pregnancies are twin pregnancies making them high risk pregnancies
    Each twinis in his or her individual gestational sac.

b. There are differences. Twin in 7.9a have the lambda sign. This is a DC/DA
    twin pregnancy. There is anterior and posterior placenta. They are not prone
    to TTTS later in the pregnancy.

Twin in 7.9b-c, have thin dividing membrane(arrow head in 7.9c) and no lambda
sign but a T sign. This is a MC/DA twin pregnancy. This twins are more likely to
be identical in gender and look alike and should they share the same placenta are
prone to TTTS.

Ultrasound Services in an Early Pregnancy and Acute Gynaecological Unit. Book 2

309

7.10

a.   There is an intrauterine gestational sac, yolk sac and embryo (7.10a-c).
     There is embryo heart beat (7.10b). CRL = 6.8mm = 6+3/40 (7.10c).

b.   It may be due to the patient not being sure of her LMP and so the one she gave
     was a guess work
     She might have conceived on the pill
     She might have irregular periods
     She might have conceived whilst breastfeeding
     She might have had a possible menstrual period earlier in the pregnancy

c .   Re date the pregnancy by CRL
     Perform the NT screening scan at CRL 45 -84mm if the woman wants
     Perform the anomaly scan.
     Perform any other ultrasound examinations that may be required e.g. growth
     scans.

7.11

a. No it's not an ectopic pregnancy. It is an intrauterine pregnancy in a retroverted
uterus (7.11a-b)

b. There are multiple small and similar in size follicles with peripheral distribution
giving each ovary a "string of pearls" appearance. There is central stromal
brightness (7.11c-d) ovarian and follicular measurements not included. There
seem to be a corpus luteum in the left ovary (a in 7.11c). Ultrasound appearances
is suggestive of PCO.

c. No obvious ultrasound cause for RIF pain in the right ovary has been
demonstrated.

d. GIT problems such as appendicitis hss not been excluded. Should this be the
case, If the Sonographer is not trained to examine the appendix or does not have
the linear probe for such examination, the patient may have to be referred to the
main ultrasound department for this.

Ultrasound Services in an Early Pregnancy and Acute Gynaecological Unit. Book 2

310

7.12

a. a. Ultrasound findings: An intrauterine gestational sac, (7.12a- c) yolk sac (7.12g – arrow, 7.12a, c, f -g), embryonic pole (7.12c, d, f, g) and embryonic heart beat– 177bpm (7.12d) . CRL = 18.7mm = 8+4/40 (7.12f.) In the cervical area of the uterus and covering the os is an approx. 67 x 57 x 71 mm solid heterogenous mass (7.12 a,b, e). Ultrasound features is suggestive of a fibroid.
    Impression: On going pregnancy with a cervical fibroid.

b. The mass which is most likely to be a fibroid. It may cause pains in the pregnancy and its location and size will require monitoring.

c. If the patient wants - Perform the NT screening scan at CRL 45- 48mm or 11+4 – 14+1/40.
    Perform the anomaly scan.
    Perform any other ultrasound examinations that may be required e.g. growth scans especially to monitor the growth of the baby, fibroid and position of fibroid as it relates with the delivery of the baby.

This fibroid would need to be monitored for size and position as this will influence type or mode of delivery – vaginal delivery or caesarian section.

7.13

a. **Ultrasound findings:** Retroverted uterus with an intrauterine pregnancy. There are at least two linear echogenic structures in the cervical canal measuring approx. 15 and 5mm, they both have posterior acoustic shadowing. Both entities do not have the typical IUCD configuration. (13a-b)There is a uterine synechiae (arrow 13c), embryonic pole and FHB with a CRL = 12.4mm = 7+4/40 (7.13e). EHB = 158 bpm (7.13f). There is an approx. 20 x 17 x 20mm corpus luteum and another 14 x 13 x 14mm echogenic structure. This is likely to be a dermoid (7.13g-h).

Impression: Single Intrauterine pregnancy with EHB. Echogenic linear foci in the cervical canal and inferior to the GS. Uterine synechiae (differentials – subchorionic haemorrhage.
  Right corpus luteum and probably dermoid. The left ovary has not been shown.

Uterine synechiae is a term that means adhesions or fibrous scars.
It may be secondary to curettage, previous caesarian section or myomectomy and sometimes there is no known cause for it.

Ultrasound Services in an Early Pregnancy and Acute Gynaecological Unit. Book 2

311

At other times it can be rarely secondary to uterine infections such as chlamydia, tuberculosis and schistosomiasis and the presence of foreign body.

Uterine synechiae is believed to cause amenorrhea, hypomenorrhea, habitual abortion and secondary infertility.

    * The pregnancy was on going at the 11+4/40 scan.

7.14

Ultrasound findings: An anteverted uterus that does not appear bulky (measurements not included). Some fluid and multiple echogenic materials or areas are seen in the endometrial cavity and in the area of the caesarean scar. Endometrial thickness measurement has not been included.

Impression: RPOC.

7.15

a. ***Ultrasound findings:*** There is a correctly positioned Copper T IUCD shaft in the endometrium (7.15a-b). The endometrial thickness is 15.4mm (7.15a). The left ovary is measuring has 2.7 x 2.9 x 3.2cm = a volume of 13.1 cc (7.15e) . There is an approx. 5.7 x 6.4 x 4.8cm smooth in outline, echogenic area with a calcified rim and multiple foci in the right adnexa with some ovarian tissue around it. (7.15c-d).

Impression: Copper T IUCD shaft in situ, right mature dermoid and left PCO.

b. No, this scan cannot exclude appendicitis or other GIT or KUB or ovarian torsion problems that may be causing the pain.

7.16

a. Singleton intrauterine gestation. CRL – 40.5mm = GA by LMP. FHB was claimed to have been seen. Anterior placenta. There is oedema especially around the fatal head and neck up to 5.9mm.
b. Yes the patient will be offered another scan but this time with a CVS or later after 16/40 amniocentesis to check the chromosomal status of the fetus and a fetal cardiac scan at 16/40 so as to confirm or exclude cardiac abnormality.

Ultrasound Services in an Early Pregnancy and Acute Gynaecological Unit. Book 2

312

Depending on the result and the wishes of the couple, anomaly scan may be performed to exclude any structural abnormality.

c. With CVS, an anterior placenta is an advantage. With amniocentesis, an anterior placenta may be challenging for the obstetrician.

7.17

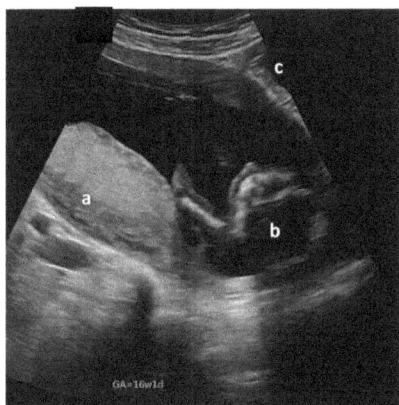
7.17a

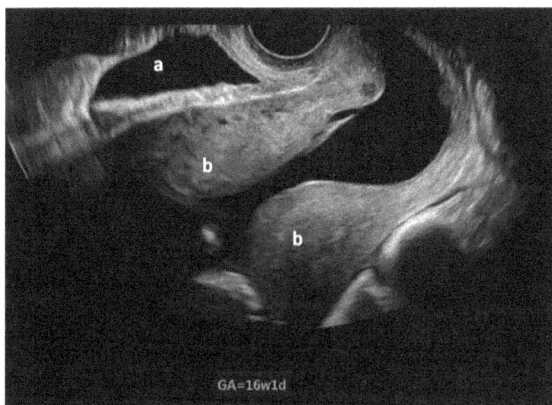
7.17i

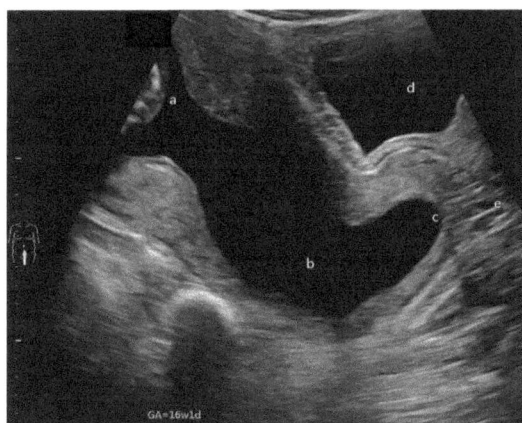
7.17j

7.17a

a-posterior placenta, b-fetal head, c-maternal urinary bladder

7.17i

Ultrasound Services in an Early Pregnancy and Acute Gynaecological Unit. Book 2

313

a- maternal urinary bladder, b- contractions

7.17j
a-buldging membrane, b-open internal os, c-open external os, d-maternal urinary bladder, e-vagina

8.17d
Images 7.17 a,b and 7.17j are images of TAS and the other images were obtained by TVS.

8.17e
Singleton pregnancy. (7.17a-b). FHR = 153 bpm (7.17b). The cervix is open, there is no measurable cervix seen and the membrane is buldging through the cervical canal. There is a 17 x 13 x 5mm non vascular hyperechoic structure in the posterior lateral wall of the cervix (7.17c-e). Cervical contractions are also noted (7.17 c-j)
Impression: Open cervix with buldging membrane in it.

7.18
a. HCG is human chorionic gonadotropin.
In pregnancy it is produced by the embryo and placenta. It is the embryo's signal to the mother that a pregnancy has occurred.
HCG can also be made from tumours that come from an egg or sperm (germ cell tumours).
It can be seen in tumours of the uterus, ovaries and testicles.
HCG can be measured in the urine or in a blood test.

b. It is a blood test to measure the level of the beta HCG in the blood.
c. Qualitative beta HCG is expressed as mIU/ml.
d. To confirm a pregnancy

In a non pregnant woman the value is usually less than 10 mIU/ml.
-   14 days post ovulation in a singleton pregnancy the value is quoted to be about 100mIU/ml. This should double every 48 – 72 hours in a healthy pregnancy in the first 42days of gestation.

Ultrasound Services in an Early Pregnancy and Acute Gynaecological Unit. Book 2

314

- To confirm or refute a molar pregnancy and monitor same.
- To confirm or refute a failing pregnancy
- To confirm or refute an ectopic pregnancy together with an ultrasound examination especially in pregnancies of unknown location. (PUL).
- If the test result is negative, normal and abnormal pregnancy including ectopic are excluded.
- Ectopic pregnancy usually shows less than 66% increase in b -hCG level within 48 hours.
- Detection of β-hCG in the serum by ELISA or radioimmunoassay are more sensitive and can detect very early pregnancy about 10 days after fertilisation i.e. before the missed period.
- In multiple pregnancy, the levels increase but it is lower in failing or ectopic pregnancy.
- It can also be done as part of a screening test for birth defects.

19

a. An intrauterine gestational sac, yolk sac, embryonic pole and EHB. CRL = 4.4mm =5+6/40. Adjacent to the GS is a cystic area measuring approximately 6 x 6 x7mm which had no YS or FP within it. A vanishing sac cannot be excluded. There is discrepancy between the patient's date and the pregnancy size.

b. Couple will be or not be brought back depending on the departmental protocol and couple's wishes.

Whilst the 12 weeks screening scan is primarily done for NT screening programme, it is also important to note that during this scan a mini anatomy check is done on the fetus so that further testing or referral to specialists within the hospital if clinically indicated. The couple should be offered the 12 weeks scan at least for the mini anatomy check and for dating the pregnancy more accurately.

20

a. Yes there seem to be something wrong. There is an approx. 58 x 51 x 50mm complex cyst between the uterus and maternal urinary bladder. ?dermoid

Ultrasound Services in an Early Pregnancy and Acute Gynaecological Unit. Book 2

315

but other pathology cannot be excluded.

Just above this and on the same side is an approx. 103 x 67 x 95mm septated cyst are two predominantly cystic entities.

b.   The presence of the ovaries and their relationship in location to the cysts.

c.   Yes to the fetal medicine unit for further assessment of the cysts. Further pregnancy management may include the patient having to have some blood tests to assess the Ca 125 level and MRI for further information on the nature of the cyst.

d.   Once the nature of the cysts are known, keeping an eye on the growth of the cysts especially as they could become torted.

* Both ovaries were not identified on ultrasound.
* An MRI scan reported a normal right ovary, that is superiorly and laterally displaced into the right iliac fossa. Left adnexal and left iliac fossa lesions were seen. Both appear to represent ovarian dermoids.

21

a.   The arrow is pointing to previous c/s scar (7.21a-b)which means this is not the 1st pregnancy of this patient.

b.   There is an intrauterine pregnancy that is far away from the previous c/s scar (measurement not included). Yolk sac, embryonic pole and embryonic heartbeat are demonstrated in the GS. CRL = 26.8mm = 9+4/40 (7.21c). EHB =165bpm (7.21d).
Impression: Single ongoing intra uterine pregnancy

22

a   There is an 11mm thickened endometrium with no obvious intrauterine gestational sac (22a). In 22b -22f there is a gestational sac in the right adnexa with hyperechoic ring that is vascular 'bagel or tubal ring' sign.

b.   Yes there is a significant difference in images 22g – h which were obtained

Ultrasound Services in an Early Pregnancy and Acute Gynaecological Unit. Book 2

316

some minutes later. These images show fluid around the right adnexal gestational sac.

c.   Rupturing right ectopic pregnancy.

* Right adnexal rupturing ectopic pregnancy was confirmed at surgery.

23
a. Yes the calcified yolk sac is abnormal (not measured)

b. An intrauterine pregnancy with calcified yolk sac, (7.23a-b), embryo that has a CRL = 17.7mm = 8+1/40 (7.23c) but with no EHB (7.23d). The right ovary measures 35 x 23 x 24mm and the left ovary measures 18 x 17 x 17mm

c.   Abnormally large YS > 5.6mm in diameter in GA </=10/40.
    Calcified or thick walled or irregular in outline YS

24
a. Ultrasound findings: An intrauterine gestational sac measuring 13 x 15 x 14mm (7.24a-f) and YS measuring 3 x 4 x 3mm (7.24c-d) There is a corpus luteum in the right ovary (7.24h -2nd image). Left ovary appears sonographically normal (7.24h- 1st image).
Impression: Early pregnancy – viability uncertain at this early GA.

b. A follow up dating scan should be arranged 3-4 weeks later or according to your protocol.
  It is not unusual not to be able to find the ultrasound cause of abdominal pain. GIT and KUB problems will need to be excluded.

25
a. Stretching across the uterus is a thick band or sheet. No fetal part is demonstrated above as caught in it.

b. Ultrasound findings: Singleton intrauterine pregnancy with FHB of 162bpm. CRL = 50.8mm =11+6/40 (7.25a-b). Stretching across the uterus is a thick

Ultrasound Services in an Early Pregnancy and Acute Gynaecological Unit. Book 2

317

band or sheet. No fetal part is demonstrated above as caught in it (7.25c-f).
Impression: Singleton pregnancy with FHB. There is uterine synchiae.
Note the free edge in 7.25e. Differentials will be a diamniotic pregnancy with one fetus however the lambda sign is missing in 7.25c-d, f and there is a free edge in 7.25e which is not seen in DC/DA pregnancy.

c. Uterine synechiae in pregnancy have also been referred to as "amniotic sheets" or "amniotic folds" by some experts. They are most commonly noted as an incidental finding during the ultrasound examination in pregnancy.

In general, experts claim that :
Synechiae do not interfere with the development or fetal growth, and are rarely associated with any complications.
Synechiae appear as thick bands connected to the uterine wall. In other words, a synechia has its base and a free edge.
In pregnancy, this appearance is caused by a combination of the fibrous synechia itself, and the complete wrapping of fetal membranes around the synechia.
Color Doppler shows blood flow in the majority of synechial bands.
Other experts claim that:
Uterine synechiae are associated with significant increase in the risk of preterm PROM, placental abruption, and cesarean delivery for malpresentation. These authors advised that notion of uterine synechiae as benign findings in pregnancy should be re-evaluated.

26
a. **Ultrasound findings:** An anteverted uterus with a triple line endometrium (measurement not included) 7.26a. The right ovary measures 31 x 24 x 25mm (7.26c-d). In the left adnexa is a 49 x 54 x 45 mm haemorrhagic cyst (7.26e). Adjacent to this cyst is a hypoechoic tubular (sausage shape like) structure (measurement has not been included). There is no peristalsis of the structure (7.26 b & g).
Impression: Normal mid cycle appearance of the uterus and endometrium. Normal right ovary. Haemorrhagic cyst in the left ovary. Hypoechoic tubular structure in the left adnexa is most likely hydrosalpinx.
b. He should have used Doppler – Coloured or Power to confirm that the sausage-

Ultrasound Services in an Early Pregnancy and Acute Gynaecological Unit. Book 2

318

like structure is not a blood vessel (though unlikely). If available and he is comfortable of using it, do a 3D ultrasound examination.

27

a. **Ultrasound findings:** The uterus is retroverted and the endometrium measuring 26.3 mm is filled with predominantly hyperechoic materials which may represent clots and blood (7.27a-b). Her where about in her cycle is unknown and there is an IUCD within the endometrium (7.27a-b). Both ovaries appear sonographically normal with the right ovary having a volume of 2.8 x 3.2 x 2.0 x 0.5233 = 9.4mls (7.27c) and the left ovary a volume of 2.7 x 3.1 x 1.7 x 0.5233 = 7.4mls (7.27d). There are multiple echogenic foci in the left ovary. ?significance

Impression: An IUCD that looks like Copper T is within the endometrial cavity but the materials in the endometrium makes it difficult to be more precise about it's exact location.

Whilst the 2D images in 7.27a-b shows the shaft of the iucd, it is impossible to be sure of the positon of the IUCD arms which can be visualized on a 3D image. 3D facility was not available at the time of this examination.

b. The materials within the endometrium might be the cause of the woman's pain in the absence of any GIT or KUB problems since the ovaries appear sonographically normal.

28

7.28a. What or Which question?:

The sonographer should ask how the pregnancy was achieved i.e. if it was a natural or through fertility treatment

Why?: In view of the large ovaries with multiple cysts.
Should this pregnancy be a result of fertility treatment the previously fertility unit assigned EDD must be used and documented as such.

b.

Ultrasound Services in an Early Pregnancy and Acute Gynaecological Unit. Book 2

319

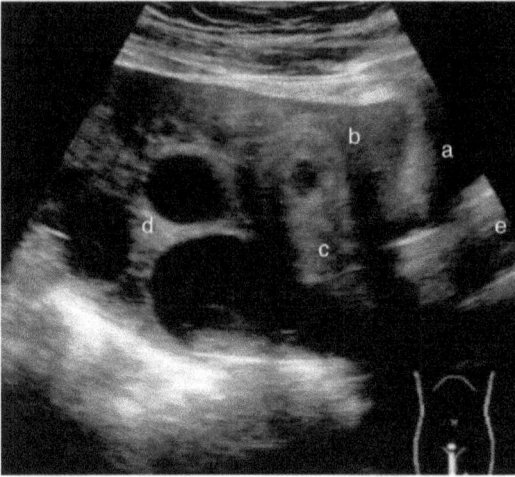

7.28a

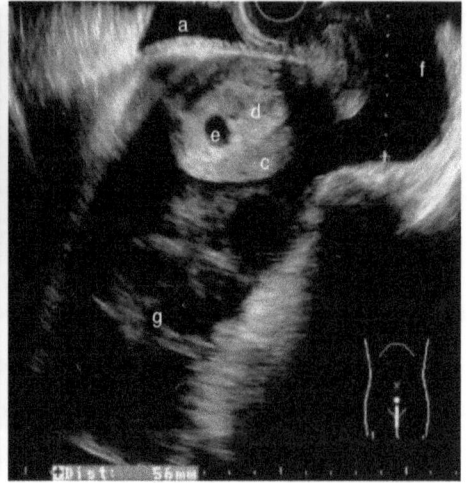

7.28b

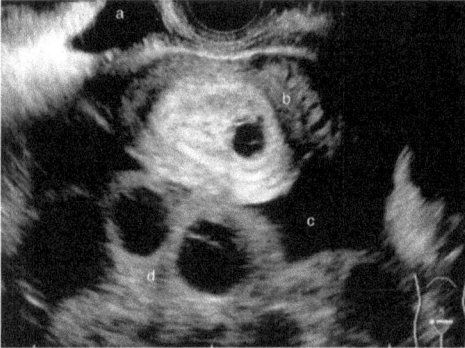

7.28e

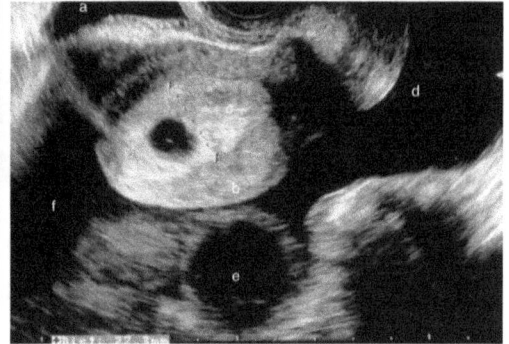

7.28f

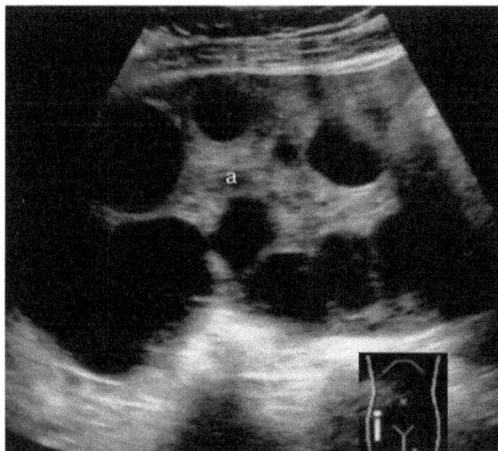

7.28g
124 x 84 x 81mm

Ultrasound Services in an Early Pregnancy and Acute Gynaecological Unit. Book 2

320

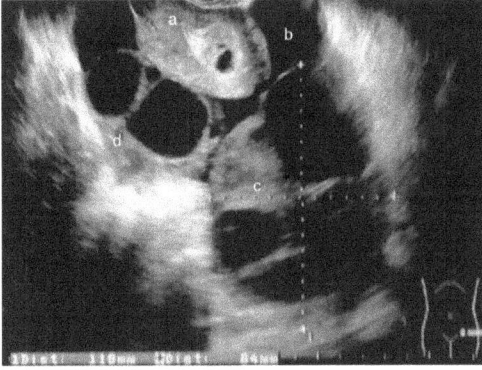

7.28i

121 x 118 x 84mm

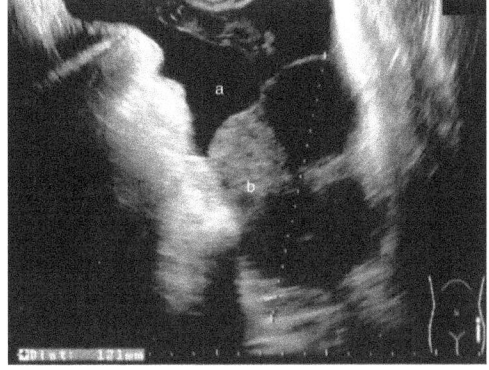

7.28j

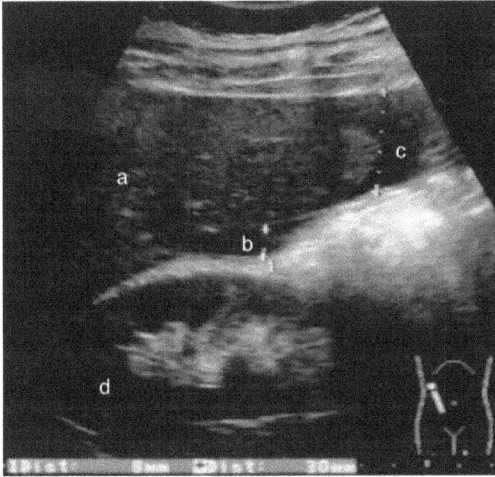

7.28k

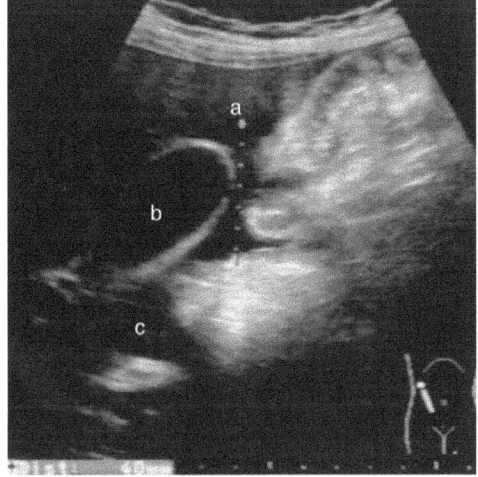

7.28l

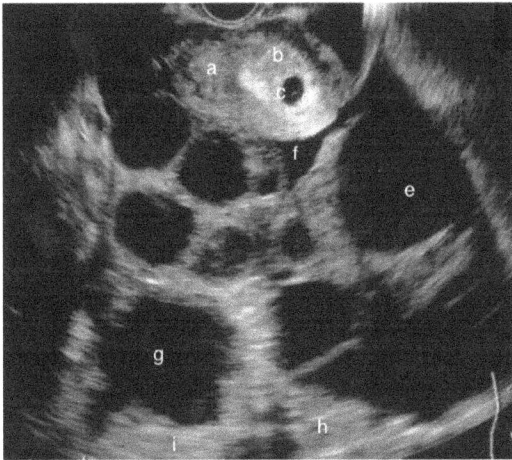

7.28m

Ultrasound Services in an Early Pregnancy and Acute Gynaecological Unit. Book 2

321

7.28a

a-maternal urinary bladder

b-anteverted uterus

c-thickened endometrium

d-enlarged ovary with multiple cysts

e-vagina

7.28b

a-maternal urinary bladder

c- posterior myometrium

d-thickened endometrium

e-intrauterine gestational sac

f-fluid in the POD

g-enlarged ovary with multiple cysts

7.28e

a- maternal urinary bladder

b-uterus

c- fluid

d- enlarged ovary with multiple cysts

7.28f

a-maternal urinary bladder

b-posterior myometrium

c-thickened endometrium

d-fluid in the POD

e-cyst

f-ascites

7.28g

a-enlarged right ovary with multiple cysts

7.28i

a-uterus

b-ascites

Ultrasound Services in an Early Pregnancy and Acute Gynaecological Unit. Book 2

322

c-enlarged left ovary with multiple cysts

d-enlarged right ovary with multiple cysts

7.28j

a-ascites

b-enlarged left ovary with multiple cysts

7.28k

a-liver

b-fluid in Morrison's pouch

c-ascites

d-right kidney

7.28l

a-ascites

b-gall bladder

c-ascites

7.28m

a-uterus

b-thickened endometrium

c-intrauterine gestatational sac

e-cyst

f-ascites

g-cyst

i-enlarged right ovary with muliple cysts

h-enlarged left ovary with multiple cysts

c. 7.28a is an image of a TAS and 7.28b is a TVS image.

d. An intrauterine gestational sac, yolk sac and embryo measuring 3.6mm
    (7.28a-d). EHB seen (7.28c) Bilaterally enlarged ovaries with multiple
    cysts. (7.28a-b, e-j)
    Right ovarian volume = 12.4 x 8.4 x 81mm x 0.5233 = 441.5mls(7.28g-h) Left
    ovarian volume = 12.1 x 11.8 x 8.4cm x 0.5233 = 628mls. (7.28i-j) . There is

Ultrasound Services in an Early Pregnancy and Acute Gynaecological Unit. Book 2

323

ascites in the pelvis, Morrison's pouch and in the abdomen.

Impression: Intrauterine pregnancy and OHSS.

The patient confirmed that this was an ICSI achieved pregnancy and she had over ten eggs removed.

It is not unusual to find bilaterally enlarged ovaries post IVF or ICSI and the cysts are normal corpus luteal cysts. The ovaries should be measured and documented so that the progress can be monitored during the pregnancy.

* Please note that finding an intrauterine pregnancy cannot exclude a co-existing heterotopic pregnancy in this patient unless it was ONLY one embryo that was transferred.

e.   Role of ultrasound in the future of this pregnancy:
-    Monitor the OHSS as per unit protocol.
-    Exclude a co-existing heterotopic pregnancy if more than one embryo was replaced in the uterus.
-    May be used if ultrasound guided aspiration of ascites is required.
     In the 12weeks NT screening program if the couple opts for screening.
     In anomaly scan and any other scan required as per the unit protocol

f. 'Kissing ovaries'.

*Patient went on to have a normal singleton pregnancy at the NT Screening scan. However the ovaries were still found to be enlarged with multiple corpus luteal cysts.

29

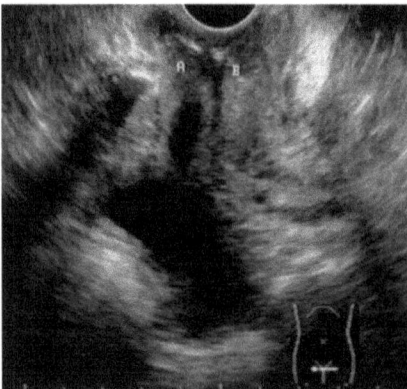 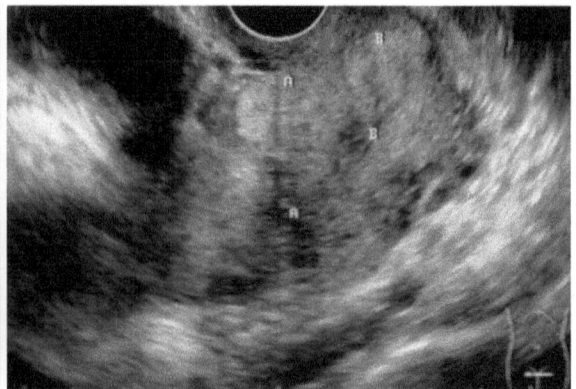

7.29a	**7.29b**

Ultrasound Services in an Early Pregnancy and Acute Gynaecological Unit. Book 2

324

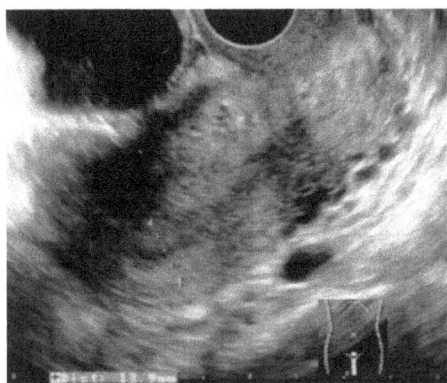

7.29c

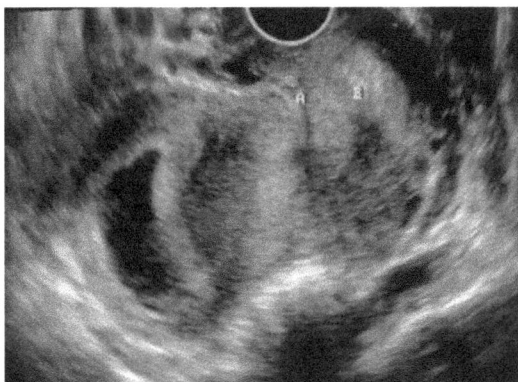

7.29d

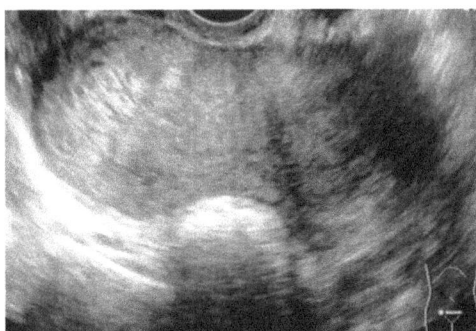

7.29e

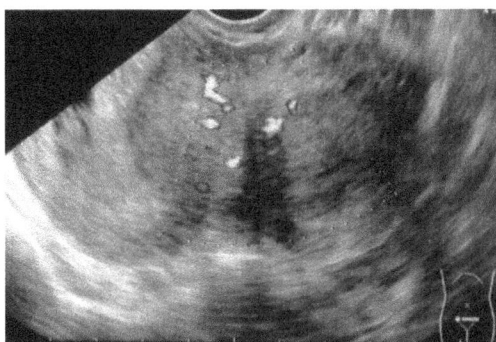

7.29f

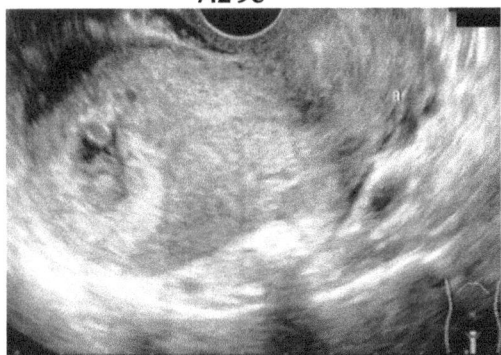

7. 29g
CRL = 26.5mm= 8+3/40

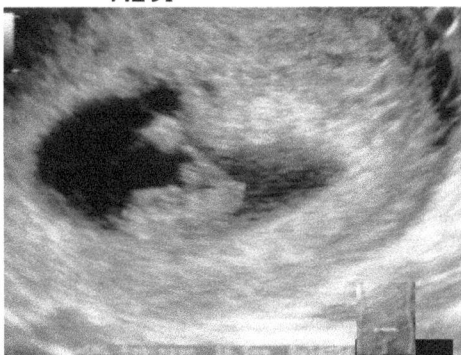

7.29h

Ultrasound Services in an Early Pregnancy and Acute Gynaecological Unit. Book 2

325

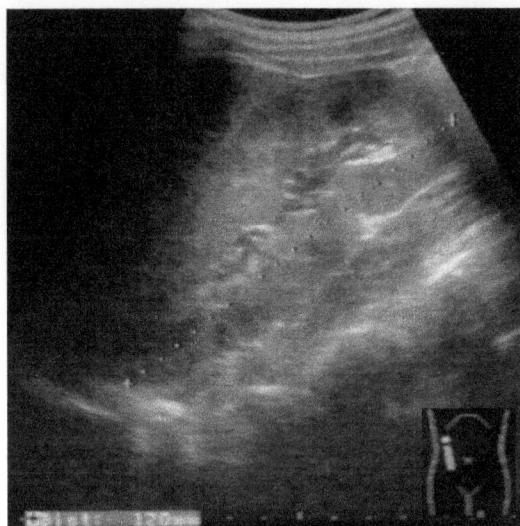 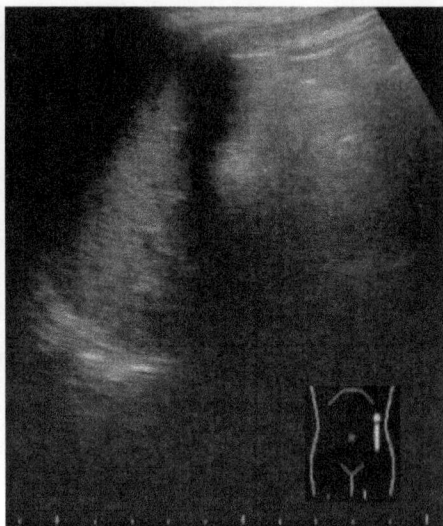

7.29i   **7.29j**

a

7.29a-b - show two cervices

7.29c- shows the pregnant uterus with a gestational sac

7.29d - shows non pregnancy uterus with a 13.8mm endometrium

7.29e - shows the embryo and EHR

7.29f - shows the embryo and CRL

7.29g-h - shows the uterus in the TS view with two uterine horns

7.29gi - shows an IUGS, embryo, yolk sac in one of the uterine horns

7.29j - shows normal maternal right kidney

7.29k - shows maternal spleen but no left kidney

b. Yes there is maternal anatomical abnormality. She has two cervices, two uterine cavities. didelphys uterus with the differentials of ?bicornuate uterus. She has the right kidney but no left kidney.

c. There are two cervices, two uterine horns/cavities. There is an intrauterine gestational sac, YS, EP and EHB in the right uterine cavity, CRL = 26.5mm = 8+3/40. The endometrium in the left horn measures 13.9mm in thickness. The patient has only one kidney on the right. The left kidney is missing in the normal left renal fossa.

Impression: Uterine didelphys with a single intrauterine pregnancy on the right. Only the right kidney is identified and it appears sonographically normal.

Ultrasound Services in an Early Pregnancy and Acute Gynaecological Unit. Book 2

326

* Differentials - bicornuate uterus.

d. Whilst a woman with didelphys uterus can carry a baby to term, experts claim that such a woman is prone to complications including miscarriage, incompetent cervix, pre term labour, premature birth, mal presentation of the baby, and uterine rupture. It is claimed that women with double uteruses have miscarriage rates of 43% compared to a miscarriage rate of 25% in women without the condition. Such a woman's pregnancy will have to be closely monitored.

30

a. There is an IUGS, yolk sac, embryonic pole with a CRL = 8.1mm = 6+5/40 (7.30a) EHB = 129 bpm (7.30b.) There is a corpus luteum in the right ovary – note the 'ring of fire' (7.30c). Left ovary (not shown) appeared sonographically normal.

b. It is 120bpm. Experts say at 6.3 – 7/40 GA, EHB should not be less than 120bpm. *Ultrasound appearances is suggestive of a threatened abortion or miscarriage.

31

An intrauterine pregnancy with a embryonic pole measuring 23.3mm (7.31c), no EHB (7.31a). Both ovaries appear sonographically normal and there is a 11 x 8 x 12mm cyst in the right ovary. 97.31e-f).

b. Missed miscarriage or missed abortion. This is because:
The pregnancy had been dated before hence the GA by previous scan is 12+2/40. CRL is less than expected (23.3mm = 9+1/40) 7.31c, No embryonic heart beat **7.31a.** rudimentary lower limb buds are seen which corresponds to about 9/40 when normally limb buds begin to be visible.
Conclusively: There is no EHB, CRL is very much less than dates. Embryonic anatomy is at least 3 weeks less than expected.

Both ovaries appear sonographically normal. There is a 12 x 11 x 8mm cyst in the right ovary

_____

Ultrasound Services in an Early Pregnancy and Acute Gynaecological Unit. Book 2

327

32

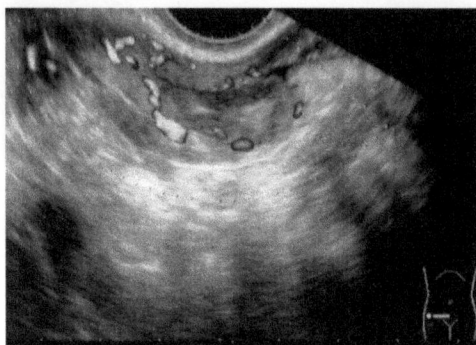
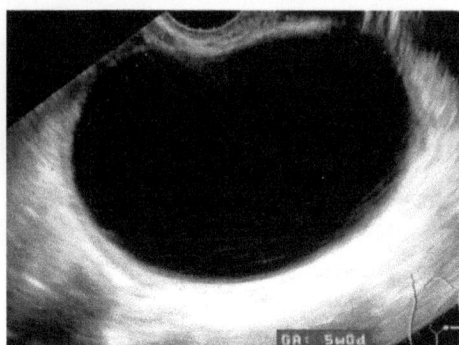

7.32e
note the 'ring of fire'

7.32h
no vascularity around this cyst

a. The cyst in 7.32e is a normal pregnancy related corpus luteum cyst whereas the 74 x 80 x 56mm avascular cystic entity posterior to the uterus and on the left is not 7.32d -h

b. The cyst on the left

c. Left ovarian torsion and cystadenoma

d. Ultrasound signs of an ovarian torsion include:
Midline ovary
Unilateral Enlarged hypo or hyperechoic ovary
Free pelvic fluid which may be seen in >80% of cases
Peripherally displaced follicles with hyperechoic central stroma or string of pearls sign
Long-standing infarcted ovary may have a more complex appearance with cystic or haemorrhagic degeneration

Doppler findings in torsion can be widely variable:
- little or no intra-ovarian venous flow (common)
- absent arterial flow (less common, but poor prognostic sign)
- absent or reversed diastolic flow
- normal vascularity does not exclude intermittent torsion

Ultrasound Services in an Early Pregnancy and Acute Gynaecological Unit. Book 2

328

- normal Doppler flow can also occasionally be found due to dual
- supply from both the ovarian and uterine arteries
- whirlpool sign of twisted vascular pedicle

e. **Ultrasound findings** – An IUGS and YS. No embryonic pole is demonstrated. There is a CLC on the right. There is an approx. 74 x 80 x 56mm avascular cystic entity posterior to the uterus and on the left. There is some ovarian tissue in the lateral wall of this cyst. The left ovary is not shown separately from this cystic entity.
Impression – An early IUP appropriate for GA. CLC on the right and an avascular cyst on the left.

f. A follow up scan in 2-3weeks later with the intention of dating the pregnancy and re-assessing the cystic entity on the left is recommended.
It is important that the left cystic entity be checked at subsequent ultrasound examination and measured so as to see if it gets bigger or otherwise.
Should this patient's LIF pain gets worse in the pregnancy an ovarian torsion will have to be excluded as the cause of the pain.
The pregnancy will need to be monitored in line with the departmental protocol.

33
a. **Ultrasound findings:** No obvious intrauterine gestational sac is demonstrated in the uterus (7.33a-c). Endometrial thickness is 21mm (7.33c). Both ovaries appear sonographically normal- measurements are not included (2nd image in 7.33f). Between the right ovary and the uterine fundus, there is an approx. 8 x 7 x 7mm gestational sac, yolk sac, embryonic pole and EHB (7.33f-i). There is mixed echo fluid in the POD up to 38mm in depth, this is likely to be haemoperitoneum(7.33c). A previous c/s scar is demonstrated in 7.33a &c)
b. Diagnosis: A live pregnancy in the RIF and haemoperitoneum in the POD

* Right ectopic pregnancy was confirmed at surgery.

34
a. No obvious intrauterine gestational sac or yolk sac or embryonic pole is seen rather the uterine cavity is distended with cystic areas which is suggestive of a

Ultrasound Services in an Early Pregnancy and Acute Gynaecological Unit. Book 2

329

molar pregnancy. The right ovary is measuring 49 x 25mm (7.34f) and there is a 46 x 36mm cyst in the left ovary (7.34g).

b. **Ultrasound diagnosis:** molar pregnancy.
*Histology report confirmed the appearances of a complete hydatidiform mole.

35
a. This patient is likely to be pregnant in view of the 3.8 x 1.7 x 3.2mm hypoechoic area in the thickened endometrium.

b. The cystic, tubular structure in 7.35 c & e arrow head

c. An anteverted uterus with a thickened endometrium (measurements not included- 7.35 a&b). There is an approx. 3.8 x 1.7 x 3.2mm hypoechoic entity in the endometrium. No obvious free fluid is seen in the pelvis. Both ovaries though the measurements have not been included appears sonographically polycystic. Images c- e. In image e is an approx. 19 x 11mm non vascular hypoechoic area adjacent to the right ovary. There is a hypoechoic tubular non vascular structure adjacent to the left ovary (measurement not included.. Should there be no peristalsis movement in both structures, then tubal pathology such as hydrosalpinx cannot be excluded.

d. TS of both ovaries with multiple follicles <10mm in diameter and a strong stroma. Ultrasound features of both ovaries is suggestive of bilateral PCO although the measurements of the ovaries have not been included.

e. Yes. Depending on the protocol some days later to check if the tiny hypoechoic area in the endometrial is bigger in size. Subsequent scans will be requested to check if the pregnancy is ongoing and date it appropriately in line with the departmental protocol.

36
a.7.36a-c were done as TAS whilst 7.36d-g were done as TVS.

b.There is an approx. 12 x 11mm hypoechoic area adjacent and to the left of the

Ultrasound Services in an Early Pregnancy and Acute Gynaecological Unit. Book 2

330

intrauterine gestational sac. (7.36g)

c. An intrauterine gestational sac, yolk sac, embryonic pole. embryonic heartbeat are demonstrated (7.36 a-e). CRL = 8.3mm =6+5/40 (7.36f). EHB of 126bpm (7.36e) There is an approx. 12 x 11mm hypoechoic area adjacent and to the left of the intrauterine gestational sac. (7.36g). There is a 84 x 85 x 93mm to the right of the gestational sac, ?fundal fibroid that is displacing the endometrium posteriorly.

d. In addition to the routine pregnancy scans as per hospital protocol, the fibroid size and appearance will need to be monitored as well.

37

a. There is no obvious ultrasound cause for pv spotting shown in any of the images.

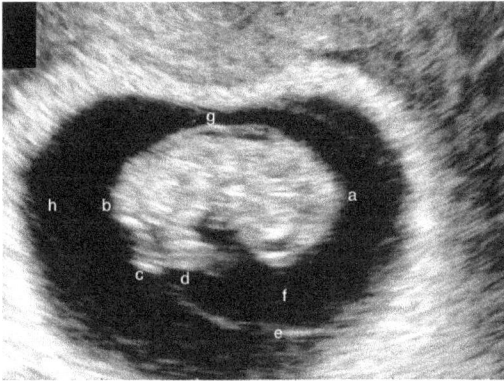
7.37c

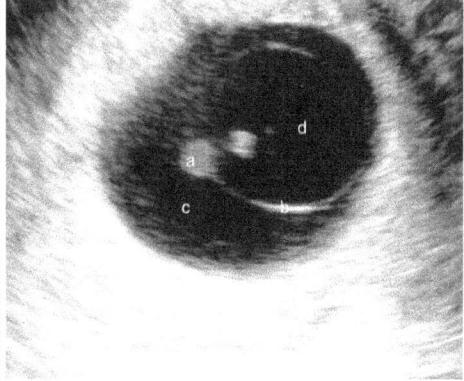
7.37d

b

7.37c
a-crown or head
b-rump or bum or bottom
c-lower limb bud
d-lower limb bud
e-amniotic membrane or amnion
f- amniotic cavity
g-embryo back
h-chorionic cavity

7.37d

Ultrasound Services in an Early Pregnancy and Acute Gynaecological Unit. Book 2

331

a-yolk sac

b-amnion or amniotic membrane

c-chorionic cavity

d-amniotic cavity

c. An intrauterine gestational sac, yolk sac, embryonic pole. Embryonic heartbeat and movement are demonstrated (note the lower limbs positioned in 7.37b &d to confirm this).

CRL = 24.4mm = 9+1/40 . FHR = 177 bpm

d. A threatened abortion or miscarriage.

It is not unusual not to find any ultrasound evidence or cause for pv spotting in women experiencing a threatened abortion or miscarriage.

38

a. It is a form of fertility treatment where the patient is asked to take 50 or 100 or 150mg of clomid tablet 1 per day from day 2 – day 6 of her cycle. Experts believe that about a quarter of women with female cause of infertility is as a result of ovulation problems. Compared to other fertility drugs, Clomid is cheaper and is believed to help with stimulating ovulation in 80% of the cases. The clomid is given to help get one but not more than 3 eggs to grow to maturity in the treatment cycle. Usually the dose starts from 50mg per day but may be increased in subsequent cycles if clinically indicated.

b. A woman with no known tubal problems.

c. A clomid treatment only involves taking 5 tablets from day 2 to day 6 or day 3 to 7 of the treatment cycle and intercourse between the couple at the appropriate time or have IUI (Intrauterine insemination). The aim is not to have more than three matured follicles (size) per cycle. It is a non invasive treatment.

Whereas with IVF the woman is given some injections over a period of time till as many as possible follicles grow in that treatment cycle and the follicles are big enough for egg retrieval. The mature eggs are retrieved, they are mixed with sperm in the test tube and 48 hours or more later, the fertilized egg(s) is /are now passed through a fine tube into the womb of the patient. IVF is an invasive and

Ultrasound Services in an Early Pregnancy and Acute Gynaecological Unit. Book 2

332

more expensive procedure although it is useful for patients with tubal problems or previous tubal surgery or unexplained infertility or previous failed intrauterine insemination or recurrent pregnancy loss or genetic conditions or male factor infertility or endometriosis and advanced maternal age.

d. **Ultrasound findings:** An Intrauterine gestational sac, yolk sac, embryonic pole and EHB (7.38a-c). CRL = 10.2mm = 7+1/40 (7.38b). The right ovary appears sonographically normal (7.38d ist image). In the left ovary is an approx. 42 x 40 x 37mm cyst (7.38d -2nd image, e-f).

e. The pregnancy will be monitored like any other pregnancy in line with the departmental protocol.

39

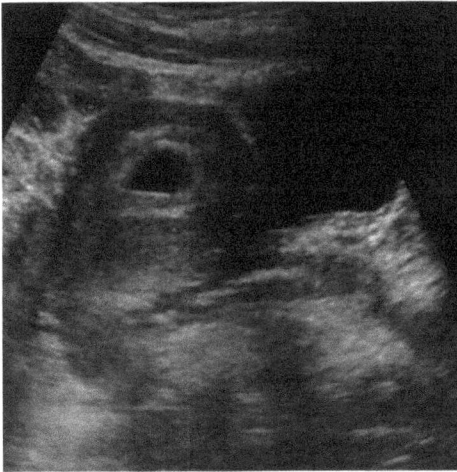 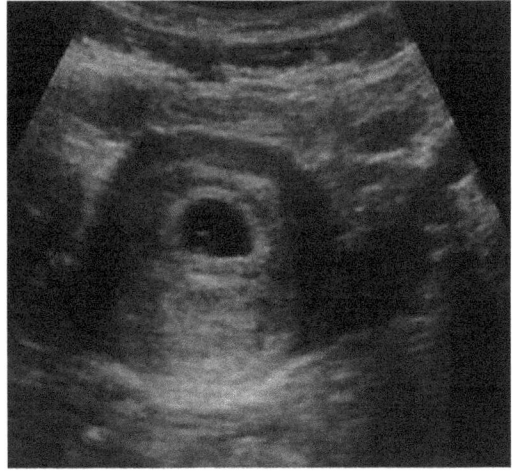

7.39a	**7.39b**

Ultrasound Services in an Early Pregnancy and Acute Gynaecological Unit. Book 2

333

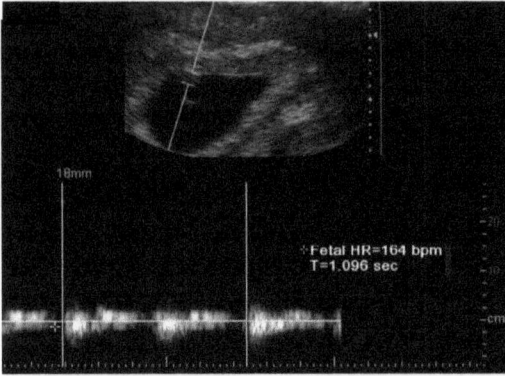

7.39c

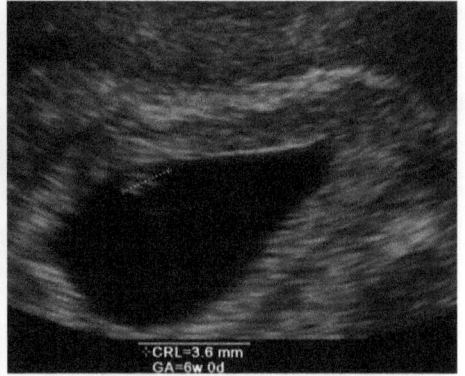

7.39d

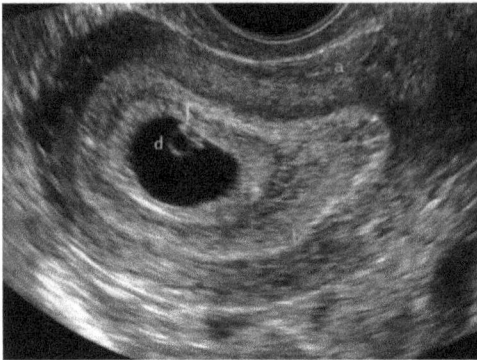

7.39e

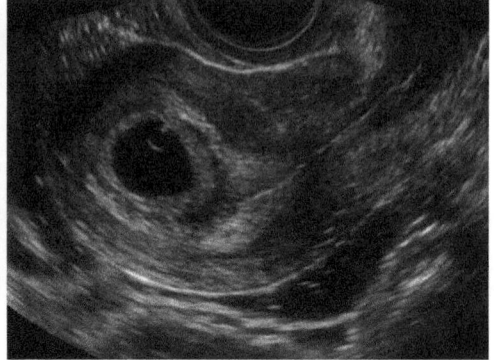

7.39f

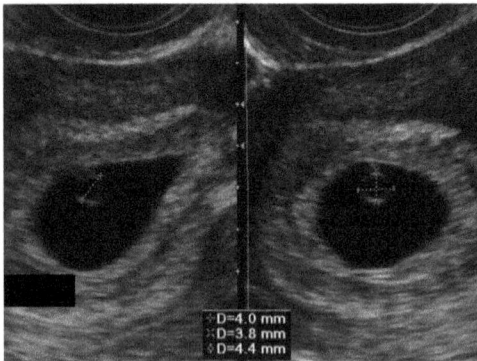

7.39g

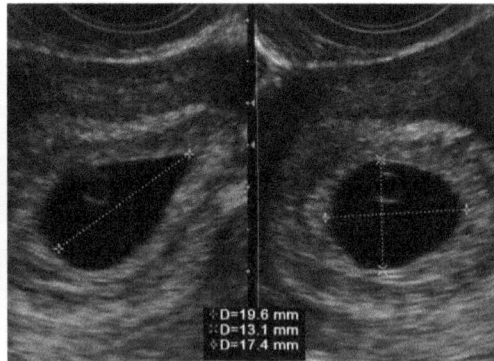

7.39h

Ultrasound Services in an Early Pregnancy and Acute Gynaecological Unit. Book 2

334

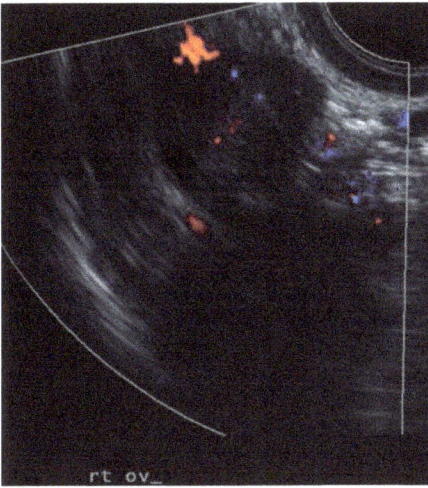
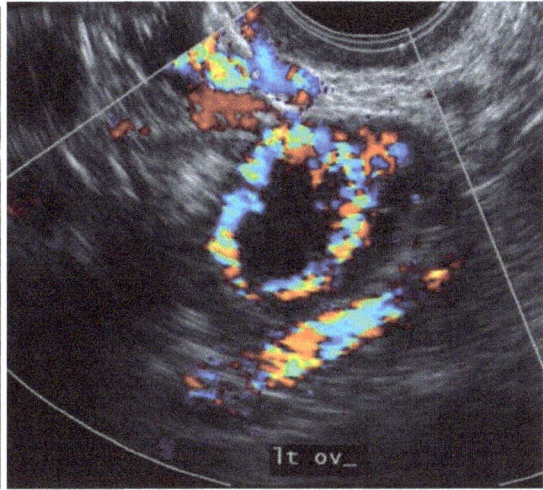

| 7.39i | 7.39j |

a. TAS (7.39a-b). TVS (7.39c-j)

b. a- anterior myometrium, b-endometrium, intrauterine gestational sac, d-yolk sac, l - embryonic pole

c. 7.39c shows the EHB = 126bpm

7.39d shows the CRL = 3.6mm =6+0/40

7.39g shows the yolk sac measurements = 4 x 3.8 x 4mm

7.39h shows the gestational sac measurements = 19.6 x 13.1 x 17.4mm

To obtain the volume manually = 19.6 x 13.1 x 17.4mm x 0.5233 = 2.4cc

d. An intrauterine gestational sac (7.39a-f) with a yolk sac (7.39e-h), embryonic pole (7.39d) with a CRL of 3.6mm. EHB =126bpm (7.39c). The right ovary (7.39i) shows normal morphology and there is a corpus luteum with a 'ring of fire' (7.39j) in the left ovary(7.39j).

Impression: Normal ongoing early intrauterine pregnancy

e. This will depend on the departmental protocol, If the dating scan was done pre NIPT test she may need another scan in 2-3 weeks time to date this pregnancy more accurately. If she is asymptomatic she may have to wait for the routine NT Screening scan.

f. Reasons for unknown LMP:

▪ Might have conceived on the pill

▪ Might have recently stopped the pill

Ultrasound Services in an Early Pregnancy and Acute Gynaecological Unit. Book 2

335

- Patient might have forgotten the date
- May not have a regular menstrual cycle
- Might have conceived while breast feeding
- Might have conceived after a recent miscarriage
- Might have bled earlier in the pregnancy thus thinking she was not pregnant

7.40

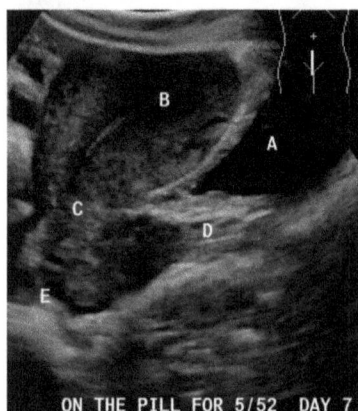

7.40a

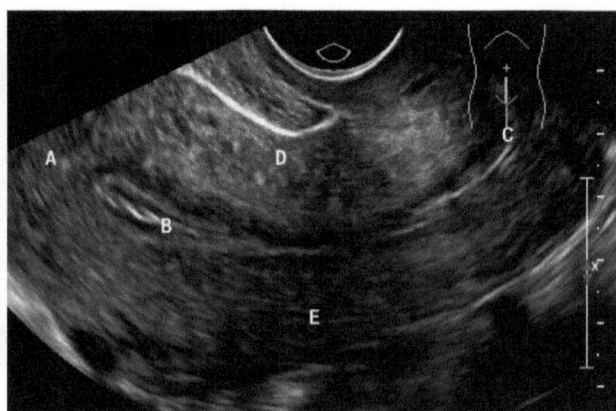

7.40b

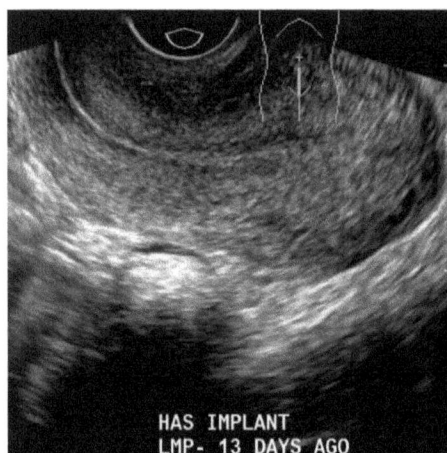

7.40c

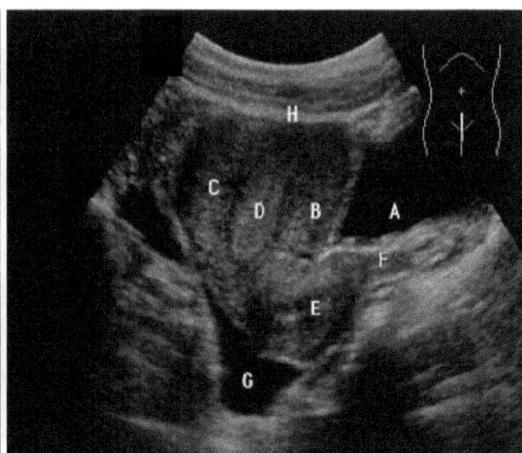

7.40d

7.40a

A-urinary bladder

B-anteverted uterus

C-cervix

Ultrasound Services in an Early Pregnancy and Acute Gynaecological Unit. Book 2

336

D-vagina
E- POD

7.40b
A-fundus
B-triple line endometrium
C-fluid in the cervical canal
D-anterior myometrium
E-posterior myeometrium

7.40d
A-urinary bladder
B-anterior myometrium
C-posterior myometrium
D-thickened endometrium
E-cervix
F-vagina
G-fluid in the POD

b. 7.40a & d was obtained by TAS. 7.40b-c were obtained by TVS.
c. 7.40b shows an anteverted uterus, with a triple line endometrium whilst 7.40c is a retroverted uterus with a thin endometrium.
d. 7.40a The endometrium is very thin

7.40d the endometrium is thick and there is fluid in the POD.
Both are anteverted uteri scanned with the TA approach.

e. There are two kinds of contraceptive pills:

Ultrasound Services in an Early Pregnancy and Acute Gynaecological Unit. Book 2

337

Type of Pill	Content of Pill	How it Works
Combined pill	Synthethic versions of oestrogen and progesterone	- Stops the user from producing FSH & LH. This prevents the ovaries from producing an egg as the eggs are not ripened or ovulated. - the synthetic progesterone thickens the mucus at the cervix thus preventing the sperm to get through. - it makes the endometrium to be too thin for any fertilised egg to be able to implant itself.
Mini pill	Synthetic progesterone	it thickens the cervical mucus making it difficult for the sperm to get through to fertilise the egg. It makes the endometrium lining too thin for implantation The popular brand –Cerazette prevents ovulation

f.   The contraceptive implant works by steadily releasing progesterone hormone into the body. The progestogen: stops the woman releasing an egg every month (i.e. prevents ovulation) thickens the mucus from the cervix, making it difficult for sperm to pass through to the womb and reach any unfertilised egg makes the lining of the womb thinner so that it is unable to support a fertilised egg

g.   A contraceptive pill is a tablet that is taken daily in order to avoid an unwanted pregnancy. The contraceptive implant is a small flexible about 40mm long tube that is inserted under the skin of the upper arm by a trained professional. It lasts for three years.

41

a.   An intrauterine gestational sac in a retroverted uterus measuring 21 x 23 x 10mm. No obvious yolk sac or embryonic pole or fetal pole is demonstrated (7.41a- c)

b.   Anembryonic pregnancy. (some refer to it as a Blighted ovum)

c.   With missed miscarriage or abortion there will be a embryoni or fetal pole but with no heartbeat

Ultrasound Services in an Early Pregnancy and Acute Gynaecological Unit. Book 2

338

d. To assess the endometrium and ovaries post miscarriage when she has stopped bleeding

42

a. Lack of amniotic fluid around the fetus (7.42a-f).
b. 7.42d – both kidneys. 7.42f – urinary bladder.
c. Fluid depth in one of the quadrants. As it was the only measurement obtained, the AFI = 1.9cm = less than the expected for GA.
d. Renal agenesis as both kidneys and urinary bladder have been demonstrated (7.42d &f).
e. ***Ultrasound findings:*** Single intrauterine pregnancy. FHB seen (7.42g). oligohydramnios. Posterior placenta not low.

Impression: Oligohydramnios. Single intrauterine pregnancy.
*Though this fetus was alive at the time of the scan the prognosis is bad.
* Unfortunately the patient later miscarried.

43

a. Yes, there is a coil shaft in the endometrium (43a &c). The string is seen in cervical canal (43b).
b. Mirena coil (43a)
c. A normal sized anteverted uterus with a mirena coil shaft correctly positioned in the endometrium(43a &c). The coil string is in the cervical canal and there is some fluid in the cervical canal (43b). Both ovaries appear sonographically normal with the right ovary having a volume of 7.5cc (43.e) and the left ovary 12.5cc (43.g). In the left ovary is an 22 x 18 x 21mm corpus luteum (43d- 2nd image, f). There is some fluid in the POD (43b).
    Impression: Mirena coil shaft correctly positioned in the endometrium and the string is in the cervical canal. Normal ovaries with a corpus luteum in the left ovary.
d. Experts claim that women using the Mirena coil are more likely to develop functional cysts. Such cysts usually burst and disappear within 2 to 3 months without treatment.

Ultrasound Services in an Early Pregnancy and Acute Gynaecological Unit. Book 2

339

44

a. There is an intrauterine slightly irregular in outline gestational sac measuring approx. 43 x 18 x 22mm, an oversized yolk sac measuring approx. 12 x 12 x 13mm but no embryonic or fetal pole. There is some irregular in outline perhaps with cystic component in the anterior wall.

b. Missed abortion or miscarriage but a hydatidiform mole cannot be excluded.

c. The body is perhaps beginning to know that the pregnancy is not going well and so the uterus is trying to get rid of the pregnancy. There is a small ?area of bleed in image 7.44d.

45

a. Given the clinical history of previous appendicectomy and IBS, there is a lot of overlying bowel gas in images 45c, e -f. The pregnancy is rightly implanted, both ovaries appear sonographically normal and that rules out a co-existing ectopic. The bowel gas is most likely the cause of this patient's RIF pain.

b. Yes to monitor the progress of the pregnancy and to date the pregnancy as the CRL is less than GA by LMP.

c. An intrauterine gestational sac, yolk sac and embryonic pole (45a-b). CRL = 2.8mm. EHB not shown here was said to have been seen. Both ovaries appear sonographically normal. The right measuring 20 x 19 x 21mm = 4.2mls (45c). Measurement of the left ovary is not included (45.d). There is a small amount of fluid in the POD up to 11mm. (47.5 b).

46

a. Mid cycle. Images 7.46c- d shows a triple line endometrium, with a small fluid in the cervical canal. 7.46 a shows a cystic entity measuring 20 x 17 x 20mm that does not have a ring of fire. This is probably a matured follicle.

b. Yes there is an approx. 13 x 5mm hyperechoic structure in the lower endometrial cavity. This is most likely to represent an endometrial polyp. See chapter 6. Applying Colour Doppler on the hyperechoic structure in the endometrium may likely show the feeding vessel.

c. A normal sized anteverted uterus with a triple line endometrium (measurement not included). There is some fluid in the cervical canal. (arrow in 7.46d) There is an approx. 13 x 5mm hyperechoic structure in the

Ultrasound Services in an Early Pregnancy and Acute Gynaecological Unit. Book 2

340

lower endometrial cavity. There is a 20 x 17 x 20mm follicle in the right ovary. The left ovary measures 25 x 28 x 14mm. Both ovaries appear sonographically normal.

Impression: Ultrasound appearance is suggestive of a normal mid cycle. There is a polyp in the endometrium.

47

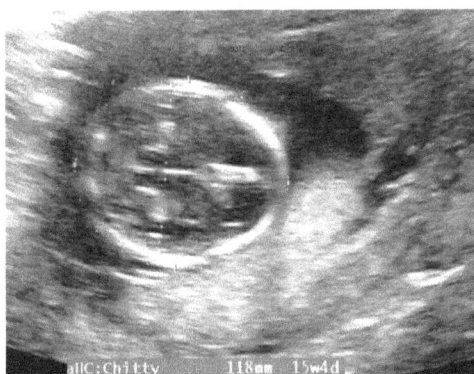

7.47a.

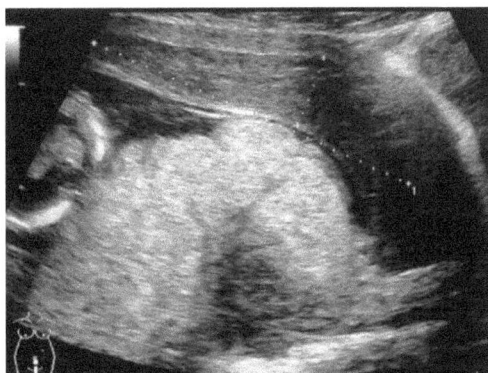

7.47b. ++86.7mm, 17.8mm

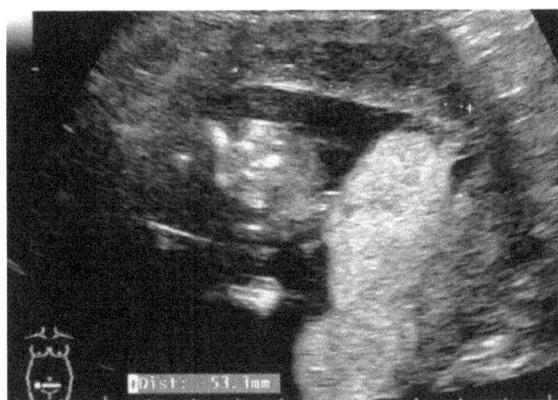

7.47c.

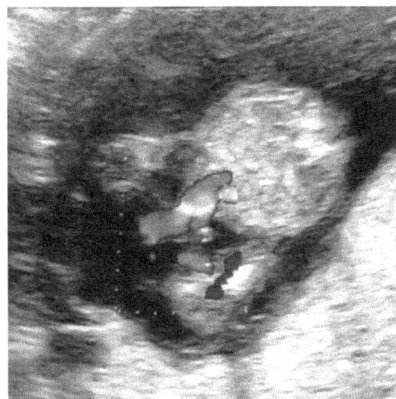

7.47d.

Ultrasound Services in an Early Pregnancy and Acute Gynaecological Unit. Book 2

341

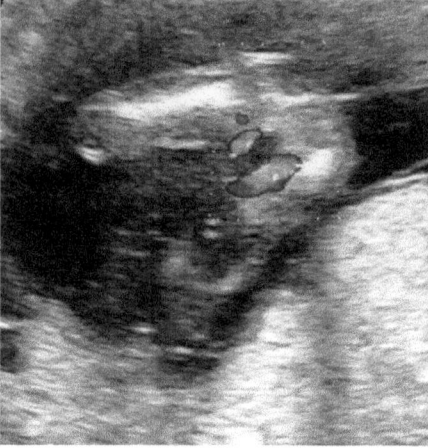

7.47e.

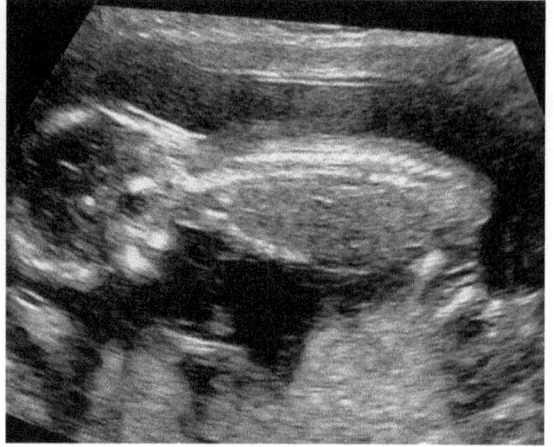

7.47 f

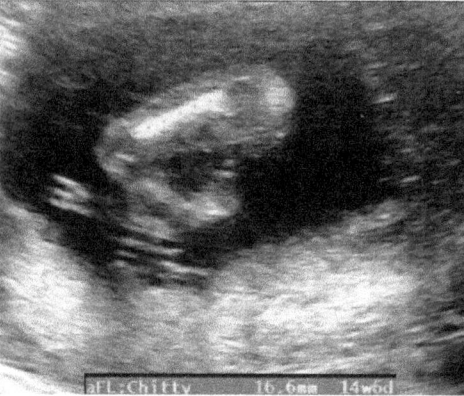

7.47g.

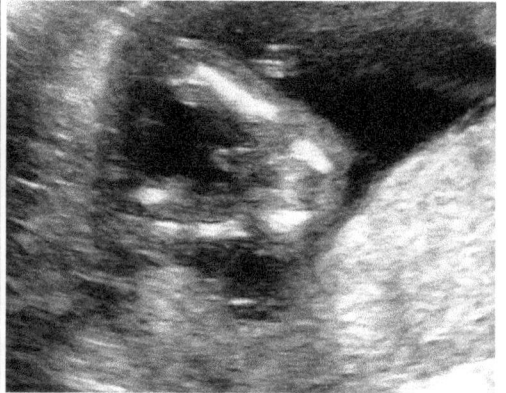

7.47h.

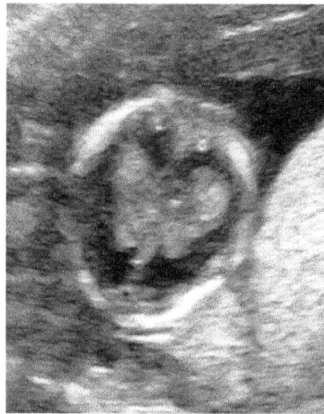

7.47 i.

b.   No not at present as it would be checked at the anomaly scan some weeks

Ultrasound Services in an Early Pregnancy and Acute Gynaecological Unit. Book 2

342

later. There is subchorionic haemorrhage or bleed in the anterior wall measuring 87 x 53 x 18mm (7.47b-c)

c. XY – a boy. Image 7.47h.

d. A single intrauterine gestational sac, fetus, posterior low placenta. There is an anterior wall subchorionic haemorrhage measuring approximately 87 x 53 x 18mm (7.47b-c). BPD = 118mm = 15+4/40 (7.47a). FL = 17mm = 14+6/40 (7.47g)

Impression: On going single intrauterine pregnancy. Anterior wall subchorionic haemorrhage.

48

a. Missed abortion or miscarriage. 7.48a-b, d-e shows an irregular in outline gestational sac. 7.48d shows no EHB hence the diagnosis.

b. The CRL = 17.9mm = 7+5/40, 7.48d confirms no EHB hence the diagnosis

c. Image 7.48a is a TAS image whilst Images 7.48 b-e are TVS images

49

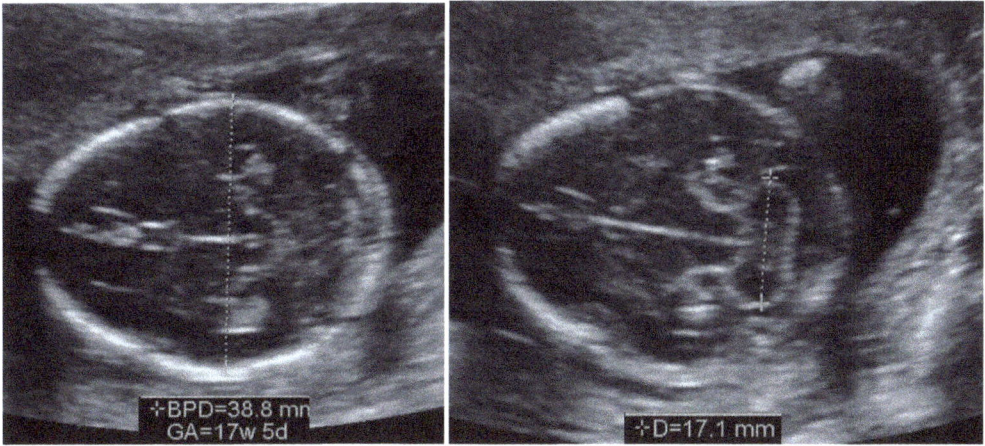

7.49a   7.49b

7.49.a – BPD section showing the cavum septum pellucidum and thalami

7.49.b – TS view of the head showing the cerebellum,
          Trans cerebellum distance, cisterna magna

Ultrasound Services in an Early Pregnancy and Acute Gynaecological Unit. Book 2

343

7.49.c - View measuring FL. FL is more reliable after 14/40 GA. Beam of insonation should be perpendicular to the shaft excluding the distal femoral epiphysis

7.49.d- AC section. TS view of the abdomen at the level of the umbilical vein which is about a third from the anterior wall, it should show TS spine, descending arota, one rib, short umbilical vein and the stoma

b.
Both are TS views of the fetal brain.7.49a is obtained at the level of BPD and 7.49b is obtained at the level lower showing the TCD

c. The fetus is at least 17+1/40.+/- 5days . (7.49b).
- Experts believe that up till 24/40, 1mm measurement of the TCD = 1/40 or one week gestational age. After 24/40, the measurement is said not to be as accurate so it not used for dating purposes.
- There are reporting packages available that can work the GA out with the measurements obtained. E.g. viewpoint.
- Please note that the fetal AC measurement is never used for dating a pregnancy.

50
a. Yes, there is, an approx. 58 x 53 x 38mm predominantly hyperechoic structure but with two hypoechoic areas and tip of the iceberg appearance within it. (7.50e-h).The left ovary has not been shown separate from this entity.

b. 7.50c-d shows a normal right ovary with a 16 x 13 x 18mm corpus luteum with the "ring of fire' whilst 7.50 e-h shows a left adnexa mass as earlier described in a.

c. An intrauterine gestational sac, embryonic pole with a CRL = 9.9mm = &+1/40 and EHB. (7.50a-b). The right ovary appears sonographically normal with a corpus luteum in it. (7.50c-d) In the left adnexal is a predominantly hyperchoic structure but with two hypoechoic areas within it. (7.50c- f)The left ovary has not been shown separate from this entity.

Ultrasound Services in an Early Pregnancy and Acute Gynaecological Unit. Book 2

344

Ultrasound Impression: Single on going pregnancy with EHB, normal right ovary and a probably a dermoid cyst in her left ovary. Other left ovarian pathology cannot be excluded.

*entity in the left adnexa turned out to be a dermoid cyst.

51

a. In both images there is a single intrauterine gestational sac and a fibroid.

b. In 7.51 a, the fibroid is in the cervical area, in 7.51b, the fibroid is fundal.

c. Could cause pain in pregnancy. The location of the fibroid as in 7.51 a. could affect the mode of delivery.
* fibroid location and size measurement are paramount at every scan if in any way it is affecting the pregnancy.

52

a. In the right adnexa there is an approx. 57 x 61 x 34mm low level echoed cyst with hyperechoic wall foci (7.52a-b)

b. An anteverted uterus with a triple line endometrium measuring 5.7mm (7.52d)
The left ovary is measuring 23 x 33 x 18mm (7.1mls). The right ovary is not demonstrated but in the right adnexal is an approx. 57 x 61 x 34mm predominantly low level echoed cyst.

c. Right endometrioma.

Ultrasound Services in an Early Pregnancy and Acute Gynaecological Unit. Book 2

345

53.

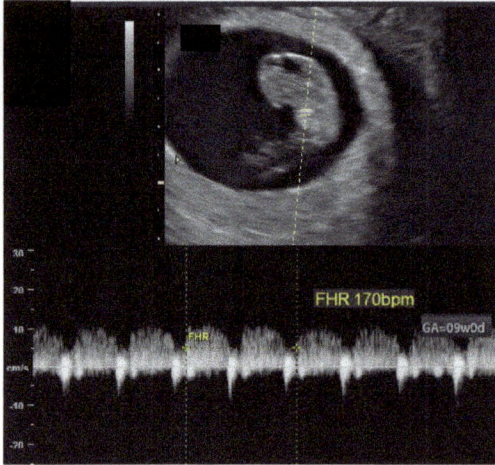

53a

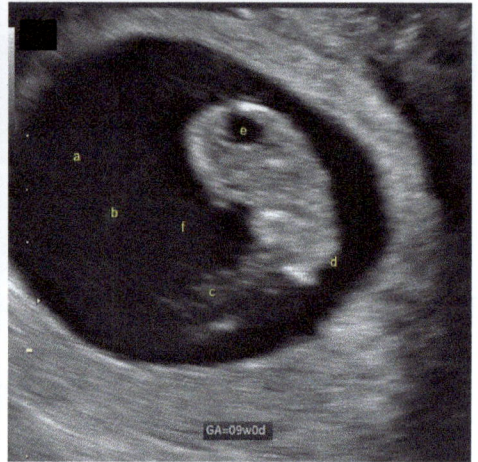

53b

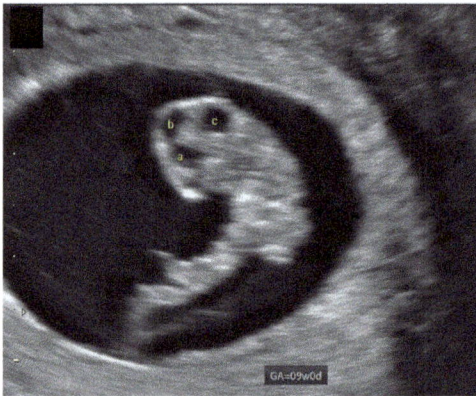

53c

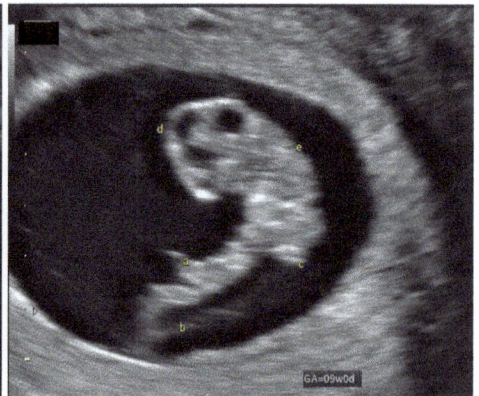

53d

53.b

a- amniotic fluid, b- amniotic membrane, c- cord, d- rump or bottom
e- embryonic rhombencephalon (normal brain finding at 8-10/40)
f- chorionic fluid in chorionic cavity.

53c

a-diencephalon, b-mesencephalon, c-rhombencephalon

Ultrasound Services in an Early Pregnancy and Acute Gynaecological Unit. Book 2

346

53d

a- cord, b- vitelline duct, c- bum or bottom, d -head or crown, e- back

53.b   The fatal heart rate is normal for the gestational age.
Normal FHR at 9-10 GA is 170bpm

53c.   Further investigations would be required if it has not been done before e.g. blood test such as Ca125 and MRI to assess the complex cyst in the left adnexa.

53d.   An intrauterine gestational sac with an embryo measuring 18.7mm = 8+3/40. (53e) EHB = 170bpm (53a). The right ovary is measuring approximately 37 x 24 x 43mm = 20mls and it appears polycystic with a possible corpus luteum (53i-j). in the left adnexa there is an approx. 95 x 65 x 48mm multiseptated, irregular in outline predominantly cystic area that has ?projections into it, ?tiny hyperechoic area in it with ?flow on Dopplers in the septa (53.f-j). No normal left ovary has been demonstrated (53f-h)
Impression: Normal ongoing IUP, Complex cyst in the left adnexa. Left ovarian pathology cannot be excluded.

54

a.   Yes, there is an irregular in outline gestational sac, with some echogenic area in it. Content of the uterus is being expelled as heavy pv bleeding. 7.54a,-c & e

b.   An intrauterine irregular in outline gestational sac measuring approx. 44 x 38 x 23mm. No obvious yolk sac is demonstrated but there is an approx. 14 x 8mm echogenic area that had no blood flow on Dopplers. (7.54a) Normal physiological appearances of the left ovary (7.54e).

c.   *Ultrasound impression:* Incomplete miscarriage with RPOC in utero.

55

a.   Fetal head position in the maternal pelvis is not favourable and may make assessing and measuring the fetal head impossible except the fetus changes the position during the examination (7.55b-d). There is not enough amniotic fluid around the fetus (7.55b).

Ultrasound Services in an Early Pregnancy and Acute Gynaecological Unit. Book 2

347

b.   There is no kidney in the normal maternal left renal bed (7.55f), instead there
      is a maternal kidney in the LIF (7.55d-e). As there has been no previous history
      of abdominal surgery, this is likely to be the normal residence of the left
      kidney. Also there is not enough amniotic fluid around the fetus (55d)
      Fetal head could not be assessed or measured.
      * *This patient was unaware of her left pelvic kidney.*

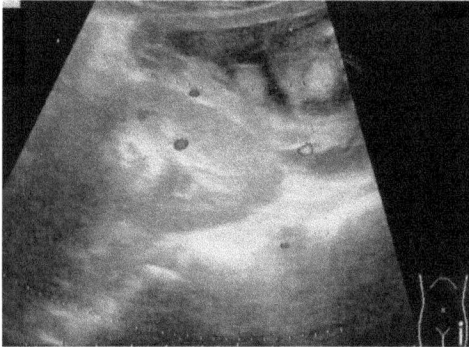 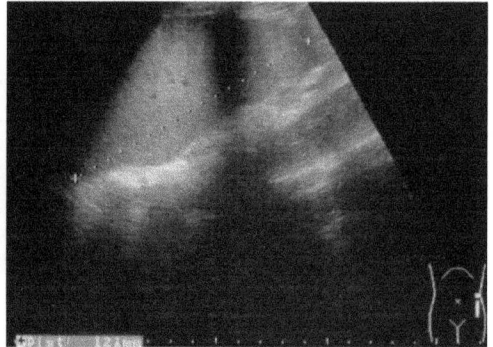

| 55e | 55f |

56

a.   a- maternal internal os, b-pear shaped hypoechoic mass that is different
      from the placenta., c- placenta, d- fetal part

b.   There is an approx. 41 x 42 x 44mm pear shaped predominantly hypoechoic
      area that does not show any flow on Dopplers, it is also not part of the fetal
      placenta. (7.56a-c,e-f, h). This is most likely to be an area of bleeding.

c.   Experts believe that hematomas or subchorionc bleeding when seen on
      ultrasound, that the fetal outcome is dependent on size of the hematoma,
      maternal age and gestational age. Miscarriage risk increases with the size
      of the hematoma and increase in maternal age. There is also increase in the
      risk of abruption placentae, stillbirth and preterm labour.

57

a.   **What:** The type of fertility treatment
      Why: If clomid sonographer can work out GA by LMP

Ultrasound Services in an Early Pregnancy and Acute Gynaecological Unit. Book 2

348

If it was by IVF or ICSI the fertility unit will have assigned the EDD which should be used in calculating the GA.

What: If it was by IVF or ICSI etc. how many embryos were transferred

Why: To exclude heterotopic pregnancy

b.   There is an approx. 32 x 18 x 23 mm area of bleed superior and posterior to the gestational sac.

c.   Co-existing heterotopic pregnancy. if it was an IVF or ICSI conception with more than one embryo transfered.

d.   An anteverted uterus with a gestational sac, yolk sac, embryonic pole and EHB (57a). CRL = 3.5mm (57f). There is an approx. 32 x 18 x 23 mm area of bleed superior and posterior to the gestational sac. No obvious free pelvic fluid is demonstrated.

Impression: Single IUP with areas of bleeding as described above.

* this patient will be followed up in line with the department protocol.

58

a.   There is an approx. 18 x 11mm slightly irregular in outline eccentrically placed gestational sac to the right of the uterus (7.58a, e-f) with a yolk sac, embryonic pole and EHB. CRL = 3.8mm. (7.58a-c). There is a corpus luteum in the right ovary (7.58g-h)and the left ovary appears sonographically normal (7.58i-j). There is some free fluid in the POD. (7.58e)

b.   Right interstitial pregnancy.

Right interstitial pregnancy was confirmed at surgery.

59

a. There is a large intrauterine gestational sac (measurements not included) that is irregular in outline, containing a hyperechoic structure and two cystic entities of various sizes (4 x 14mm and 7 x 6mm). No obvious fetal pole is demonstrated. There is an approx. 41 x 41mm fundal fibroid.(7.59c) The right ovary appears sonographically normal and there are few cystic entities in the left ovary (7.59d).

Ultrasound Services in an Early Pregnancy and Acute Gynaecological Unit. Book 2

349

b. Missed miscarriage, ? hydatidiform mole. Fundal fibroid.
* *Follow up laboratory findings – partial hydatiform mole confirmed.*

60

a.   Yes, the right ovarian size (53mls) and appearance. (7.60c)

b.   An anteverted normal size uterus with a 7mm endometrium. The left ovary appears sonographically normal with a volume of 3.7mls (7.60d). The right ovary is oedematous and has a complex appearance with a volume of 53mls (7.60c). No obvious free fluid is seen in the POD.
   Impression: Right ovarian torsion cannot be excluded.

c.   Ultrasound features of ovarian torsion include:
   - Enlarged ovary with heterogenous central stroma which is secondary to infact or oedema
   - Abnormal midline location of the ovary.
   - Peripherally displaced follicles or cysts with no flow within the ovary on Colour Doppler
   - Twisted pedicle between the ovary and the uterus – whirlpool sign on Colour Doppler
   - Target sign.
   - Assymetric thickening of the ovarian cyst wall
   - Look for an underlying mass

Check for arterial flow with the ovary – may have to use Colour and Power or Spectral Doppler.
Check for free pelvic fluid.
*Patient does not necessarily have to present with acute pelvic pain.

d. MRI or CT.

61

a.   No obvious normal uterine myometrium is demonstrated. Rather there is a complex in appearance entity measuring 58 x 69 x 59mm. In this entity are hypoechoic areas that is very vascular and irregular in outline hyperechoic component.(7.61a-d). There is a ?6.8mm endometrium (7.61e). Both ovaries

Ultrasound Services in an Early Pregnancy and Acute Gynaecological Unit. Book 2

350

appear sonographically normal with the right ovarian volume is 1.45mls and the left ovarian volume is 1.67mls (7.6g-h)

b.   The patient does need immediate follow up because of the uterine findings. MRI or CT should be suggested.

62

a. This patient's ovaries should appear sonographically normal. This is because her ovaries will not have been stimulated.

b. Monochorionic diamniotic pregnancy. They will be of same sex.

c. An intrauterine gestational sac with two yolk sacs (6.62 f) two amniotic sacs with a thin dividing membrane (6.62 c-e & h), two embryos seen with embryos' CRI's 22.4mm and 22.5mm. (6.62 g and h). Heartbeats are noted in both embryos. (6.62 a & b, rate not included). Tiny hypoechoic areas superior to the GS. ?area of bleed (6.62i).

d. Performing the routine scans if the patient agrees (NT screening scan and anomaly scan later) plus additional growth scans as this pregnancy is classified as a high risk pregnancy (multiple and monochorionic MC).
if the patient opts for the NT screening, then the age of the ovum or egg donor is used for the calculations and NOT that of this patient. That has to be documented in her report.

63a. The patient is pregnant. There is an IUGS and YS (63a-e)

b. *Ultrasound findings:* A retroverted uterus with a 22.4mm diameter intrauterine gestational sac(63c). There are two cystic entities within this IUGS, the smaller one measuring 4 x 4 x 4mm is the YS. The larger cystic entity is measuring 12x 12 x10mm and this is the amniotic membrane or amnion. No obvious embryonic pole is demonstrated. Ultrasound appearances is suggestive of an 'empty amnion sign'. There is a left ovarian cyst is measuring 13 x 13 x 19mm (63.g) and a right corpus luteum cyst measuring 12 x 12 x 8mm (63.f). Ultrasound findings are not consistent with a 11+1/40 pregnancy.

Ultrasound Services in an Early Pregnancy and Acute Gynaecological Unit. Book 2

351

Impression: Missed abortion or miscarriage. Corpus Luteum in the right ovary and a small cyst in the left ovary.

c. An 'empty amnion sign' is a sonographic observation where there is the visualization of an amniotic sac without associated visualization of an embryo. It is believed to be an indicator of pregnancy failure regardless of the mean sac diameter and is considered to have a sufficiently high positive predictive value.

64

a. There is no ultrasound identifiable intrauterine pregnancy looking through 6.64 a & b.

b. Challenges from the multiple cysts in the pelvis may make assessing the pelvis difficult.

c. Urine and blood pregnancy tests.

d. An anteverted uterus with no obvious intrauterine gestational sac. (6.64 a &b.) Endometrial measurement has not been included.
In both adnexal and superior to the uterine fundus are multiple septated cystic entities, (6.64 c – g) a mixture of some low level echoed (64a), some purely cystic entities, there is multiple echogenic foci in 64c, the largest septated cyst in the RIF is approx. 72 x 46 x 53mm and in the left 54 x 43 x 63mm (64c-h)

Ultrasound impression: Bilateral endometriomas.
* Pregnancy test in this patient was later found to be negative.

65

a. Patient's pelvic pain, overlying bowel gas (65a-b & e) and ?lack of known landmark - uterus. No LMP to work out in which menstrual phase the patient should be in.
b. Ultrasound findings: Previous hysterectomy noted. Left ovary contains two cystic areas (65c-d) the larger one measuring 20 x 24 x 21mm. In the midline and right adnexa, there is a mixed echo collection with fluid up to 19mm in depth (65a-b & e). There is a ?clublike, ?tubular hypo echoic structure with flow on Dopplers

Ultrasound Services in an Early Pregnancy and Acute Gynaecological Unit. Book 2

352

(stated with no peristalsis was noted in as well 65a). Hydrosalpinx cannot be excluded.

c. Hydrosalpinx is a fluid filled dilatation of the fallopian tube.

d. Causes include:
- PID
- Tubal ligation
- Tubal malignancy
- Ovulation induction e.g. secondary to IVF treatment
- Endometriosis (often haematosalpinx)
- Post hysterectomy without salpingo-oophorectomy – this may be unilateral or bilateral

e. Distinct from the uterus and ovary. May be proximal to the ovary Elongated or folded, tubular, serpiginous, C-shaped, or S-shaped fluid- filled structure
Thin- or thick-walled (in chronic cases)
Will not demonstrate any peristalsis (so it is not a bowel loop) or flow on Colour Dopplers (not a blood vessel) i.e. no internal reflection or vascularity.

f. May be non symptomatic or present with pelvic pains or infertility.

g. Hydrosalpinx – as described above
Pyosalpinx – Fallopian tube that is filled, and often distended, with pus.
May be secondary to PID or be part of a tubo-ovarian abscess.
On ultrasound may be seen as a dilated serpentine or tubular structure in the pelvis, thick walled, filled with fluid and debris or low level echoed content with no peristalsis or internal vascularity. Distinct from the uterus and ovary. May be proximal to the ovary Hydro or pyosalpinx may be unilateral or bilateral.

66

a. **Ultrasound findings:** No obvious IUGS is demonstrated (7.66.a-b, d-e).
Endometrial thickness is 12.6mm. (7.66e). Left ovary is 27 x 18 x 36mm.
(66.f). Right ovary is 28mm other measurements are not shown. (7.66g &

Ultrasound Services in an Early Pregnancy and Acute Gynaecological Unit. Book 2

353

j) Adjacent to the right ovary and sandwiched between the right ovary and the uterus is an approx. doughnut ring/sign or bagel sign. (7.66.c, h, i) measuring approx. 24 x 29 mm. There is some fluid around it and in the POD. (short arrow in 7.66e)

Impression: Ectopic pregnancy in the right adnexa.

b. The bagel or doughnut ring sign in pregnancy is that of a gestational sac in the adnexa (outside the uterus) with hyperechoic ring. Depending on the GA, it may contain the YS or and embryo. This confirms an ectopic pregnancy.

c. Rate of ectopic pregnancy in the UK is 11:1000 and mortality rate is 1:10,000. Rate of ovarian pregnancy is less than 2%
*At surgery : Right ovarian ectopic pregnancy was found.

67

a. Turn the gain on the equipment down and or adjust the contrast on the printer settings.

b. Yes the large yolk sac measuring approx. 10 x 8 x 9.6mm (7.67b)and the hyperechoic area in the lateral wall of the gestational sac measuring approx. 15 x 15 x 12mm (7.67f,h,j).

c. An IUGS measuring 29 x 22 x 26mm, a yolk sac measuring approx. 10 x 8 x 9.6mm (Embryo with a CRL = 3.4mm with no EHB). In the lateral wall of the gestational sac is a hyperechoic area measuring approx. 15 x 15 x 12mm.

d. Depending on the Unit protocol, it would be nice to bring the patient back in 7 -14days time to re-assess the ultrasound findings.
* Patient later miscarried .

68

a. Yes, there is a unilocular low leveled echoed slightly irregular in outline cyst in the left adnexa with hyperechoic wall plus an hyperechoic focus.

b. An anteverted uterus with a 11mm endometrium (7.68b). In the left adnexa is an approx. 77 x 40 x 70mm slightly irregular in outline ?low level echoed ? solid area. Echogenic focus is seen in this structure and some posterior echogenic rim. Interlacing linear hypoechoic area and multiple hyperechoic

Ultrasound Services in an Early Pregnancy and Acute Gynaecological Unit. Book 2

354

areas are shown within the mass (7.68c-e). No obvious blood flow is noted in this structure. The left ovary was not seen separate from this structure. This entity is probably displacing the uterus anteriorly (7.68b).

Ultrasound impression: A left endometrioma but other ovarian pathology cannot be excluded.

c.   Ovarian torsion

69

a.   In the area of this patient's pain is an approx. 54 x 56 x 64mm (7.69 a & d) avascular (7.69 e), predominantly solid mass with central necrosis (7.69 a-e).

b.   Ultrasound findings is suggestive of an anterior degenerating fibroid. when a patient is to be scanned due to pain during pregnancy, it is a good idea to ask the patient to point with one finger the area of the worst pain. This will help to focus on that area during the examination. Asking the patient to tell you if and when she experience the pain during the scanning is another useful way of focusing the examination to the request.

70

a.   Yes there is a low level echoed cystic structure in the RIF.

b.   A poorly demonstrated uterus. The endometrium has not been clearly shown nor the measurements of same . In the RIF, is an approx. 117 x 110 x 88 mm slightly irregular in outline, avascular, predominanantly low level echoed cyst. There are a few echogenic foci in this entity (7.70e-f). The right ovary is not demonstrated. The left ovary measuring approximately 35 x 21 x 29mm and appears sonographically normal. Ultrasound appearance is suggestive of right endometrioma. Differentials : right haemorrhagic cyst.

c.   A follow up scan in six weeks from this scan or in another menstrual phase will help to monitor the size and echopattern of the cyst. If it is a haemorrhage cyst, the size and appearances will have changed in line with the menstrual phase. Whereas an endometrioma will not change its echopattern but may now be bigger especially if there has been further bleeding into it.

Ultrasound Services in an Early Pregnancy and Acute Gynaecological Unit. Book 2

355

71

a. Ask the patient why she is on Zoladex. This is because Zoladex is used in treating many diseases or conditions.

b. Goserelin whose brand name is Zoladex may be used to prevent the production of certain types of hormones in the body. Zoladex is used in women who are having surgery or other procedures to treat uterine fibroids or other uterine problems. Zoladex is also used to treat endometriosis or as part of a programme of fertility treatment in women.

c. Yes there is a lot of overlying bowel gas (7.71 e,f and i)

d. An anteverted uterus with a 2.8mm endometrial thickness. (7.71 b, d & h). There is up to 19.8mm free fluid in the POD (7.71 c). The left ovary appears sonographically normal measuring approx. 23 x 20 x 18mm (7.71a).
7.71g shows a 7 x 7mm hyperechoic area within the hypoechoic mass (measurement not included) 'dermoid plug'. There is a lot of free fluid in the RIF measuring more than 13mm (7.71 e, f & i)
*"dermoid plug" sign, which has the appearance of one or more hyperechoic areas within a hypoechoic mass.
* This patient's endometriosis was being treated with Zoladex.

72

a. Yes at least in one of the ovaries, the image of the right ovary shown in 7.72e. it is difficult to confirm or refute PCO in the left ovary at present because of corpus luteum in it. (7.72 a,b,d and e).

b. No, he should not. The CRL is more accurate and should be used to date the pregnancy. With known PCO, the menstrual period may be irregular or longer than 28days and ovulation may not occur on day 14 as in a normal menstrual cycle.

c. There is an intrauterine gestational sac, yolk sac and embryonic pole. EHB not shown here was claimed to have been seen. CRL = 6.4mm = 6+3/40. The right ovary appears polycystic (measurements not included). There is a 33 x 28 x 31mm corpus luteum in the left ovary.

Ultrasound Services in an Early Pregnancy and Acute Gynaecological Unit. Book 2

356

PCO may be unilateral or bilateral.

73

a. Yes, 7.73 a, b, d & f shows a predominantly avascular hypoechoic mass with echogenic rim in the same gestational sac with the fetus. (measurements not included)

b. An intrauterine gestational sac with a yolk sac, fetus and FHB. FHR = 184 bpm (7.73c). CRL = 37.4mm = 10+4/40. (7.73 e). Anterior to the placenta is a predominantly avascular hypoechoic mass with echogenic rim in the same gestational sac with the fetus. (measurements not included (7.73 a-b,d & f) There is an approx. 25 x 27 x 6mm possible area of bleed posterior to the amniotic membrane. (7.73 b &d) The bulk of the placenta is fundal and anterior (7.73b, d &f).

c. Yes to monitor the worringsome findings described above. This could be done at the time of the NT screening examination.
    * *Abnormal blood clots may mimick an embryo, asking the patient to roll over may show the blood clot movement.*

74

a   The patient was scanned trans abdominally (74a- c) and transvaginally (74 d- g)

b. An anteverted uterus (measurements not included). The endometrial cavity to the cervix is filled with low level echoed fluid. ? blood (long arrow in 74.d). C/s scar is noted (short arrow) in 74.d. A 24 x 21 x 27mm posterior subserosal fibroid is noted. (74d –f). The cervix is closed.
Impression: Low level echoed filled endometrial cavity with a closed cervix.

c. Depending on departmental protocol. Another scan could be performed after she has bled so as to confirm or refute any RPOC or fluid in the endometrial cavity which if left could cause infection.

Ultrasound Services in an Early Pregnancy and Acute Gynaecological Unit. Book 2

357

75

a. Images 75a-b were obtained by TAS whilst images 75c-f were obtained by TVS.

b. An anteverted uterus with a thickened endometrium and posterior intramural fibroid (measurements which has not been included c-d). Superior to the uterus and on the right is a gestational sac, fetus with a CRL of 40.7mm and FHB = 118 bpm (75a-b). Note myometrium does not completely surround the gestational sac nor is there any communication between the gestational sac and the cervix. (75e-f)

c. An on going ectopic pregnancy in the right adnexa due to the facts that:
- there is no IUP, there is a gestational sac in the right adnexa with myometrium that was not completely surrounding the gestational sac nor is there any communication between the gestational sac and the cervix.

d. The ectopic pregnancy is the cause of the woman's pain.

Symptoms of an ectopic pregnancy usually develop between the 4th and 12th weeks of the pregnancy. Often, the first warning signs of an ectopic pregnancy are pain or vaginal bleeding. There might be pain in the pelvis, abdomen, or even the shoulder or neck (if blood from a ruptured ectopic pregnancy builds up and irritates the diaphragm). The pain can range from mild and dull to severe and sharp.

* At surgery a pregnancy was seen in a rudimentary horn on the right. Patient made a good recovery post surgery.

76

a. An anteverted normal size uterus with an endometrium that is smooth and thin- (subjective assessment as the measurements have not been included (7.76 a, b, j & k). Posterior to the uterus and extending to the POD is an approx. 72 x 31mm predominantly hypoechoic tubular structure with a 3.4mm wall and posterior to the uterine fundus is another 74 x 44mm ?tubular ?circular mixed echo structure (7.76 a, b, j & k). Both ovaries are multicystic in appearance. The left ovarian volume is 40 x 29 x 40mm - 24.3mls and the right ovarian volume is 27 x 31 x 37mm - 16.2mls (7.76e and f). Separated from the ovaries are various

Ultrasound Services in an Early Pregnancy and Acute Gynaecological Unit. Book 2

358

cystic entities in the pelvis, some of which are low level echoed and others that are purely cystic (7.76 c-f, g, j, h). No obvious free fluid has been demonstrated in the pelvis.

Ultrasound impression: Bilateral multi cystic ovaries. ?bilateral endometriomas, ?bilateral hydro or pyosalpinx, ?bilateral tubo-ovarian abscess.

b. This patient will benefit from follow up scans either following any gynaecology treatment she receives or in another phase of her menstrual cycle if clinically indicated.

Post treatment to confirm if the treatment has worked and to what extent.

*Sometimes the ultrasound appearances of the pelvis is difficult to interprete and what the Sonographer can do is to describe what is seen and as best seen.

77

a. There is an approx. 24 x 14 x 8mm slightly irregular and elongated in outline gestational sac in the cervical area, with a yolk sac and embryo with a CRL of 2.9mm (77a-d). There is no ultrasound documentation of EMB or not. There is a 20 x 12mm cyst in the right ovary. Left ovary is not shown. (77.h)

b. Ultrasound appearances is suggestive of an ongoing threatened or inevitable miscarriage or a cervical pregnancy.
* Unfortunately the patient miscarried.

78

a. No, there is no need to check the upper abdomen in this case.

b. Since there is no free fluid in the POD or pelvis, there will be no ascites in the abdomen.

c. An intrauterine DC/DA twin pregnancy with CRLs of 38.5mm and 37.4mm. (78a-c). Heart beats were noted in both twins (not shown here), gestational sac with two embryos. Bilateral enlarged ovaries with multiple cysts within them, the right ovary measuring 103 x 83 118mm (528mls)and the left ovary measuring 101 x 114 x 87mm (524mls)

Ultrasound Services in an Early Pregnancy and Acute Gynaecological Unit. Book 2

359

d. Impression: DC/DA Twins. Spontaneous hyperstimulation syndrome. (Mild OHSS)

e. The bilateral enlarged ovaries are most likely cause of the patient's pelvic pain.

f. Monitor the Spontaneous hyperstimulation syndrome, perform the screening ultrasound examinations if the patient wants and monitor the pregnancy in line with the hospital or departmental policy.

Spontaneous hyperstimulation syndrome. Experts believe:

That it is rare and mostly seen during pregnancy.

It develops between 8 and 14 weeks of amenorrhoea whereas iatrogenic OHSS usually starts between 3-5 weeks of amenorrhoea

Can be seen with single or multiple pregnancies or hydatiform mole

May be associated with hypothyroidism

May be seen in non pregnant, non ovulation induction patient

79

a. A normal sized anteveted uterus with a 4.7mm endometrium (79.a). Both ovaries especially the right one have a solid stroma and multiple peripheral follicles which gives the impression of polycystic ovaries. The right ovarian volume is 12.6mls and the left is 9.8mls (79.g). Adjacent to and eccentric to each ovary is a cystic entity with no internal echoes or septations (79.b-i). The right cyst measures 38 x 34 x 35mm and the one on the left measures 40 x 40 x 41mm. Some fluid is seen in the POD and between the cystic entities.

Impression: Bilateral cysts, ? bilateral paraovarian cysts, ?PID, ?torsion.

b. Yes , she is likely to benefit from an MRI scan.

c. Post treatment ultrasound can be repeated to re-assess the current ultrasound findings. Alternatively this patient could be re scanned in 6 weeks from the initial scan. The next menstrual period will help in the interpretations of the scan examinations, as both findings could then be compared.

*MRI was done few days after this scan and the findings were very similar. Ovarian torsion could also not be excluded.

Ultrasound Services in an Early Pregnancy and Acute Gynaecological Unit. Book 2

360

80
a.

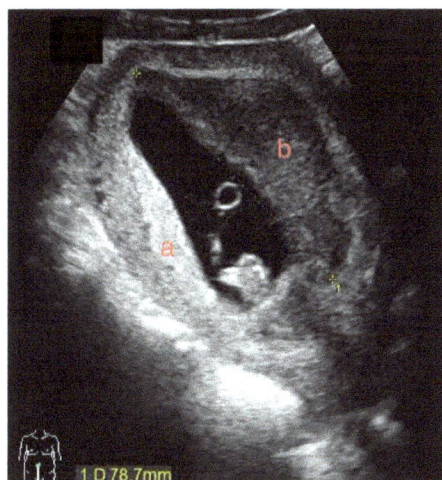

a – is the placenta, b is an area of bleed.

b. Images 80a- f were obtained by TVS whilst images 80g- j were obtained by TAS.

c. Singleton intrauterine pregnancy with FHB of 172bpm (80.c). CRL = 51.2mm = 11+5/40 (80.g). Posterior placenta (80.d, i,h). There is an approx. 79 x 84 x 52mm hematoma in the anterior and left lateral wall of the gestational sac. (80.a,b,d-i). Impression: This is a case of threatened miscarriage.

d. Experts claim that threatened miscarriage—vaginal bleeding before 20 gestational weeks—is the commonest complication in pregnancy, occurring in about a fifth of cases. Miscarriage is 2.6 times as likely and 17% of cases are expected to present complications later in pregnancy.
Others claim that it does not affect the pregnancy outcome.

81
a. Posterior to the previous c/s scar in the cervical area is an elongated , slightly irregular in outline sac measuring 26 x 7 x 7mm. (81a, c-h). The gestational sac is 11mm from the internal os (81f). The endometrium thickness is 1.3mm (81a). There seem to be two yolk sacs and tiny embryonic poles without heart beats, CRL measured = 1.8mm (81b, e-f). In the left ovary is a corpus luteum measuring 15 x

Ultrasound Services in an Early Pregnancy and Acute Gynaecological Unit. Book 2

361

14 x 17mm and a 8 x 7 10mm hyperechoic area ?dermoid cyst (81i-j) . There are cysts in the right ovary the largest one measuring 26 x 18 x 18mm (81l-m).

b. Impression: Threatened miscarriage. Differentials - cervical pregnancy.
   Bilateral ovarian cysts, ?drmoid in the left ovary.
* Unfortunately the woman miscarried.

82
a. Singleton intrauterine pregnancy with FHB. (82a-b). There is an approx. 32 x 22 x 29mm retro placental fluid collection. ? hematoma (82i). Within the gestational sac is another approx. 48 x 53 x 33mm mixed echo area with no vascularity seen on Colour flow Doppler (82c-d, f-h). Left lateral placenta (82e). Fetal measurements = dates.
Impression: on going pregnancy with retro placenta fluid collection, ?hematoma and hematoma within the gestational sac.

b. Subchorionic hematoma could increase the chance of miscarriage – depending on its size and maternal age. Ultrasound identified subchorionic hematoma in the late 1st trimester or 2nd trimester increases the risk of miscarriage, abruption placenta, preterm labor   secondary to PROM and stillbirth. Retroplacental hematomas are found in 5% of all placentae and in 15% of women with pregnancy induced hypertension. Retroplacental bleeding with premature placental separation is thought to be due to rupture of a maternal uteroplacental artery. They are often accompanied by infarction of the overlying villous tissue and decidual necrosis.

c. To confirm if the pregnancy is still ongoing, assess the previously noted subchorionic hematoma, assess fetal growth and well being, assess the cevix to see if it is open or closed.

83
a. The presence of anterior and posterior fibroids plus the fetal position in the maternal pelvis (83b).
b.   An intrauterine single gestation (83a-b) with FHB. (i). CRL = 76.8mm = 13+6/40 (83a). There is an abdominal wall defect that seems to demonstrate the liver and bowel outside the abdomen (83b, e-h, j). The placenta is posterior (83i-j).

Ultrasound Services in an Early Pregnancy and Acute Gynaecological Unit. Book 2

362

There is an approximate 54 x 49 x 50 mm anterior cervical fibroid and another 88 x 64 x 78mm posterior fibroid (83a, c-d).

c. The diagnosis is exomphalos. Differentials is body wall stalk. However in body wall stalk the fetal abdomen will be attached to the placenta or uterine wall (83b, e – j).

d. Further scans including a CVS or amniocentesis will be offered to the patient to exclude any chromosomal abnormality.

84

a. There is some generalized oedema around the fetus measuring up to 2.3mm around the abdomen and more around the fetal head (84a-d).

b. An IUGS with a fetus with FHB (84a-e) FHB = 152 bpm. CRL – 35.3mm = 10+3/40 (84.a). There is some generalized oedema around the fetus measuring up to 2.3mm around the abdomen and more around the fetal head (84a-d)

c. CVS would or may be offered to this patient. NT Screening and other routine ultrasound examination in line with the departmental protocol.

85

a. There is no evidence of RPOC.

b. An intrauterine gestational sac and fetus with FHB (85.a-c). CRL = 32.6mm =10+1/40.

Impression: An ongoing intrauterine pregnancy.

Ultrasound Services in an Early Pregnancy and Acute Gynaecological Unit. Book 2

363

86

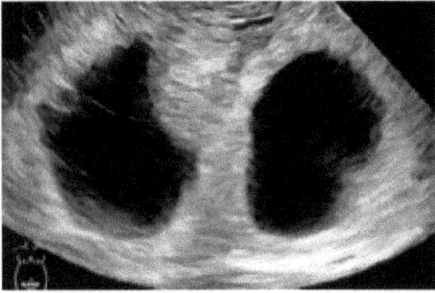

a. There is a yolk sac in the right gestational sac but none in the left gestational sac.

b. There are two intrauterine gestational sacs - Dichorionic/diamniotic pregnancy (DCDA) (7.86a-d). The thick dividing membrane (not measured)(7.86b-c). The fact that the pregnancy on the right is ongoing but the one on the left not.

c. Two intrauterine gestational sacs approx. of same size (subjective assessment} and thick dividing membrane (7.86c) There is an embryo in the gestational sac on the right with EHB= 162bpm (7.86f). CRL = 13.8mm = 7+6/40 (7.86e). There is no yolk sac or embryo in the left gestational sac (7.86b-c). Posterior to the gestational sacs is a heart shaped hypo echoic area. ?possible area of bleed (7.86g). There is a cyst in one of the ovaries.

d. NT Screening and other routine ultrasound examination in line with the departmental protocol.

87

a. Measuring an accurate CRL in view of the absence of the calvarium.

b. 'Frog's eye view' or "mickey mouse" appearance . This may be seen when fetus is in the coronal plane due to absent cranial bone or brain and bulging orbits.

c. An intrauterine pregnancy with a fetus. There was no ossified bony structure at the upper part of fetal head and brain tissue is exposed to amniotic fluid i.e. Fetus has no calvarium (skull bones) 7.87a-e). CRL = 62mm = 12+4/40. (7.87e). FHB =

Ultrasound Services in an Early Pregnancy and Acute Gynaecological Unit. Book 2

364

154bpm (7.87b)

d. Acrania or exencephaly is suspected.

e. It is fatal.

f. If the head is too low in the maternal pelvis and it is not examined or assumed to be normal. Poor technique, High BMI, poor image resolution

88

a. There is no obvious intrauterine gestational sac or placenta demonstrated in the uterus. Instead the uterus is filled with a predominantly hyperechoic mass with multiple, tiny hypoechoic or cystic areas. The is suggestive of a 'snow storm' appearance (7.88a - 7.88c).

b. Molar pregnancy

c. Molar pregnancy (as explained above in 88.a). In a missed miscarriage, the fetus is seen but with no heartbeat. CRL may be = or < dates.

89

a. Yes, the size of the placenta compared to the size of the embryo.

b. An intrauterine pregnancy with an embryo with heartbeat. EHB = 144 bpm. (7.89c) CRL = 16.2mm = 8+0/40 (7.89d). The placenta is large compared to the size of the embryo measuring 44 x 19 x 16mm.
The right ovary is measuring 45 x 25 x 3 0mm. The left ovary was not identified.

c. ? partial mole however the embryo has a heartbeat.
*Partial molar pregnancy confirmed and the pregnancy went to term.

Ultrasound Services in an Early Pregnancy and Acute Gynaecological Unit. Book 2

365

90

a

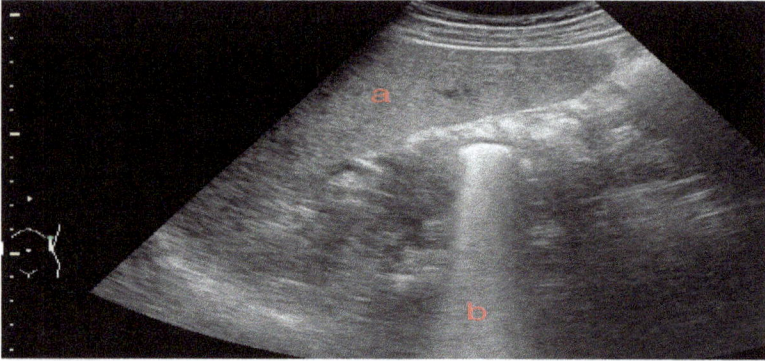

a. a-spleen, b- bowel gas

b. OHSS, ectopic pregnancy and heterotropic pregnancy

c. To confirm or exclude ascites secondary to OHSS which could have caused the abdominal distension and abdominal pain.
However there is no evidence of free fluid in the upper abdomen (90.i-l).

d. An anteverted uterus with a 21mm thickened endometrium. No obvious ultrasound evidence of an IUGS is demonstrated. (7.90a-b). There is bilateral multiple corpus luteum cysts and bilateral enlarged ovaries. The left ovarian volume is 64.8mls and the right ovarian volume is 142mls. There is some fluid in the POD up to 44mm deep.
Impression: OHSS. Pregnancy wise –inconclusive. Further scan to be determined by the beta hCG levels.

e. Monitoring the OHSS and the pregnancy – to ascertain if it is in utero or otherwise, how many embryos, EMB, for NT and anomaly screening and other ultrasound examinations as per hospital protocol.
*Follow up scans showed a normal DC/DA twin pregnancy.

Ultrasound Services in an Early Pregnancy and Acute Gynaecological Unit. Book 2

366

91

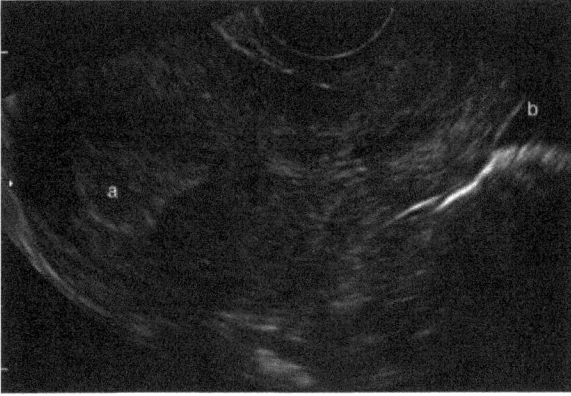

a

a. a- thickened endometrium, b-some fluid in the POD

b. An anteverted uterus with a 12.4mm endometrium with no obvious intra uterine gestational sac (91.a-b). Both ovaries appear sonographically normal with the right ovarian volume measuring 6mls (91.f), left ovarian measurements have not been included (91e-f). Adjacent to the left ovary in the left adnexa is a 20 x 25mm gestational sac (91.e) with 2 yolk sacs (91 c-d), 2 embryonic poles (91.j CRL's 1.5mm and 1.6mm) and 2 sets of embryonic heart beats. (91.g-h). Peritrophoblastic flow is demonstrated around the gestational sac. (91.i). Small fluid in the POD (91.b)

c. Monochorionic twin ectopic pregnancy in the left adnexa. The incidence of twin ectopic pregnancies is estimated to occur in 1 in125,000 pregnancies, and twin tubal ectopic 1 in 200 of ectopic pregnancies.
* At surgery a left adnexa ampullary ectopic pregnancy was seen.

92

a. This is a monochorionic but diamnotic pregnancy (MCDA). One gestational sac and one yolk sac (92a) with a very thin dividing membrane (Tsign)92a-h.

b. An intra uterine gestational sac, (measurements not included) single large yolk sac measuring 10 x 8 x 8mm (92b). There is a very thin dividing membrane and two embryonic poles with CRL measuring 19.1mm and 16.7mm = 8+1 /40 (92c, e-f). Calculated GA was 9+3/40. There is no embryonic heartbeat demonstrated in

Ultrasound Services in an Early Pregnancy and Acute Gynaecological Unit. Book 2

367

twin 1 or twin 2 (92d,g-h).

c. Ultrasound diagnosis: Missed miscarriage in a monchorionic, diamniotic twin pregnancy.

93

a. To confirm that the pregnancy is ongoing or not and re-assure the patient if possible.

b. An intrauterine pregnancy with a embryo with a CRL = 25mm = 9+2/40 (93a). EHB = 168bpm (93.b). The left ovary appears sonographically normal (93.c). There are two cystic lesions with a thick and vascular septum in the right adnexa (93d-j) The cysts measure 30 x 24 x 25mm and 50 x 38 x 49mm.

Impression: An ongoing intrauterine pregnacy. Multicystic lesion in the right adnexal with septal vascularity.

94

a. By caesarean section./// in 7.94a shows it.

b. An anteverted uterus with a TS measuring approx. 107mm (other measurements not included). No obvious fluid collection is demonstrated around the uterus. The endometrium measures 7.1mm (94.b) and the endometrium is filled with predominantly echogenic material (94.a-d) Caesarean section scar is noted /// (94.a).

Impression: RPOC. No obvious fluid collection is seen around the uterus or in the POD.

95

a. There is an IUGS (95a), yolk sac measuring 5 x 4 x 5mm (95b). There is an embryo with a CRL of 2.3mm (95c) with EHB (95d). The right ovary appears sonographically normal. (95e). The left ovary appears sonographically normal (95f). Sandwiched between the left ovary and the uterus is a 45 x 24 x39mm predominantly heterogenous mass ? with 'doughnut ring' appearance (95j-k). There is some fluid around this mass (95f – l).

b. Heterotopic pregnancy. The ectopic pregnancy is in the LIF.

_____
Ultrasound Services in an Early Pregnancy and Acute Gynaecological Unit. Book 2

368

c. Monitoring the IUP post surgery, performing the screening ultrasound examinations in line with the departmental protocol if the patient agrees.

*An ectopic pregnancy was found on the isthmic portion of the left tube at surgery.
*Post surgery, the IUP continued to grow normally.

Heterotopic pregnancy:
Otherwise referred to as a combined ectopic pregnancy, multiple-sited pregnancy, or coincident pregnancy -
Is a rare occurrence where there is an intrauterine and extrauterine pregnancy in the same patient and at the same time.
Experts belief that incidence in the general population with natural conception is 1:30,000 but in patients who have had assisted reproduction could be around 1-3:100.
It is estimated that up to 70% of heterotopic pregnancies are diagnosed between 5-8 weeks of gestation, 20% between 9-10 weeks and only 10% after the 11th week.
Causes or risk factors of heterotopic pregnancy include:
* prior tubal surgery
* history of pelvic inflammatory disease
* history of a previous ectopic pregnancy
* use of an intrauterine contraceptive device .

96
a. Image 96c is a TVS showing a LS view of an anteverted uterus
   Image 96d is a TVS showing a TS view of the anteverted uterus

Ultrasound Services in an Early Pregnancy and Acute Gynaecological Unit. Book 2

369

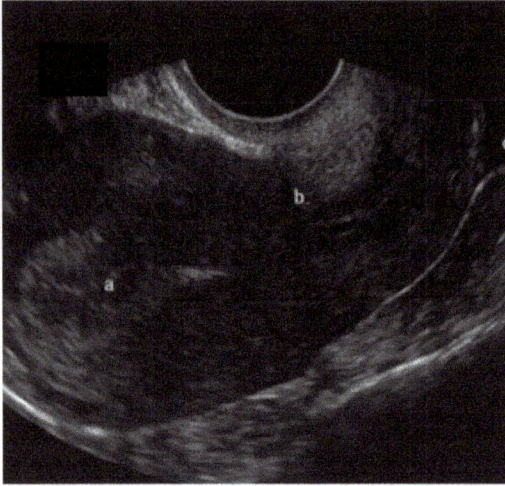

96c

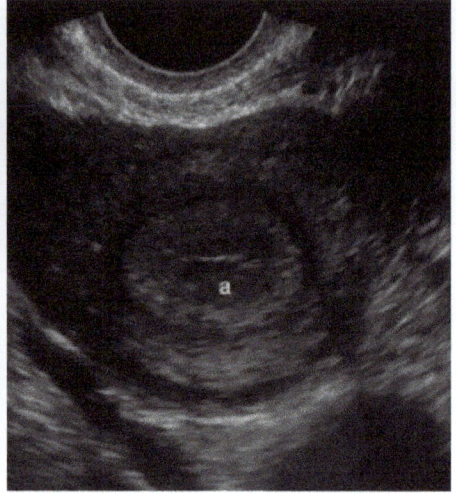

96d

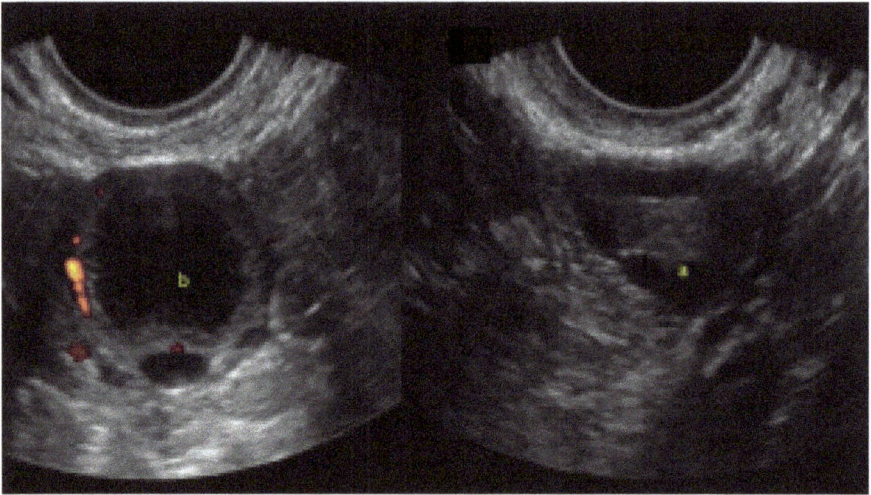

96h

b.   (c) a- endometrium, b- previous C/S scar, c- fluid in the POD.

(d) TS endometrium normal ovulation

(h) b-corpus luteum, a-follicle

c.   This is a luteal phase findings. Thickened triple line endometrium (96a-d), fluid in the POD (96b-c), corpus luteum in the right ovary (96e-f).

d.   An anteverted uterus with a 16.5mm luteal phase endometrium (96a).

Ultrasound Services in an Early Pregnancy and Acute Gynaecological Unit. Book 2

370

Previous c/s scar is noted (b in 96c). Both ovaries appear sonographically normal. The left ovary appears measures 23 x 17 x 28mm (5.7cc) (96g). The right ovary measures 29 x 29 x 28mm (12.3cc) **(96f)** and in it is a corpus luteum measuring 17 x 17 x 18mm (96e). There is some fluid in the POD up to 15mm(96b-c).

Ultrasound impression: Normal luteal phase findings.

97

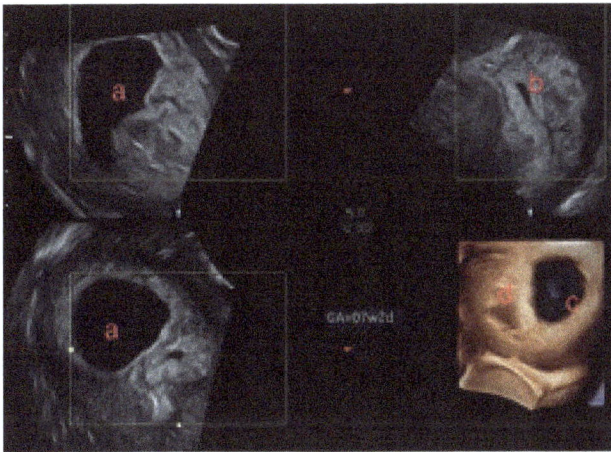

a.
a-intrauterine gestational sac.
b- thickened endometrium in rudimentary horn
c - intrauterine gestational sac
d- rudimentary horn

b. An intrauterine gestational sac, yolk sac and embryo (97a-d). Superior to the left and adjacent to the gestational sac is a rudimentary horn with thickened endometrium and a 7 x 5mm hypoechoic area in it. (7.97b)

c. The gestational sac appears intact with no obvious area of bleed. The pvb is most likely to come from the rudimentary horn.

98

a. To confirm or rule out abnormality of the renal tract which is common with Mullerian duct anomalies.

Ultrasound Services in an Early Pregnancy and Acute Gynaecological Unit. Book 2

371

b. There are uterine horns in the uterus and two endometrial cavities one of which is 9.8mm thick (98k). The other LS endometrial measurement has not been included (98j). There is one cervix. (98i, o). The left ovary is measuring 34 x 22 x 24mm- 9.4mls (98p) and in it is a 21 x 17 x 14mm cyst (98q). There is a 44 x 39 x 53mm haemorrhagic cyst in the right ovary (98g,h,n). No free fluid in the POD. Both kidneys are seen and they appear sonographically normal (98l-m).

c. Subseptate uterus. Differentials – bicornuate uterus.

   Haemorrhagic cyst in the right ovary.

99

a. There are two retroverted uteruses with two cervical canals and two endometrial cavities (99a-d). The endometrial thickness on the right is 7.2mm and on the left 4.5mm (99d). Right ovarian volume is 26mls and the left ovarian volume is 23.6mls. Multiple small peripheral follicles with strong stoma is seen in the ovaries. (99d).

The right kidney measures 10.5cm and the left kidney measures 11.4cm. Both kidneys appear sonographically normal. (99.h-i)

b. Ultrasound diagnosis or impression: Normal kidneys, didelphys uterus and bilateral PCO.

MRI Report – Congenital uterine malformation with configuration of uterine didelphys. Two separate non communicating endometrial cavities and cervical canals. Bilateral PCO,

Ultrasound Services in an Early Pregnancy and Acute Gynaecological Unit. Book 2

372

100
A

	Ultrasound image	What is it?	Clinical significance
a		Calcified cystic lesion in the ovary. This is either calcified dermoid or ovarian fibroma with rim calcification	
b		A dermoid cyst	
c		Haemorrhagic cyst	Will most likely disappear, change it's appearance or change size after the next menstrual period or in another menstrual phase
d		Paraovarian cyst	Can become torted otherwise of no clinical significance

Ultrasound Services in an Early Pregnancy and Acute Gynaecological Unit. Book 2

373

e		Polycystic ovaries	May affect the regularity of menstrual period, Can cause female related cause of infertility. Can cause miscarriage where there is no luteal phase support especially in early pregnancy
f		Haemorrahgic post ovulation cyst	Will most likely disappear, change it's appearance or change size after the next menstrual period or in another menstrual phase.
g		Multicystic ovaries.	May be female related cause of infertility.

Ultrasound Services in an Early Pregnancy and Acute Gynaecological Unit. Book 2

374

h		Homgenous, low level echo cyst or chocolate cyst' or Endometrioma. pelvic structures, alteration of the immune system functioning, changes in the hormonal environment of the eggs impairing the implantation of a pregnancy, and altering the egg quality.	Can cause pain, get bigger become torted. It may cause subfertility, causing infertility in up to 30-50% cases. it may cause infertly by distorting the anatomy of the pelvis, causing adhesions, causing fallopian tube scarring, inflammation of the pelvis structures, alteration of the immune system functioning.

Ultrasound Services in an Early Pregnancy and Acute Gynaecological Unit. Book 2

375

| i | | Mature teratoma | Cystic Teratomas or Dermoids account for 10% to 15% of all ovarian tumors and are bilateral in 10% of the cases
They are composed of mature epithelial elements: a combination of skin, hair, sebum, desquamated epithelium, and teeth. Dermoids range in size and echogenicity. Depending on the extent and admixture of their epithelial elements, the ultrasound patterns can vary markedly, even within a single mass. |

Ultrasound Services in an Early Pregnancy and Acute Gynaecological Unit. Book 2

376

j		Predominantly cyst with complex appearance.	Needs immediate further imaging.
k		Haemorrhagic cyst	Will most likely disappear, change it's appearance or change size after the nest menstrual period or in another menstrual phase.
l		Dermoid	Rarely malignant. See i above.
m		Dermoid	Rarely malignant. See i above. Large dermoid cyst can undergo torsion or leak when it hurts

Ultrasound Services in an Early Pregnancy and Acute Gynaecological Unit. Book 2

377

100b

	Image	What?	Where?	Clinical Significance
i		Fibroid posterior to a gestational sac.	In the cervical area.	May have implications on the mode of delivery at term. May cause pain in the pregnancy.
Ii		Calcified posterior intramural fibroid	In the uterus	
iii		Fibroid within the endometrium. Note the posterior acoustic shadowing which is not seen with polyps	Fibroid within the metrium.	Can be a reason for Menorrhagia and. Infertility

Ultrasound Services in an Early Pregnancy and Acute Gynaecological Unit. Book 2

378

iv		Anterior submucousal fibroid.	Anterior fibroid displacing the endometrium posteriorly.	As it may buldge into the dometrium
v		Pedunculated anteriorfibroid	Outside the uterus in the anterior wall	None but large pedunculated fibroid may twist and cause severe pain.

■

Ultrasound Services in an Early Pregnancy and Acute Gynaecological Unit. Book 2

379

7.101

a.   This is a DCDA twin pregnancy – 7.101a-d and 7.101g
b.   Yes there are: anhydramnios and no FHB in fetus 1. Having to break some bad news to the woman or couple

c.   Ultrasound findings: There are two gestational sacs. F1 – who is twin 1 and presenting has no FHB as documented in 101c -l01d.

	Fetus 1	Fetus 2
BPD	3.2cm	3.6cm
HC	13.2cm	13.6cm
AC	9.6cm	11.2cm
FL	Not shown	2.2cm
Maximum fluid depth	Anyhydramnios	5.45cm
FHB	Absent	Present (not shown)
	See 7.101a, c-d	

The placenta is anterior.

d. Ultrasound diagnosis: DC/DA Twins. Missed miscarriage in fetus 1. Fetus 2 is ongoing with FHB not shown

e. The pregnancy will be monitored in line with the departmental protocol
 in performing anomaly scan and growth scans as will be requested by the Consultant.

Ultrasound Services in an Early Pregnancy and Acute Gynaecological Unit. Book 2

380

Chapter Conclusion

The various cases that have been presented in this chapter are examples of what happens in a typical EPAGU. It can be challenging especially when the identified pelvic pattern on ultrasound does not fit into a known condition. In such an instance, the Sonographer should provide a detailed ultrasound description of what had been seen.

Ultrasound Services in an Early Pregnancy and Acute Gynaecological Unit. Book 2

381

The role of the Sonographer in EPAGU includes:
(in no particular order)

Arriving at a diagnosis i.e. being able to answer the question or reason for the scan and where the diagnosis is not straight forward being able to describe the ultrasound appearances as clearly as possible.

Reassuring the patient where possible e.g. a confirmed single intrauterine pregnancy cannot change and become an ectopic pregnancy subsequently.

Educating the patient or and relatives e.g. weekly scan cannot guarantee no miscarriage.

Departmental protocols need to be adhered to in order to avoid unnecessary repeat scan examinations.

Showing good quality care in communication and empathy.

Be humble and comfortable to ask for a second opinion with the patient or couple's consent as some situations are 1 in many thousands.

Be willing to learn from others - no one knows it all or have seen it all.

Follow up interesting cases - it is a good way of learning and getting better

Attend MTD meetings when and where available

As a Sonographer working in EPAGU be prepared to (not in any particular order) :
- Perform TAS and interpret it
- Perform TVS and interpret it
- Communicate 'bad news'
- Get a second opinion
- Be flexible in technique

Ultrasound Services in an Early Pregnancy and Acute Gynaecological Unit. Book 2

382

- Refer to the Consultant
- Suggest further imaging where applicable
- Identify fetal abnormality relative to fetal GA
- Identify gynaecology abnormalities or pathologies
- Perform and interpret 3D imaging where available
- Comfortably access hospital counseling services if he needs it
- Identify serious maternal problems e.g. complex ovarian cyst or mass.
- Have his own suitable way of dealing with work related stress especially that which is related to many times repeatedly having to communiicate 'bad news' to patients.

Ultrasound Services in an Early Pregnancy and Acute Gynaecological Unit. Book 2

383

Book Conclusion
(not in any particular order):

The Sonographer:
- Should have and demonstrate good communication skills
- Should be familiar with department protocols and policies
- Should be humble enough to ask for a second opinion if need be
- Should be comfortable with performing and interpreting TAS or and TVS
- Should be familiar with the ultrasound appearances of a normal female pelvis
- Shoud be able to identify gynaecology abnormalities or and pathologies
- Should be able to answer the question on the request form in the ultrasound report
- Should be familiar with the normal ultrasound appearances of the embryo or fetal anatomy at each GA
- Should be able to communicate nicely and clearly ultrasound findings that are 'bad news' to the patient or couple or family
- If possible he should be familiar with performing and interpreting 3D ultrasound where the facility is available
- Not every ultrasound finding is straight forward, when a diagnosis or impression is unclear, he should at least be able describe what he has seen during the ultrasound examination.
- Have a good rapport with the other multidisciplinary team members. In our experience this makes the work easier.
- Should attend relevant MTD meetings and keep abreast of latest information and technique as this is an essential quality for good practice.
- Working in EPAGU for the Sonographer could be challenging, keeping calm under pressure and following one's routine pattern of scanning will help in not missing pathology or abnormalities.
- Workflow could be heavy or busy and demanding but he should not neglect his health - stretch regularly during the session, hydrate himself and find time to visit the toilet if need be.

Ultrasound Services in an Early Pregnancy and Acute Gynaecological Unit. Book 2

384

Chapter 7 & 8
Further Reading:

Articles:

Alice. How do birth control pills work? http://goaskalice.columbia.edu/answered-questions/how-do-birth-control-pills-work

American Pregnancy Association. Human Chorionic Gonadtropin (HCG): The Pregnancy Hormone. http://americanpregnancy.org/while-pregnant/hcg-levels/

Beta HCG levels – and how to interpret them. http://www.drmalpani.com/articles/betahcglevels/

Cabar F. R Ovarian hyperstimulation syndrome in a spontaneous singleton pregnancy. https://www.ncbi.nlm.nih.gov/pmc/articles/PMC4943359/

Cerekja A, Piazze J, Uterine synechiae. https://sonoworld.com/Fetus/page.aspx?id=2780

Chhabra A, Lin E. C et al. Subchorionic Hemorrhage. http://emedicine.medscape.com/article/404971-overview

Czarniecki M and Weerakkody Y et al. Pyosalpinx. https://radiopaedia.org/articles/pyosalpinx
doi: 10.4103/0974-1208.117164 PMCID: PMC3778607

Countdown My Pregnancy. Baby's Heartbeat. http://www.countdownmypregnancy.com/pregnancy/heartbeat.php

Ectopic pregnancy – Symptoms at: http://www.nhs.uk/Conditions/Ectopic-pregnancy/Pages/Symptoms.aspx
Ectopic pregnancy at: http://kidshealth.org/en/parents/ectopic.html

Ultrasound Services in an Early Pregnancy and Acute Gynaecological Unit. Book 2

385

El Gezeiry I Anencephaly - Case Presentation. https://radiopaedia.org/cases/anencephaly-7

EI-Mowafi D. Obstetrics Simplified - Ectopic Pregnancy. http://www.gfmer.ch/Obstetrics_simplified/Ectopic_pregnancy.htm

Farinde A, Staros E.B. Human Chorionic Gonadotrophin (hCG) https://emedicine.medscape.com/article/2089158-overview

Feride Söylemez. J Turk Ger Gynecol Assoc. 2014; 15(4): 239–242. Published online 2014 Dec 1. doi: 10.5152/jtgga.2014.14170 PMCID: PMC4285213 Available at: Https://www.ncbi.nlm.nih.gov/pmc/articles/PMC4285213/

FPA. Contraceptive implant. http://www.fpa.org.uk/contraception-help/contraceptive-implant

Gaillard F et al. Ectopic pregnancy. https://radiopaedia.org/users/frank

Govindarajan MJ and Rajan R . Heterotopic pregnancy in natural conception. J Hum Reprod Sci. 2008 Jan-Jun; 1(1): 37–38. https://www.ncbi.nlm.nih.gov/pmc/articles/PMC2700683/

Hennessey C. How does the pill work? Lloyds Pharmacy Online Doctor. https://onlinedoctor.lloydspharmacy.com/uk/info/how-does-the-contraceptive-pill-work

Human Chorionic Gonadotropin (HCG). http://www.webmd.com/baby/human-chorionic-gonadotropin-hcg#1

Ilanchezhian S, Mohan S V, Ramachandran R, et al. Spontaneous ovarian hyperstimulation syndrome with primary hypothyroidism: Imaging a rare entity. Https://www.ncbi.nlm.nih.gov/pmc/articles/PMC4921160/

Jones J, Weerakkody Y et al. Fetal heart rate . https://radiopaedia.org/articles/

Ultrasound Services in an Early Pregnancy and Acute Gynaecological Unit. Book 2

386

fetal-heart-rate

Knipe H, Gaillard F. et al. Anencephaly. https://radiopaedia.org/articles/anencephaly

Management guidelines for OHSS as per Green-top Guidelines no. 5. http://www.rcog.org.uk/womens-health/clinical-guidance/management-ovarian-hyperstimulation-syndrome-green-top-5.

Morgan M .A and Weerakkody Y et al .Physiological gut herniation https://radiopaedia.org/articles/physiological-gut-herniation

Morgan M and Weerakkody Y et al. Heterotopic pregnancy. https://radiopaedia.org/articles/heterotopic-pregnancy

National Collaborating Centre for Women's and Children's Health Commissioned by the National Institute for Health and Clinical Excellence. Pain and bleeding in early pregnancy: assessment and initial management of ectopic pregnancy and miscarriage in the first trimester. https://www.nice.org.uk/guidance/cg154/documents/pain-and-bleeding-in-early-pregnancy-draft-guideline.

NHS choices. Combined pill. http://www.nhs.uk/conditions/contraception-guide/pages/combined-contraceptive-pill.aspx

NHS choices. Contraceptive implant. http://www.nhs.uk/Conditions/contraception-guide/Pages/contraceptive-implant.aspx

Nogueira AB, Nogueira AB, Gemi FR.. Two consecutive intrauterine pregnancies following transperitoneal ovum migration. https://www.ncbi.nlm.nih.gov/pubmed/21971904

Nogueira A. B et al., Sao Paulo Medical Journal, Print version ISSN 1516-3180, Sao Paulo Med. J. vol.129 no.4 São Paulo 2011, http://dx.doi.org/10.1590/S1516-31802011000400012 http://www.scielo.br/scielo.php?script=sci_arttext&pid=S1516-31802011000400012

Ultrasound Services in an Early Pregnancy and Acute Gynaecological Unit. Book 2

387

Patel M. S. Ectopic pregnancy case contribution. https://radiopaedia.org/cases/17698/studies/17441

Sotiriadis A, Papatheodorou S and Makrydimas G. Threatened miscarriage: evaluation and management https://www.ncbi.nlm.nih.gov/pmc/articles/PMC478228/

Sridev S and Barathan S. Case report on spontaneous ovarian hyperstimulation syndrome following natural conception associated with primary hypothyroidism. J Hum Reprod Sci. 2013 Apr-Jun; 6(2): 158–161. doi: 10.4103/0974-1208.117164Published online 2014 Dec 1. doi: 10.5152/jtgga.2014.14170, http://www.fetalultrasound.com/online/text/33-013.htm

Şükür, Y. E, Göç G, Köse O et al. The effects of subchorionic hematoma on pregnancy outcome in patients with threatened abortion . https://www.ncbi.nlm.nih.gov/pmc/articles/PMC4285213/
Turk J. Ger Gynecol Assoc. 2014 Dec 1;15(4):239-42. doi: 10.5152/jtgga.2014.14170. eCollection 2014. The effects of subchorionic hematoma on pregnancy.

The Ectopic Pregnancy Trust . Symptoms of ectopic pregnancy at: http://www.ectopic.org.uk/patients/symptoms-and-diagnosis/

The Ultrasound of life. Ultrasound of placental hematoma, ultrasound of placenta abruption. http://www.fetalultrasound.com/online/text/33-013.htm

Patel M. S. Ectopic pregnancy Case contribution. https://radiopaedia.org/cases/17698/studies/17441

Shah C . Hydrosalpinx. Https://sonoworld.com/CaseDetails/Hydrosalpinx.aspx?ModuleCategoryId=468

Sridev S and Barathan S. Case report on spontaneous ovarian hyperstimulation syndrome following natural conception associated with primary hypothyroidism . J Hum Reprod Sci. 2013 Apr-Jun; 6(2): 158–161.

Ultrasound Services in an Early Pregnancy and Acute Gynaecological Unit. Book 2

388

Sotiriadis A, Papatheodorou S, Makrydimas G. Threatened miscarriage: evaluation and management https://www.ncbi.nlm.nih.gov/pmc/articles/PMC478228/

Tuuli MG1, Shanks A, Bernhard L et al. Uterine synechiae and pregnancy complications. Obstet Gynecol. 2012 Apr;119(4):810-4. doi: 10.1097/AOG.0b013e31824be28a. Available at: Https://www.ncbi.nlm.nih.gov/pubmed/22433345

Vohra S, Mahsood S, Shelton H et al. Spontaneous live unilateral twin ectopic pregnancy – A case presentation . Ultrasound. 2014 Nov; 22(4): 243–246. https://www.ncbi.nlm.nih.gov/pmc/articles/PMC4760554. Published online : 2014 Oct 16. doi: 10.1177/1742271X14555565 PMCID: PMC4760554

WebMD. Pregnancy tests. https://www.webmd.com/baby/guide/pregnancy-tests

Wheeler JM, Dodson MG. Transperitoneal migration of the ovum. A case report. https://www.ncbi.nlm.nih.gov/pubmed/4078825 J Reprod Med. 1985 Nov;30(11):895-8.

Wheeler JM, Dodson MG. Transperitoneal migration of the ovum. A case report. J Reprod Med. 1985 Nov;30(11):895-8. https://www.ncbi.nlm.nih.gov/pubmed/4078825

Weerakkody Y and Radswiki et al. Hydrosalpinx .radiopaedia.org/articles/hydrosalpinx

Worrall J. A & Dubose T. Recognizing Intra-amniotic Band-like Structures on Obstetric Ultrasound July 14, 2011 http://www.obgyn.net/articles/recognizing-intra-amniotic-band-structures-obstetric-ultrasound

Yeo, L, Ananth, C, et al. Global Library of women's Medicine. Placental Abruption, (ISSN: 1756-2228) 2008; DOI 10.3843/GLOWM.10122. https://www.glowm.com/section_view/heading/Placental%20Abruption/item/122

Ultrasound Services in an Early Pregnancy and Acute Gynaecological Unit. Book 2

389

Appendix

Ultrasound Services in an Early Pregnancy and Acute Gynaecological Unit. Book 2

390

Sample of an Ultrasound Request

An example of an ultrasound examination request form that could be used in EPAGU.

- Hospital/GP details:
- Patient's details:

• Surname:	• LMP:
• First Name:	• Menstrual Cycle: regular / Irregular
• Date of Birth:	• Average length of Cycle: days
• Hospital Number:	• Pregnancy test result: Positive/Negative
• View Point Number if known:	• ß-HCG level if known:

- Reason for today's scan. Please tick or circle all that applies.
- Bleeding: Yes ☐   No ☐
- Spotting ☐ Light bleeding ☐ Heavy bleeding ☐ Since when (date)?
- Abdominal/Pelvic pains: Yes ☐ No Localised ☐ Generalised ☐
- Since when date?
- Nausea ☐ Vomiting ☐ Hyperemesis ☐
- Missing IUCD: Which type: Mirena ☐ Copper T ☐ No idea ☐
- ? Ectopic:
- Maternal anxiety
- Post-miscarriage:
- Previous miscarriage
- Conceived on the pill
- Recommended follow-up
- Unknown or unsure of LMP
- Conceived with the coil in situ
- Post-fertility treatment: Yes ☐ No ☐
- Which type: Clomid ☐ Metformin ☐ IUI ☐ IVF ☐ ICSI ☐ SUZI ☐
- How many embryos were transferred?
- What date was the embryo transfer done?
- Other reasons and relevant history. Please specify:
  Referring clinician & Designation: Date:--/--/--

Ultrasound Services in an Early Pregnancy and Acute Gynaecological Unit. Book 2

391

Sample of an Early Pregnancy Ultrasound Report

Our reference no.:
Date: 1.11.201

Patient: **Patient Test**, DOB 1.1.1997

Indication:
light bleeding from 18.11.2018 to 20.11.2018. Uncertain dates.

History:
Maternal age: 21 years.

EDD by ultrasound: 31.5.2019 .
Gestational age: 9 weeks + 6 days.

Early Pregnancy Assessment:
Transvaginal US with Voluson E6. Ultrasound view: good.
Singleton pregnancy.
Gestational Sac: present. Gestational sac size: 40 mm x 44 mm x 20 mm.
Yolk Sac: present. Yolk sac size: 5.0 mm x 5.0 mm x 6.0 mm.
Amniotic Sac: present.
Embryo present. Fetal heart activity present. Frequency 175 bpm.

Gestational Sac (Mean)	34.7	mm	-
Gestational Sac Volume	18.4	ml	
Yolk Sac (Mean)	5.3	mm	-
CRL	29.9	mm	-

Right ovary: Visibility: clearly seen. Normal morphology. Outline smooth.
Size: 35 mm x 20 mm x 25 mm. Volume: 9.2 ml.
Left ovary: Visibility: clearly seen. Normal physiological changes. Outline smooth.
Size: 40 mm x 25 mm x 30 mm. Volume: 15.7 ml.
Corpus luteum: 16 mm x 20 mm x 22 mm.
Pouch of Douglas: free fluid: none seen.
Diagnosis based on ultrasound findings: intrauterine pregnancy with fetal heartbeat .
Please refer to ANC so that 12 - 14 week scan can be arranged.

Probe cleaned using Tristel Duo Batch Number 734108. Expiry Date 30.09.2019.

Ultrasound Services in an Early Pregnancy and Acute Gynaecological Unit. Book 2

392

Gestational sac diameter

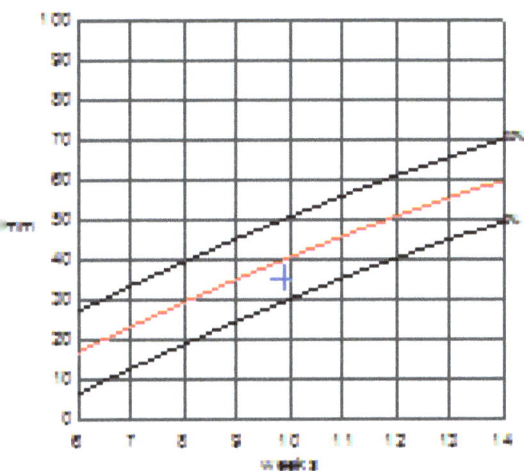

Yolk Sac Diameter

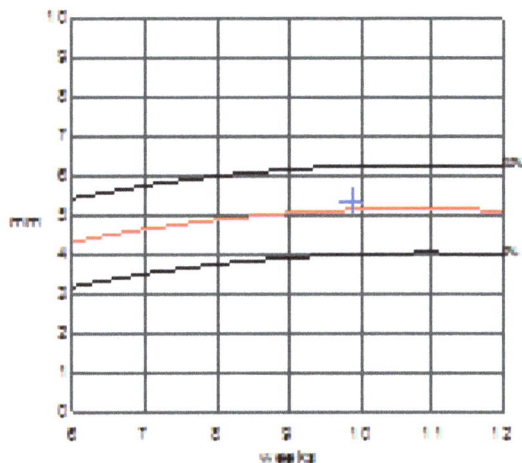

Crown-rump length

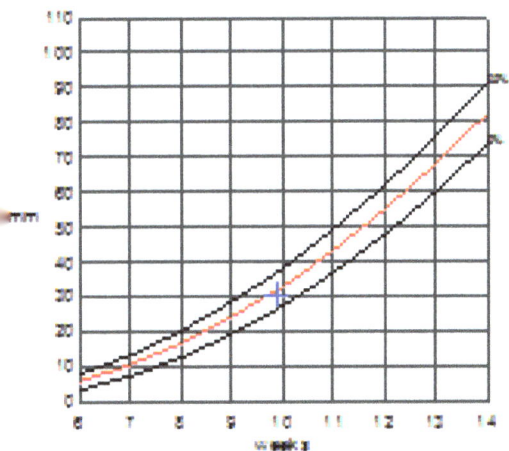

Fetal heart rate

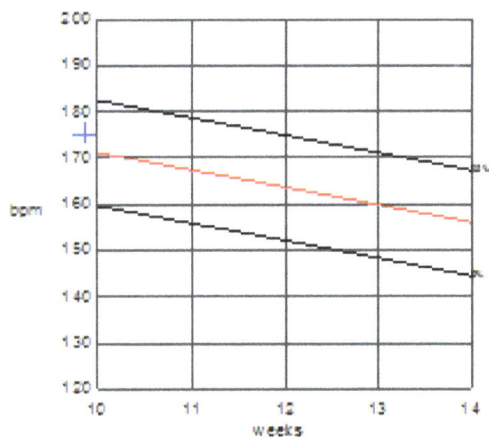

Operator: - Sonographer

Ultrasound Services in an Early Pregnancy and Acute Gynaecological Unit. Book 2

393

Sample of an Emergency Gynaecology Ultrasound Report

Acute Gynaecology & Early Pregnancy Unit

Our reference no.:
Date: 20.11.2018

Patient: **Patient Test**, DOB 2.2.1996

Indication:
Sudden and severe LIF pain for 3/7. Known 30 days cycle.
Pelvic pain.

Relevant history: last period 3.11.2018 (day of cycle 18).

Gynaecological Ultrasonography:
Method: Voluson E6, transvaginal ultrasound, transabdominal ultrasound, colour Doppler, 2 D, view: suboptimal - restricted because of increased bowel gas or activity.
Uterus: retroverted, longitudinal 75 mm, AP 32 mm, transverse 40 mm, Volume 50.3 ml. Uterine anomalies: none.
Myometrium: normal homogeneous echotexture.
Endometrium: endometrium clearly visualised, thickness (total) 13.2 mm, structure: secretory, endometrial cavity: shows normal appearences.
Pouch of Douglas: free fluid: present, largest pool 8.0 mm x 5.0 mm x 7.0 mm, volume 0.1 ml, appearances: anechoic. Findings consistent with physiological changes (e.g.ovulation).
Right ovary: Visibility: clearly seen. Normal morphology. Outline smooth.
Size: 25 mm x 25 mm x 22 mm. Volume: 7.2 ml.
Left ovary: Visibility: clearly seen. Normal physiological changes. Outline smooth.
Size: 30 mm x 28 mm x 27 mm. Volume: 11.9 ml.
Corpus luteum: 22 mm x 20 mm x 21 mm.

Summary of ultrasound features: Normal pelvic scan
Diagnosis based on ultrasound findings: Normal Pelvic Scan
The corpus luteum was seen in the area of the patient's pain.

Probe cleaned using Tristel Duo Batch Number 734108 Expiry Date 30.08.2019.

Diagnosis:
Normal Pelvic Scan.

Operator: - Sonographer

Ultrasound Services in an Early Pregnancy and Acute Gynaecological Unit. Book 2

394

Sample of Obstetrics Charts

Obstetric graphs   **GSD**

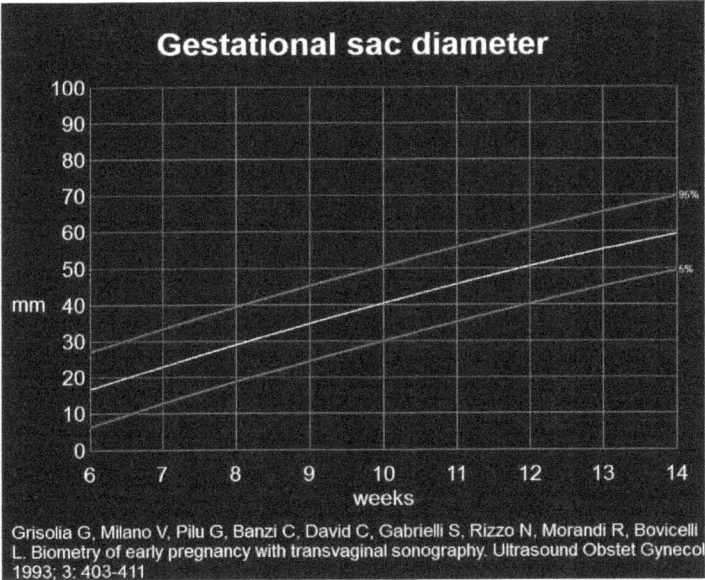

Gestational sac diameter

Grisolia G, Milano V, Pilu G, Banzi C, David C, Gabrielli S, Rizzo N, Morandi R, Bovicelli L. Biometry of early pregnancy with transvaginal sonography. Ultrasound Obstet Gynecol 1993; 3: 403-411

YSD

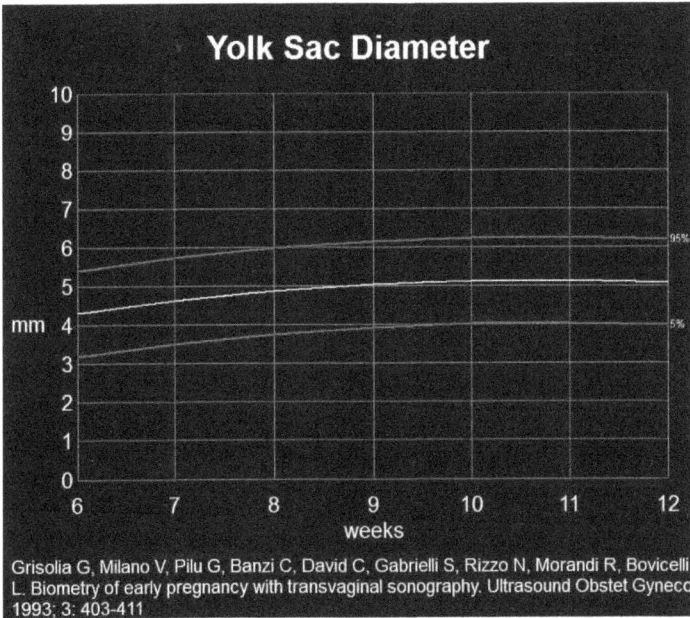

Yolk Sac Diameter

Grisolia G, Milano V, Pilu G, Banzi C, David C, Gabrielli S, Rizzo N, Morandi R, Bovicelli L. Biometry of early pregnancy with transvaginal sonography. Ultrasound Obstet Gynecol 1993; 3: 403-411

Ultrasound Services in an Early Pregnancy and Acute Gynaecological Unit. Book 2

395

CRL

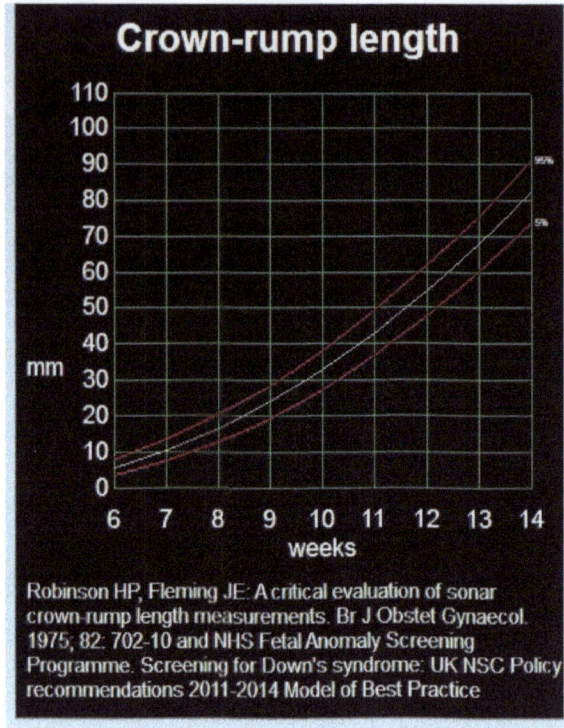

Crown-rump length

Robinson HP, Fleming JE: A critical evaluation of sonar crown-rump length measurements. Br J Obstet Gynaecol. 1975; 82: 702-10 and NHS Fetal Anomaly Screening Programme. Screening for Down's syndrome: UK NSC Policy recommendations 2011-2014 Model of Best Practice

FHR

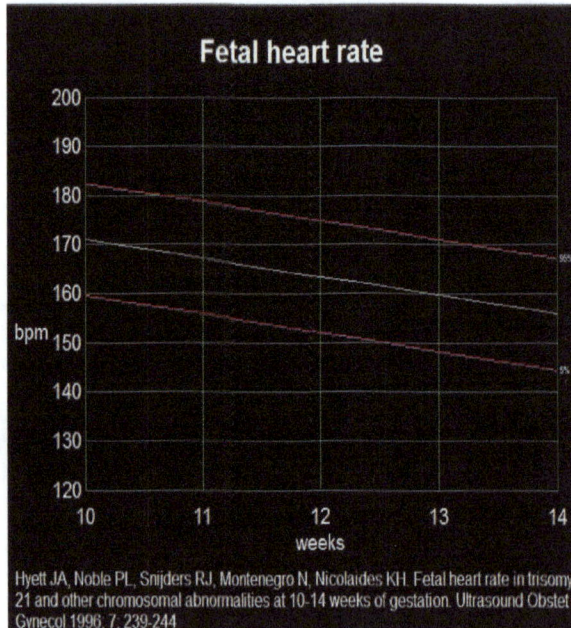

Fetal heart rate

Hyett JA, Noble PL, Snijders RJ, Montenegro N, Nicolaides KH. Fetal heart rate in trisomy 21 and other chromosomal abnormalities at 10-14 weeks of gestation. Ultrasound Obstet Gynecol 1996; 7: 239-244

Ultrasound Services in an Early Pregnancy and Acute Gynaecological Unit. Book 2

396

BPD

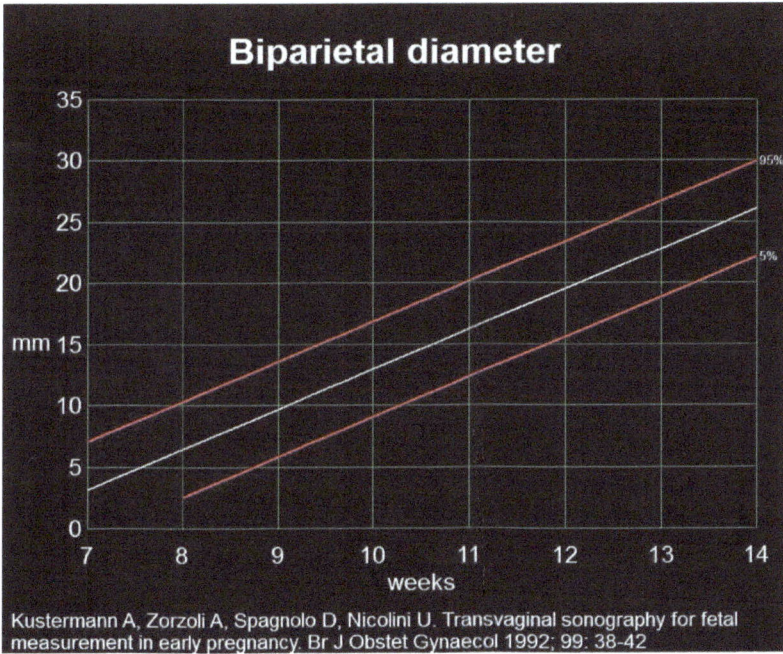

Biparietal diameter

Kustermann A, Zorzoli A, Spagnolo D, Nicolini U. Transvaginal sonography for fetal measurement in early pregnancy. Br J Obstet Gynaecol 1992; 99: 38-42

HC

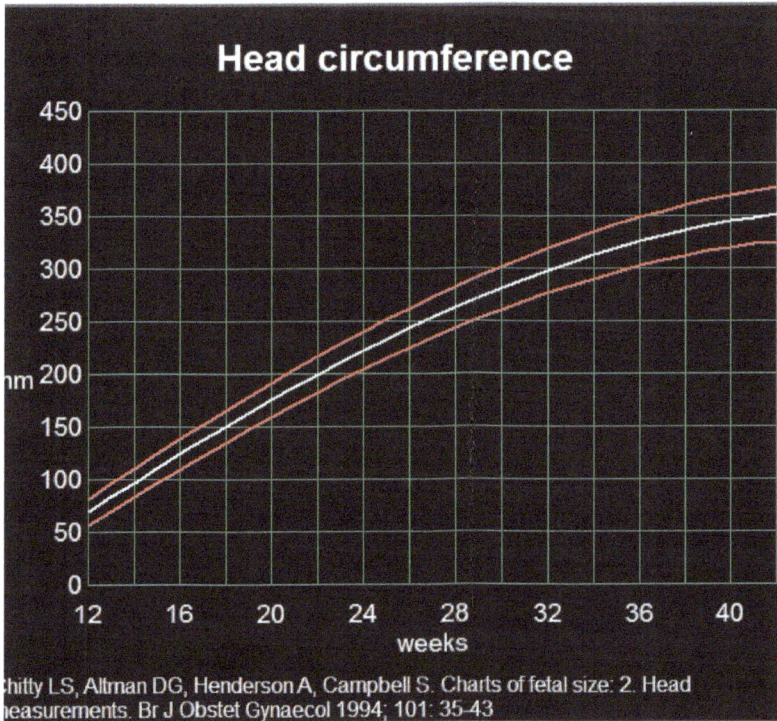

Head circumference

Chitty LS, Altman DG, Henderson A, Campbell S. Charts of fetal size: 2. Head measurements. Br J Obstet Gynaecol 1994; 101: 35-43

Ultrasound Services in an Early Pregnancy and Acute Gynaecological Unit. Book 2

397

FL

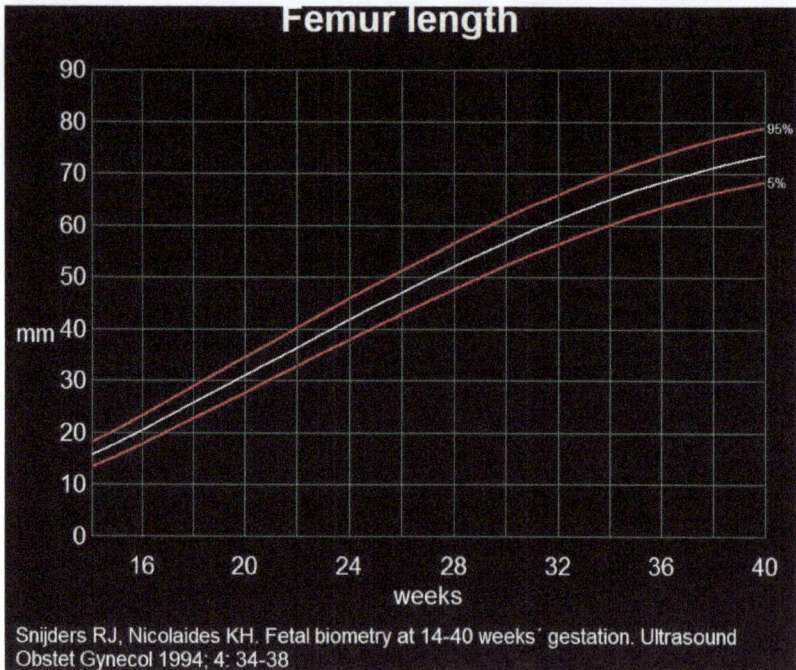

Femur length

Snijders RJ, Nicolaides KH. Fetal biometry at 14-40 weeks' gestation. Ultrasound
Obstet Gynecol 1994; 4: 34-38

AC

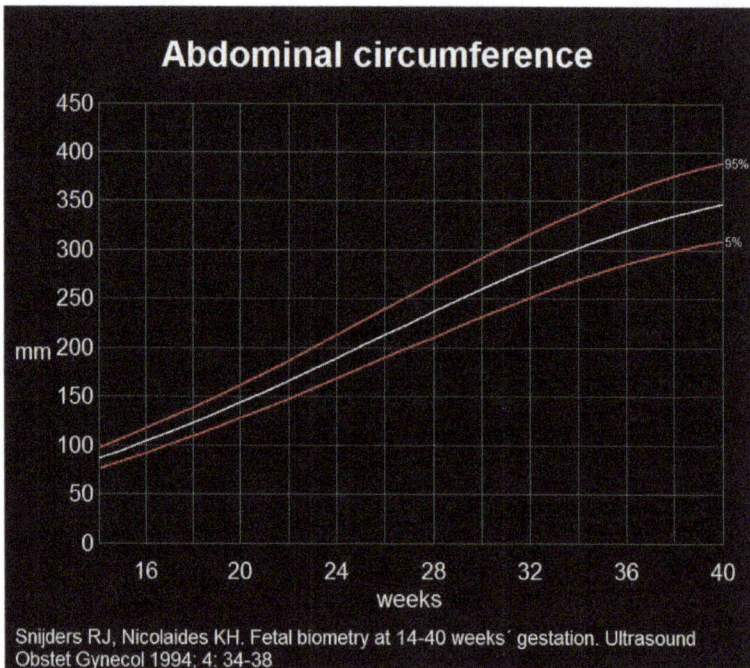

Abdominal circumference

Snijders RJ, Nicolaides KH. Fetal biometry at 14-40 weeks' gestation. Ultrasound
Obstet Gynecol 1994; 4: 34-38

Ultrasound Services in an Early Pregnancy and Acute Gynaecological Unit. Book 2

398

Useful websites and addresses

American Institute of Ultrasound in Medicine: http://www.aium.org

The American Institute of Ultrasound in Medicine (AIUM) is a multidisciplinary organisation dedicated to advancing the art and science of ultrasound in medicine and research through its educational, scientific, literary and professional activities. The website contains a useful menu selection on Standards for the Performance of Ultrasound Examination.

British Medical Ultrasound Society

36 Portland Place

London W1B 1LS

Tel: 020 7636 3914

http://www.bmus.org

The British Medical Ultrasound Society (BMUS) includes amongst its aims the advancement of the science and technology of ultrasonics as applied to medicine, as well as the provision of advice and information regarding ultrasound to the general public. It also provides links to affiliated societies concerned with the science and application of ultrasound.

The Ectopic Pregnancy Trust,

3rd floor

28 Portland Place

London

W1B 1LY

http://www.ectopic.org.uk

Tel: 020 7733 2653

Supporting people who have experienced an early pregnancy complication and the healthcare professionals who care for them

European Federation of Societies for Ultrasound in Medicine and Biology:

http://www.efsumb.org

The Federation's (EFSUMB) purpose is to promote the exchange of scientific knowledge and development in the medical and biological professions as applied to ultrasound, proposing standards and giving advice concerning criteria for the

Ultrasound Services in an Early Pregnancy and Acute Gynaecological Unit. Book 2

399

optimum apparatus and techniques together with presentation and interpretation of results.

http://www.jultrasoundmed.org:
The Journal of Ultrasound in Medicine (JUM) is dedicated to the rapid, accurate publication of original articles dealing with all aspects of medical ultrasound, particularly its direct application to patient care but also relevant to basic science, advances in instrumentation, and biological effects. The journal is an official publication of the American Institute of Ultrasound in Medicine and publishes articles in a variety of categories, including original research papers, review articles, pictorial essays, technical innovations, case series, letters to the editor, and more, from an international bevy of countries in a continual effort to showcase and promote advances in the ultrasound community.

http://209.217.125.17/SOGCnet/sogc docs/common/guide/pdfs/ps30.pdf
This website links the guidelines for the Performance of Ultrasound Examination in obstetrics and gynaecology with the policy statement document prepared by the Diagnostic Imaging Committee of the Society of Obstetricians and Gynaecologists of Canada. It outlines a standard for practitioners performing ultrasound studies of the female pelvis, including routine obstetrical ultrasound, fetal sex determination and use of ultrasound in delivery room emergencies.

Human Fertilisation & Embryology Authority
Paxton House
30 Artillery Lane
London E1 7LS
Tel: 0207 377 5077
http:www.hfea.gov.uk
The Human Fertilisation and Embryology Authority (HFEA), which was set up in the UK in 1991, ensures that all UK treatment clinics offering in vitro fertilisation (IVF) or donor insemination (DI), or storing eggs, sperm or embryos, conform to high medical and professional standards and are inspected regularly. They collect comprehensive data about such treatments, and provide detailed advice and information to the public. The publications section offers links to patient guides,

Ultrasound Services in an Early Pregnancy and Acute Gynaecological Unit. Book 2

400

code of practice and information leaflets.

International Federation of Gynecology and Obstetrics (FIGO) is a worldwide organisation of obstetricians and gynaecologists. The aims of FIGO are to promote the well-being of women and to raise the standard of practice in obstetrics and gynaecology. The website provides information about FIGO's activities, events and projects together with access to some of its publications including the FIGO newsletter, ethical guidelines and annual reports. http://www.figo.org/

The Miscarriage Association,
c/o Clayton Hospital
Northgate
Wakefield
West Yorkshire WF1 3JS
Tel (helpline): 01924 200799; admin: 01924 200795
Scottish helpline: 0131 334 8883 (answerphone with names of local contacts)
http://www.miscarriageassociation.org.uk
The Miscarriage Association publishes leaflets, fact sheets and audiotapes and has online information about miscarriage, ectopic pregnancy and molar pregnancy, including what is currently known about possible causes and the different treatments available. The association can provide information on the hospital provision of specialist services relating to pregnancy loss and it maintains a directory of other organisations which may also be of help.

Organising Medical Networked Information (OMNI) and Nursing, Midwifery and the Allied Health Professions (NMAP) are gateways to internet resources in medicine, biomedicine, allied health, health management and the Social Sciences. They aim to provide comprehensive coverage of the UK resources in both areas and provide access to the best resources worldwide.
http://www.omni.ac.uk and http://nmap.ac.uk/

Radiopaedia.org
The site provides a free educational radiology resource with one of the web's largest collections of radiology cases and reference articles. The site is targeted at medical and radiology professionals, and contains user contributed content and

Ultrasound Services in an Early Pregnancy and Acute Gynaecological Unit. Book 2

401

material that may be confusing to a lay audience.

Royal College of Midwives
15 Mansfield Street
London W1G 9NH
Tel: 020 7312 3538
http://www.rcm.org.uk/
The Royal College of Midwives (RCM) is the only trade union and professional organisation run by midwives for midwives. It is the voice of midwifery, providing excellence in professional leadership, education, influence and representation for and on behalf of midwives. The RCM produces information and advice on a wide range of midwifery issues.

Royal College of Obstetricians and Gynaecologists
27 Sussex Place
Regents Park
London NW1 4RG
Tel: 020 7772 6309
http://www.rcog.org.uk/
The Royal College of Obstetricians and Gynaecologists (RCOG) states that its objectives are the encouragement of the study and the advancement of the science and practice of gynaecology. The RCOG publishes a number of guidelines on the use of ultrasound in its website Information Services section.

The Society and the College of Radiographers,
207 Providence Square
Mill Street
London SE1 2EW
Tel: 020 7740 7200
Fax: 020 7740 7205
http://www.sor.org.news.news.htm
The Society of Radiographers includes in its objectives the promotion and development of the science and practice of radiography and radiotherapeutic technology and allied subjects. It publishes the results of study and research work therein and encourages public education, and it protects the honour and interests

Ultrasound Services in an Early Pregnancy and Acute Gynaecological Unit. Book 2

402

of those working in this field.

Sonoworld
http://sonoworld.com
A website that is dedicated to training and equipping professionals in ultrasound worldwide.

United Kingdom Association of Sonographers
36 Portland Place
London W1B 1LS
Tel: 0207 636 3714
http://www.ukasonographers.org
The United Kingdom Association of Sonographers (UKAS) produces guidelines that cover many areas, including medicolegal issues, audit and quality assurance, reporting of examinations, scanning procedures, communication to the patient and relevant clinician, ultrasound equipment usage and safe use and safety of ultrasound examination.

Wikipedia
Wikipedia is hosted by the Wikimedia Foundation, a non-profit organisation that also hosts a range of other projects. They provide free information on various subjects including medical conditions.
https://www.wikipedia.org

World Federation of Ultrasound in Medicine and Biology:
http://www.wfumb.org
World Federation of Ultrasound in Medicine and Biology (WFUMB) is a federation of affiliated organisations consisting of regional federations and national societies for ultrasound in medicine and biology, including the AIUM and EFSUMB mentioned above. WFUMB organises world congresses in ultrasound every 3 years covering the whole field of diagnostic ultrasound; it also organises and sponsors workshops on safety of ultrasound in medicine. Reports are published (monthly by Elsevier Science Inc.) in the official journal of WFUMB, Ultrasound in Medicine and Biology (UMB). See also www.elsevier.com/locate/ultrasmedbio

Ultrasound Services in an Early Pregnancy and Acute Gynaecological Unit. Book 2

403

Other Ultrasound books by the Author

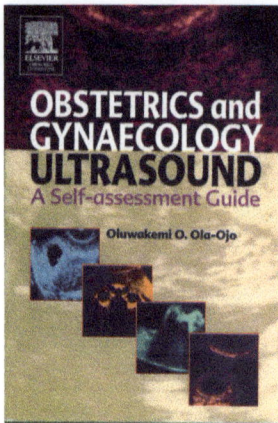

Obstetrics and Gynaecology Ultrasound-
A Self-assement Guide

Author: Oluwakemi O. Ola-Ojo.

Written by a radiographer, this excellent new book is a study guide and self-assessment tool for trainees in obstetric and gynaecological ultrasound. It will also be of interest to anyone involved in this field who wishes to keep up to date.

The book is divided into three sections: questions, answers and an appendix with further information.

Section one consists of seven systematic sets of questions which cover: essential anatomy; physics and instrumentation; gynaecology; first, second and third trimester obstetric scans; and fertility.

Each set begins with clearly laid out learning objectives and a short introduction, followed by a comprehensive range of short questions aimed at testing both knowledge and understanding. None of the questions are multiple choice and they follow a structured and logical sequence aided by division into subsections.There is a wide variety of questions on topics such as: identification of structures, making a diagnosis, differential diagnosis, pitfalls in interpreting scans,writing an ultrasound report, counselling, when to refer a patient, how cases can be managed and the role of ultrasound in the future management of conditions. The case presentation format used in many of them encourages the student to develop an understanding of the underlying clinical problem and its possible causes, the clinical significance of the diagnosis, the clinical and ethical dilemmas that can arise in some situations, and the role of the sonographer in advising or counselling women.

Good quality line diagrams and high-resolution ultrasound images are used throughout to illustrate many of the questions and aid learning.

The first set of questions deals with relevant normal anatomy. The essentials of ultrasound physics, including Doppler ultrasound and instrumentation, are thoroughly covered in the second set. The use of ultrasound in gynaecology is the subject of the third set, which includes the appropriate use of transvaginal ultrasound, preparing a woman for a gynaecological scan, normal findings, abnormal pathology and intrauterine contraceptive devices. The fourth set is devoted to obstetric ultrasound in the first trimester.

Ultrasound Services in an Early Pregnancy and Acute Gynaecological Unit. Book 2

404

The introduction contains a useful section about breaking bad news.These questions look at dating pregnancy in the first trimester, the diagnosis of pregnancy failure, ectopic pregnancy and molar pregnancy. There are comprehensive subsections on chorion villus sampling, nuchal translucency screening,multiple pregnancy and chorionicity. Good use is made of case presentations. The fifth and sixth sets are about ultrasound in the second and third trimesters.

There are questions about measurement, dating pregnancy, normal and abnormal growth, the placenta and amniotic fluid, normal fetal structural anatomy, identification of a wide range of fetal abnormalities, ultrasound 'soft markers' and their significance,multiple pregnancy and some maternal problems. The sixth set is extensively illustrated. The final, seventh, section deals with fertility, including the use of ultrasound in fertility investigations and treatment, and ovarian hyperstimulation.

Section two of the book contains the answers. These are clearly set out, concise and comprehensive.

Section three contains the centile charts which are referred to in some of the answers in section two.

There is a section containing useful addresses and websites. The list of suggested further reading begins with recommended source reading and then gives more specific lists of books and scientific articles for each of the topics covered.

This is an attractive paperback that should be essential reading for trainee obstetric and gynaecological sonographers,whether they are radiographers or radiology or obstetric trainees. It will be of particular value to those preparing for the RCOG/RCR Diploma in Advanced Obstetric Ultrasound and to specialist registrars in obstetrics and gynaecology undertaking special skills modules in fetal medicine, gynaecological ultrasound and infertility.

Reviewer Ann Harper MD FRCPI FRCOG
Consultant Obstetrician and Gynaecologist
Royal Jubilee Maternity Service, Belfast,UK
Churchill Livingstone, 2005

ISBN 0443064628
Paperback, 468 pages, £24.99
10.1576/toag.8.3.201.27260

Ultrasound Services in an Early Pregnancy and Acute Gynaecological Unit. Book 2

405

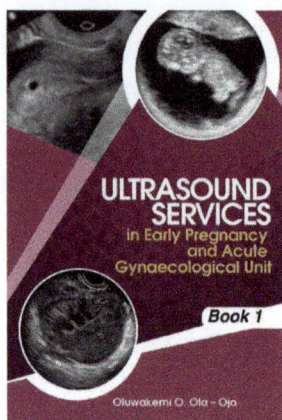

Ultrasound Services-
in an Early Pregnancy and Acute Gynaecological Unit (Book 1)
Author: Oluwakemi O. Ola-Ojo.

About the Book

Ultrasound Services in an Early Pregnancy and Acute Gynaecological Unit, Book 1 written by Oluwakemi O. Ola-Ojo, can be best described as a combined, yet comprehensive detail of contents and package.

Oluwakemi O. Ola-Ojo, a trained and practicing radiographer/ ultrasonographer with many years of experience, presents in the first chapter of this book, an in-depth assessment of the ultrasound services required in an early pregnancy and acute gynaecological unit. This chapter discusses the design of the unit, the arrangement of its facilities, infection control, quality and safety measures, as well as protocols and guidelines to be observed during and after ultrasound examinations.

Chapter 2 presents normal ultrasound appearances of the embryo, fetus and the maternal ovaries in the first trimester. It addresses pregnancy dating. Chapter 3 presents in detail, many of the clinical indications for emergency ultrasound in early pregnancy with relevant case presentations. The author also addresses the issues involved in 'communicating bad news' as well as the technicality of ultrasound reporting in early pregnancy. Book 1, chapter 4, concludes with more case presentations.

This book is primarily a resource for students, newly qualified sonographers, and trainee doctors in the field of obstetrics and gynaecological ultrasound, and would, no doubt, serve as a useful reference book for practitioners who need to stay on course and acquaint themselves with current practices.

The book, which comes highly recommended, is presented in two parts. Book 1 addresses Early Pregnancy Ultrasound, while Book 2 focuses on Emergency Gynaecology Ultrasound.

"This is a great effort and dedication on illustration of the ultrasound images and explanation of findings. The author has taken time in explaining different scenarios with the aid of ultrasound images. The case reviews are interesting and logically approached."

Mr. Khaled Zaedi
Consultant Obstetrician & Gynaecologist
EPAGU Consultant lead, Royal Free London NHS Trust

"All ultrasound trainees both medical and non-medical should get their hands on this book, which provides a comprehensive guide to gynaecology/obstetrics ultrasound and can be used as a first reader for ultrasound trainees and referred to throughout the course of training."

Phyllis Nsiah- Sarbeng
Then Radiology Registrar, Royal Free London NHS Trust

About the Author

Oluwakemi O. Ola-Ojo, an Ultrasonographer with a Master of Science degree in Radiography has obtained extensive training and practise both in the temperate and tropical regions of the world. She has also been involved in various research projects. A prolific writer, Oluwakemi has written books in other genres: children's books, poems as well as a Student's self assessment guide in her profession. She is a member of professional bodies in the UK and Nigeria and presently lives and works in England.

Ultrasound Services in an Early Pregnancy and Acute Gynaecological Unit. Book 2

406

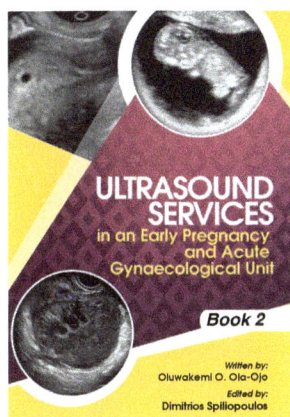

Ultrasound Services-
in an Early Pregnancy and Acute Gynaecological Unit (Book 2)

Author: Oluwakemi O. Ola-Ojo.
Editor: Dimitrios Spiliopoulos.

About the Book

Written by Oluwakemi Ola-Ojo, a seasoned practising Radiographer and Ultrasonographer. This series of two books is for professionals and trainees who provide ultrasound services in any early pregnancy unit and or acute gynaecological unit.

Chapters 1-4 of Book 1 focus on early pregnancies, address amongst other things the procedures and technicalities of setting up an ultrasound service in an early pregnancy and acute gynaecology unit. Topics covered also include Normal ultrasound recognisable embryonic and fetal development, Clinical indications for an early pregnancy ultrasound examination, The role of ultrasound in diagnosing the reason for the examination and The role of ultrasound in the management of such clinical conditions'. For each clinical indication, examples of the ultrasound findings are included.

Book 2 examines issues related to Acute Gynaecological cases. Chapter 5 discusses the normal anatomy and ultrasound appearances of the biological female pelvis and menstrual cycle. Chapter 6 addresses the clinical reasons for acute gynaecological referrals backed up by examples. Chapter 7 has 101 self-assessment questions for the practitioner or student using a case study approach while Chapter 8 provides the answers for the questions in Chapter 7.

An in-depth study in early pregnancy and acute gynaecological ultrasonography, this book comes highly recommended for trainees in the profession as well as all practitioners in the field.

"A well-illustrated and readable account of the busy area of acute gynaecological and obstetric ultrasound imaging. The case studies replicate real world situations and the excellent quiz chapter test and refresh knowledge using a wide range of pathologies. A very useful book both for those starting training in this area and those seeking to update their knowledge base."

Dr. Peter Wylie
Consultant Radiologist, Royal Free London NHS Trust

"All ultrasound trainees both medical and non-medical should get their hands on this book, which provides a comprehensive guide to gynaecology/obstetrics ultrasound and can be used as a first reader for ultrasound trainees and referred to throughout the course of training."

Phyllis Nsiah- Sarbeng
Then Radiology Registrar, Royal Free London NHS Trust

Ultrasound Services in an Early Pregnancy and Acute Gynaecological Unit. Book 2

407

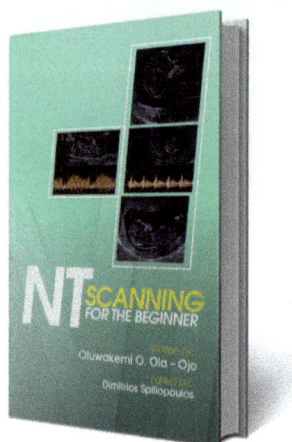

NT SCANNING
FOR THE BEGINNER

Author: Oluwakemi O. Ola-Ojo.
Editor: Dimitrios Spiliopoulos.

Review

*F*rst impressions are that this is a richly illustrated book throughout and aimed as described at the beginner new to nuchal translucency screening. It assumes no prior knowledge and takes the reader through the entire range of applications and interpretations. Examples are used with excellent quality ultrasound images and labelled in detail which provides the newcomer with clear images to use for reference.

Its systematic and structured approach makes each chapter a learning module but also it can be a reference book to dip into. The chapters comprise a greater portion of images than text, and the style is direct and concise with appropriate practical learning points throughout given by the author with extensive practical experience. The wide range of ultrasound images mean that examples of all common conditions have been collected for reference. The book would be ideally placed in the ultrasound examination room for comparisons to be made by the sonographer in training. Qualified sonographers will also find this ideal for revision and reference as will trainee doctors entering fetal medicine.

I found the book ideal as a teaching aid to use in the scan room. The title gives no hint of the more extended content of other first trimester anomalies found incidental to nuchal screening such as megacystis and omphalocoele which gives a more rounded and comprehensive picture of first trimester screening.
The inclusion of early pregnancy complications into the realm of early pregnancy assessment is useful and particularly the cases combining pregnancy with benign gynaecological pathology such as the complex ovarian cyst, fibroids and pregnancy with an IUCD. The inclusion of an IVF pregnancy and the dilemma of not redating it at the time of NT screening but using dating derived from IVF treatment is instructive as is the case of Ovarian Hyperstimulation Syndrome with co-existing pregnancy.

Ultrasound Services in an Early Pregnancy and Acute Gynaecological Unit. Book 2

408

The setting in which the author works has allowed for uncommon scenarios to be presented such as pregnancy with a transplanted kidney in the pelvis. Chapter 5 incorporates a useful section on what's wrong with these images? It's very appropriate when auditing image quality and pertinent to everyday practice The last chapter comprises of 40 case presentations all relevant to pregnancy, again well illustrated, some more common place than others.

Its size makes it a true handbook and portable to use in the work environment.

The index is limited but adequate and balanced by the clearly labelled table of content in the preliminary pages. It's the book to carry around and dip into regularly. The author describes that only the best obtainable views have be used for illustration which makes the examples all the more useful for teaching purposes. The websites referenced are limited to imaging and are pertinent to the text.

Mr William Taylor *FRCOG*
Consultant Obstetrician & Gynaecologist
Special interest Fetal Medicine
Wrexham Maelor Hospital
Wrexham
North Wales.

Ultrasound Services in an Early Pregnancy and Acute Gynaecological Unit. Book 2

409

Index

Ultrasound Services in an Early Pregnancy and Acute Gynaecological Unit. Book 2

410

Ultrasound Services in an Early Pregnancy and Acute Gynaecological Unit. Book 2

411

Ultrasound Services in an Early Pregnancy and Acute Gynaecological Unit. Book 2

412

Ultrasound Services in an Early Pregnancy and Acute Gynaecological Unit. Book 2

413

www.ingramcontent.com/pod-product-compliance
Lightning Source LLC
Chambersburg PA
CBHW050104220326
41598CB00043B/7379